Concise Encyclopedia of Periodontology

David C. Vandersall

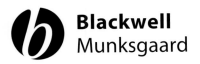

Blackwell
Munksgaard

Editorial Offices:
Blackwell Publishing Professional,
2121 State Avenue, Ames, Iowa 50014-8300, USA
   Tel: +1 515 292 0140
9600 Garsington Road, Oxford OX4 2DQ
   Tel: 01865 776868
Blackwell Publishing Asia Pty Ltd,
550 Swanston Street, Carlton South,
Victoria 3053, Australia
   Tel: +61 (0)3 9347 0300
Blackwell Wissenschafts Verlag,
Kurfürstendamm 57, 10707 Berlin, Germany
   Tel: +49 (0)30 32 79 060

First published 2007 by Blackwell Munksgaard,
a Blackwell Publishing Company

Library of Congress Cataloging-in-
Publication Data

Vandersall, David C.
   Concise encyclopedia of periodontology /
David C. Vandersall. — 1st ed.
      p.   ; cm.
   Includes bibliographical references.
   ISBN-13: 978-0-8138-2602-8 (alk. paper)
   ISBN-10: 0-8138-2602-0 (alk. paper)
   1. Periodontics—Encyclopedias.   I. Title.
[DNLM: 1. Periodontal Diseases—Dictionaries.
2. Oral Surgical Procedures—Dictionaries.
3. Periodontics—methods—Dictionaries.
   WU 13 V241 2007]
   RK361.V36 2007
   617.6′32003—dc22

                                          2006018852

0-8138-2602-8

Set in Palatino
by Data Management, Inc.
Printed and bound by C.O.S. Printers Pte. Ltd.

For further information on
Blackwell Publishing, visit our website:
www.blackwellpublishing.com

Preface

This reference book is a collection of periodontal terms, procedures, and techniques written for individuals interested in periodontology, either undergraduate, graduate and dental hygiene students, or their respective faculty. In addition, it is an atlas of periodontology for problem based learning (PBL) and literature seminars, plus a source book for researchers and clinicians.

The contents are divided into three distinct sections: the 'what,' the 'where' and the 'who' of periodontology. The 'what' portion consists of over 700 defined periodontal terms accompanied by respective literature references. The 'where' section contains the many references which are keyed from the 'what' section, directing the reader to an expansive periodontal literature. The last or Appendix section is the 'who' portion and lists the aforementioned authors with their specific contributions to periodontal literature. If a reference from the 'where' section is multi-authored, only the senior author is listed in this section. Their listed contributions can then redirect the reader to the 'what' portion for the specific definitions, thus completing the cycle of this *Concise Encyclopedia of Periodontology*.

Acknowledgments

Many individuals have assisted and worked unselfishly during the writing, editing, and production of this manuscript. A special appreciation to Sophia Joyce, Commissioning Editor at Blackwell, who had faith in my project, and to Erica Judisch, Editorial Assistant at Blackwell, for her guidance and technical advice. Gratitude to periodontists Drs. Jack G. Caton and Sebastian G. Ciancio for their technical input and to Jill Rethman, registered dental hygienist, for her positive comments and encouragement. In addition, I'd like to thank the faculty of the Department of Periodontology and Dental Hygiene at Indiana University School of Dentistry for the critical evaluation and comments. Resource information was provided by Barbara A. Gushrowski, Access Services Manager at the Indiana University School of Dentistry (IUSD) library. The production of the illustrations was effortlessly undertaken by Thomas C. Meador, photographer and graphic designer of IUSD. A deep appreciation to Kimberly J. Stuck for her technical ability, skills, and perseverance in transposing the written word into the final electronic format.

Many thanks to Barbara, my wife of 45 years, for her encouragement, patience, understanding, and gentle persuasion during the inception, writing, and editing of this manuscript. Thanks to everyone.

David C. Vandersall, DDS, MS

Figure Reprint Acknowledgments

Reprint permissions for the following figures used in this volume have been obtained from the publishers listed below.

BLACKWELL PUBLISHING

Figures H-3, H-4: From Murray PH. Periodontal diseases in patients infected by human immunodeficiency virus. Periodontology 2000 1994;6:52, figs 1, 3

Figure L-2: From Holmstrup P, Westergard J. HIV infection and periodontal diseases. Periodontology 2000 1998;18:38, fig 1

Figures G-5d, P-6: From Camarga PM, Melnick PR, Kenny EB. The use of free gingival grafts for aesthetic purposes. Periodontology 2000 2001;27:78,85, figs 11, 16

Figures P-14, S-1: From Hallmon WW, Harrel SK. Occlusal analysis, diagnosis and management in the practice of periodontics. Periodontology 2000 2004;34:152, figs 1, 2

Figure P-9: From Kerry GJ. Supportive periodontal therapy. Periodontology 2000 1995;9:177, fig 1

Figure R-6: From Pihlstrom BL. Periodontal risk assessment, diagnosis and treatment planning. Periodontology 2000 2001;25:43, fig 7b

ELSEVIER PUBLISHING

Figures P-1a,b,c,d: From Giansanti JS, Hrabak RP, Waldron CA. Palmar-plantar hyperkeratosis with concomitant periodontal destruction (Papillon-Lefevre syndrome). Oral Surg Oral Med Oral Pathol 1973;36(1):40-48, figs. 3,4,9,10

Figure B-4: From Misch CE. Bone density: A key determinant for clinical success. In: Dental Implant Prosthesis. St. Louis: Mosby 2005:134, fig 9-8

Figure C-1: From Halik FJ. The role of subgingival curettage in periodontal therapy. Dent Clin North Am 1969;13(1):21, fig 1

Figure C-6: From Pfeifer JS. The present status of bone grafts in periodontal therapy. Dent Clin North Am 1969;13(1):198, fig 2

Figures O-2, S-6: From Aleo JJ, Vandersall DC. Cementum: Recent concepts related to periodontal disease therapy. Dent Clin North Am 1980;24(4):637, figs 5,6

Figures B-2, C-3b: From Newell DH. The diagnosis and treatment of molar furcation invasion. Dent Clin North Am 1998;42(2):303, figs 4,5

Figure P-5: From Scannapieco FA. Systemic effects of periodontal diseases. Dent Clin North Am 2005;49(3):534, fig 1

AMERICAN ACADEMY OF PERIODONTOLOGY

Figures D-1a,b,G-5a: From Vandersall DC. Management of gingival recession and a surgical dehiscence with a soft tissue autograft: 4 year observation. J Periodontol 1974;45:276, figs 1,2

Figures G-3,G-6a,b: From Vandersall DC, Slade D. Periodontic/orthodontic management of diphenylhydantoin gingival hyperplasia: Case report. J Periodontol 1976;47:656,658, figs 1a,3

Figure E-1a: From Corn H. Edentulous area pedicle grafts in mucogingival surgery. Periodontics 1964;2:237, fig 4c

Figure O-1: From Pennel BM, Higgason JD, Towner JD, King KO, Fritz BD, Salder JF. Oblique rotated flap. J Periodontol 1965;36:306, fig 1b

AMERICAN DENTAL ASSOCIATION

Figures I-2a, 2b, 2c: From Vandersall DC. Localized periodontitis induced by rubber elastic: Report of case. J Am Dent Assoc 1971;83:1326–1328, figs 1,3,4

Figures I-1a,b: From Vandersall DC, Varble DL: The missing orthodontic elastic band, a periodontic-orthodontic dilemma. J Am Dent Assoc 1978;97:661-663, figs 1,3

Figure T-6a,b,c,d: From Vandersall DC, Detamore RT. The mandibular molar class III furcation invasion: A review of treatment options and a case report of tunneling. J Am Dent Assoc 2002;133:55–60, figs 2,3

Figure C-4a,b: From Arnim SS, Hagerman DA. The connective tissue fibers of the marginal gingiva. J Am Dent Assoc 1953;47:276, fig 4

Figures B-5, T-4: From Tibbetts LS Jr. Use of Diagnostic probes for detection of periodontal disease. J Am Dent Assoc 1969;78:553, fig 6

Figure I-10b: From Zwarych PD, Quigley MB. The intermediate plexus of the periodontal ligament: History and further observations. J Dent Res 1965;44:388, fig 7

INDIANA DENTAL ASSOCIATION

Figures C-9a,b, E-7a, W-1a,d: From Vandersall DC. Soft and hard tissue resection in periodontal therapy. J Ind Dent Assoc 1999;(summer):11-16, figs 3a,3b,4a,5a,5b

Concise Encyclopedia
of Periodontology

Abfraction—As teeth are moved in a facial (buccal)-lingual direction during occlusion or bruxing, cervical lesions may result from the microcracking of tooth substance by the process of physical and/or physiochemical wasting. These lesions are said to be abfractions or stress-induced noncarious lesions (Grippo 1991; Grippo et al. 2004). Supporting data suggesting that the application of occlusal loading produces the clinical entity of cervical tooth wear are not yet available (AAP 2001a; Litonjua et al. 2004). See also abrasion, corrosion, erosion.

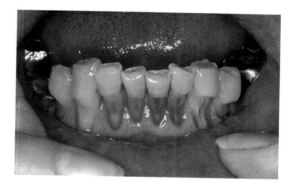

Fig. A-1

Abrasion—The wearing away of a substance or structure (i.e., teeth) through an abnormal mechanical process by an exogenous agent (Grippo et al. 2004). Examples include gingival and dental abrasions due to incorrect toothbrushing (See Fig. A-1) (Hirschfeld 1939) or through the incorrect use of dental floss (See Fig. F-3a,b) (Everett and Kunkel 1953). The incorrect and/or overzealous use of interproximal massaging aids may also produce excessive tooth wear (See Fig. A-2a,b,c). See also abfraction, corrosion, erosion.

Acellular Cementum—This type of cementum, the first to be formed, covers the cervical portion of the root and does not have cementocytes (Goldman 1957; Aisenberg 1952). See also altered cementum, cellular cementum, cementum, intermediate cementum.

Acquired Cuticle—This expression refers to the pathologic products of inflammation, salivary fluids, microbial flora, and exogenous oral debris that accumulates on the clinical crown (Wertheimer and Fullmer 1962). See also tooth accumulated material (TAM).

Active Eruption—The process by which a tooth moves from its germinative position to its functional position or contact; i.e., this term refers to actual movement of a tooth toward the occlusal line (Gottleib and Orban 1933). See also passive eruption.

Acute Necrotizing Ulcerative Gingivitis (ANUG)—An acute recurring gingival inflammation of complex etiology characterized by papillary necrosis, gingival bleeding, and pain but no loss of attachment. (See Fig. A-3) Predispositions in-

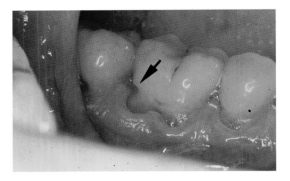

Fig. A-2a

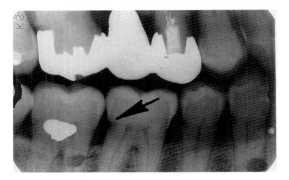

Fig. A-2b

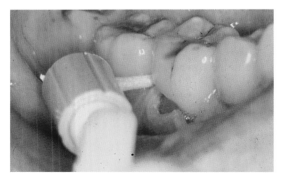

Fig. A-2c

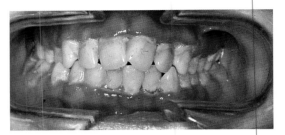

Fig. A-3

mouth, ulceromembranous gingivitis, Vincent's angina infection.

Acute Ulcerative Gingivitis—An acute gingival disease, characterized by an overgrowth of gram-negative anaerobic bacteria, occurring often in individuals with poor oral hygiene, under emotional stress, living in crowded conditions, with possible debilitating diseases, and smokers (Kowolik and Nisbet 1983). See also acute necrotizing ulcerative gingivitis (ANUG), necrotizing periodontal diseases, necrotizing ulcerative gingivitis (NUG), trench mouth, ulceromembranous gingivitis, Vincent's angina infection.

Adaptability Index (AI)—This index judges the capacity of the periodontium to adapt to excessive biting forces by comparing pronounced tooth wear and a radiographically thickened lamina dura. AI-positive teeth show less loss of clinical attachment and more bone support. AI-negative teeth show more loss of clinical attachment and less bone support (Jin and Cao 1992).

Advanced Flap—A flap that reaches its final site without rotation or lateral movement. It is used primarily in periodontal reconstructive or plastic surgery. It consists of two straight-line vertical incisions with or without cutbacks (Bahat and Handelsman 1991). See also rotational flap.

Aggressive Periodontitis—This is a new classification for highly destructive forms of periodontitis, formerly considered under the umbrella of "early-onset periodontitis"; it may further be classified as localized or generalized (Armitage 1999,

clude poor oral hygiene, smoking, emotional stress, nutritional deficiency, and systemic disease (Johnson and Engel 1986). See also acute ulcerative gingivitis, necrotizing periodontal diseases, necrotizing ulcerative gingivitis (NUG), trench

2004a; AAP 2000f). See also early onset periodontitis, generalized juvenile periodontitis (GJP), juvenile periodontitis, localized juvenile periodontitis (LJP), Papillon-Lefevre syndrome, periodontosis, precocious periodontitis, prepubertal periodontitis, rapidly progressive periodontitis (RPP).

Allogenic—This term refers to a graft obtained from the same species but having a different genetic constitution. It may also be spelled allogeneic (Wirthlin 1987). See also allograft; homograft.

Allograft—A tissue graft transferred between genetically dissimilar members of the same species (Brunsvold and Mellonig 1993). Another definition is a tissue graft between individuals of the same species but with nonidentical genetic compositions. (Mellonig 1996; AAP 2001b). See also allogenic, decalcified freeze-dried bone allograft (DFDBA), demineralized freeze-dried bone allograft (DFDBA), homograft.

Alloplast—A bone graft comprising inert (synthetic) materials. Although alloplasts have been shown to have some osteoconductive capacity, this is of insignificant degree. Examples of synthetic bone graft materials are plaster of Paris, calcium carbonate, and calcium phosphate (ceramics) (Shetty and Han 1991; Yukna 1993).

Altered Cementum—Root surface cementum that has been exposed in a periodontal pocket containing plaque products such as endotoxin, which may promote inflammation in adjacent gingival tissues (Stambaugh et al. 1981). See also acellular cementum, cellular cementum, cementum, intermediate cementum.

Altered Passive Eruption—A tooth eruption that does not progress beyond stage I or II of passive eruption. The junctional epithelium does not migrate apical to the cervical concavity of the tooth (Evian et al. 1993). See also delayed passive eruption, passive eruption.

Alveolar Bone Proper—That portion of the alveolar process which surrounds the root

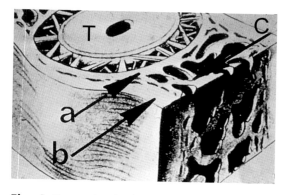

Fig. A-4: a, alveolar bone proper; b, supporting alveolar bone; C, cancellous (spongy) bone; T, tooth

of a tooth. It is made up of compact cortical bone into which the fibers of the periodontal ligament attach (See Fig. A-4) (Orban 1957). It is also considered to be the thimble of bone lining the socket of the tooth (Melcher 1976). See also alveolar process, cribriform plate, lamina dura.

Alveolar Crest Fiber Group—A group of fibers in the periodontal ligament that traverses from the cementum just apical to the "epithelial attachment" to the crest of the alveolar bone (See Fig. P-4c). Their function is to resist lateral movement of the tooth and keep the tooth in its socket (Orban 1957). See also periodontal ligament.

Alveolar Mucosa—The covering of the alveolar process extending from the fornix of the oral vestibulum and, on the lower jaw, to the sublingual sulcus (See Fig. A-5). The alveolar mucosa is thin and loosely attached to the periosteum by a well-defined submucous layer of loose connective tissue; it may contain small mucous glands (See Fig. A-6). The epithelium is thin, not cornified; the epithelial ridges and papillae are low and often entirely missing (Orban 1948a). See also attached gingiva, mucogingival junction, mucogingival line.

Alveolar Process—That portion of the maxilla and mandible which forms and sup-

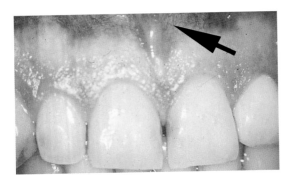

Fig. A-5: Arrow, alveolar mucosa

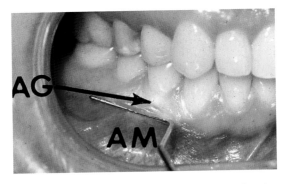

Fig. A-6: AG, attached gingiva; AM, alveolar mucosa

ports the teeth (See Fig A-4). It consists of (A) *alveolar bone proper,* which surrounds the root, is made up of bundle bone, and attaches the periodontal ligament fibers and (B) *supporting alveolar bone,* which consists of buccal and lingual cortical plates and intervening (C) cancellous bone (Orban 1957; Bhaskar 1976; Hassell 1993). See also alveolar bone proper, supporting alveolar bone.

Alveolar Ridge Deformities—These deformities of edentulous ridges fall into three groups: class I, buccolingual loss of tissue with normal ridge height in an apicocoronal dimension; class II, apicocoronal loss of tissue with normal ridge width in a buccolingual dimension; and class III, combined buccolingual and apicocoronal

loss of tissue resulting in loss of normal height and width (Seibert 1983a).

Alveolodental Ligament—This expression is synonymous with the term *periodontal ligament* (Orban 1957). See also periodontal ligament.

Alveologingival Fiber Group—These collagenous fibers, which attach the gingiva to the alveolar bone, arise from the alveolar crest and insert into the lamina propria of the gingiva (Orban 1957). See also gingival fiber group.

AmeloCemental Junction—The cementoenamel junction of the tooth (Davies et al. 1969). See also cementoenamel junction (CEJ).

Amelogenins—These are hydrophobic enamel matrix proteins that have been shown to induce cementogenesis (Hammarstrom 1997); they can stimulate recapitulation of embryonic new cementum and subsequent formation of alveolar bone and a new periodontal ligament (Brooks et al. 1995). See also enamel matrix proteins.

Anchor Suture—A variation of the interdental suture, used when one delicately positions a single papilla and chooses not to tie it into tissue on the opposite side (Morris 1965a; Dahlberg 1969). See also suture.

Angle Classification of Malocclusion—The governing criterion for this classic gross classification of malocclusion, introduced in 1907 by Edward H. Angle, is the anteroposterior relationship of the maxillary and mandibular first molars. "Divisions" are used in class II, based on the inclination of the maxillary incisors. "Subdivisions" are used to describe unilateral malocclusion characteristics of the affected posterior segmental relationships. Class I: In this malocclusion the mesiobuccal cusp of the maxillary first molar occludes the buccal groove of the mandibular first molar. Class II: This malocclusion occurs when the mesiobuccal cusp of the maxillary first molar occludes mesial to the buccal groove of the mandibular first molar, usually near the embrasure between the mandibular first molar and the second bi-cuspid. Division 1: A class II bilateral molar associated with proclined maxillary incisors with respect to the mandibular incisors. Subdivision: Unilateral distal molar associated with protruding maxillary incisors. Division 2: A class II bilateral molar associated with retruding maxillary incisors. Class III: This malocclusion typically occurs when the mesiobuccal cusp of the maxillary first molar occludes near the embrasure between the mandibular first and second molar (Angle 1907; AAO 1993).

Animalcules—A term coined by Antony van Leeuwenhoek in 1693 meaning "little animals." It refers to bacterial flora found around the teeth after 3 days of not brushing. His drawings of these "animalcules" closely resembled the spirochetes, bacilli, spirilla, and cocci of today (Dobell 1960). See also microcosm, plaque (dental).

Apical Fiber Group—This group of principal fibers of the periodontal ligament, located around the apex of a tooth, runs from the cementum to the alveolar bone (See Fig. P-4c). Its function is to resist the tipping of a tooth (Orban 1957). See also periodontal ligament.

Apically Displaced Flap—This flap results from the excision and discarding of existing gingiva and depends on a large granulating wound to obtain new gingiva (Friedman 1962a). This was originally known as the "pushback" procedure. It is considered an archaic approach to managing mucogingival defects. See also pushback procedure.

Apically Displaced Split Flap—This is a partial-thickness flap that is apically displaced in order to change the position of the mucogingival junction and increasing the width of keratinized gingiva. This procedure is intended to correct mucogingival defects (Zamet 1969). See also partial-thickness flap, mucosal flap, split-thickness flap.

Apically Positioned Flap—In the 1960s, this term was introduced to replace *apically*

repositioned flap because *repositioning* means returning the flap to its original position or location, which was not the objective of this procedure (Corn 1968). See also apically repositioned flap.

Apically Positioned Pedicle Gingival Graft—This was a synonym used when referring to the apically repositioned flap, according to Perry A. Ratcliff (1966). See also apically repositioned flap, vertical gingival pedicle graft.

Apically Repositioned Flap—Coined by Nathan Friedman in 1962, this term refers to a surgical procedure performed to eliminate the periodontal pocket where the base of the pocket approximates or is apical to the mucogingival junction, as the aim is to create a functionally adequate zone of attached gingiva (Friedman 1962a). Friedman's technique placed two vertical releasing incisions as compared to Claude L. Nabers' single vertical incision, as reported in his paper "Repositioning the attached Gingiva" (Nabers 1954). See also apically positioned flap, vertical gingival pedicle graft.

Apoxesis—The surgical removal of various substances from the surfaces of the teeth by different kinds of steel scalers (Zemsky 1926). The term has recently reappeared in the periodontal literature but is now an archaic expression for instrumentation of the root and soft tissues (Halik 1969). See also root curettage, root planing, scaling.

ASA Classification—This category, as described by the American Society of Anesthesiology (ASA), places patients into the following five classes according to their surgical risk. Class I: Normal, healthy patients with blood pressure below 140/90 mmHg. Class II: Patients with mild to moderate systemic disease, no medical consult required, consider stress reduction protocol. Class III: Patients with severe systemic disease that limits activity but is not incapacitating. Must have medical consult; stress reduction required if treated as an outpatient. Class IV: Patients with severe systemic disease that limits activity and is a constant threat to life. Emergency treatment only in office if minimal; otherwise must be performed in a hospital. Class V: Patients who are not expected to live beyond 24 hours (Saklad 1941). In 1989, during a world workshop in clinical periodontics, the American Academy of Periodontology (AAP) included only classes I to IV (AAP 1989).

Attached Epithelial Cuff—A term used by B.J. Orban, H. Bhatia, J.A. Kollar, and F.M. Wentz to describe the "union" of the epithelial attachment cells to the enamel of the tooth (See Fig J-1), refuting Jens Waerhaug's 1952 thesis that "the bottom of the clinical pocket was found to be situated consistently at the cemento-enamel junction" (Orban et al. 1956; Waerhaug 1952). See also epithelial cuff.

Attached Gingiva—Gingiva that is firmly and immovably attached to the underlying tooth and bone (See Fig. A-6). It is frequently stippled, firm, and thick, lacking a submucous layer; and it has no glands. It is separated from the alveolar mucosa by the mucogingival junction and from the free gingiva by the free gingival groove (Orban 1948a). See also free gingival groove, mucogingival junction, mucogingival line, stippling.

Attachment Apparatus—This term refers to the (1) cementum (2) periodontal ligament, and (3) alveolar bone proper; all three together provide suspensory, formative, nutritional, and sensory support to the tooth (Mellonig 1992). See also alveolar bone proper, cementum, periodontal ligament.

Attrition—The physiologic wearing away of teeth by the tooth-to-tooth friction that occurs during deglutition and clenching or bruxism (AAP 2001a; Grippo et al. 2004). See also abfraction, abrasion, corrosion, erosion.

Autogenous Bone Graft—Grafts taken from one part of a patient's body and transferred to another (Brunsvold and Mellonig 1993). The first recorded human autogenous bone graft in periodontics was reported in 1923 by Zoltan Hegedus, who grafted a portion of a tibia to the labial surface of the mandibular anteriors (Hegedus 1923). The first big impact in periodontics was the successful use of autogenous osseous bone chips in restoring the lost attachment apparatus, as reported by Claude Nabers and Timothy O'Leary (Nabers and O'Leary 1965). Synonyms for *autogenous grafts* are *autografts, autologous grafts,* and *autoplasts*. See the following for procedures in retrieving autogenous bone grafts in periodontal surgery: bone blending, bone swaging, iliac crest autograft, osseous coagulum, and osseous filtration.

B

Baer-Sumner Fat Pack—A non-eugenol-containing periodontal dressing. It consists of zinc oxide, rosin, and zinc bacitracin mixed in an ointment of zinc oxide and hydrogenated fat. The purpose is to alleviate pain in surgical areas where bone is exposed, which requires two or more weeks for maturation (Baer et al. 1960). See also periodontal dressing.

Balancing Side—In the study of occlusion, the disoccluding side of the maxillomandibular relationship when the mandible moves toward the working or chewing (bolus) side (Posselt 1968). See also nonworking side, working side.

Balancing-Side Interference—Also known as *non-working-side interference.* This term refers to tooth interferences that occur on the nonfunctioning side of the mandible when it is shifted laterally toward the working side and is applied in the study and analysis of occlusion (Posselt 1968). See also non-working-side interference.

Balneotherapy—(L., *balneum,* meaning "bath") Balneotherapy, popularized in Europe in the 1920s, was a method of treating periodontal disease by forced water irrigation using a combination of heat and mineral water or with medications such as sulfate and sulfur added to the water. This "mouth douche" mechanically cleaned the tooth surfaces and interdental spaces and pockets, massaged the gingiva, warmed the periodontal tissues, and provided a psychological benefit (Munch-Hansen 1953). It has been shown that the prolonged use of a well-recognized mouth douche does not reduce the amount of plaque. Thus, there is no valid justification for using such a procedure in periodontal therapy (Dabelsteen 1964).

Bass Toothbrushing Technique—This technique of toothbrushing, introduced by Charles Cassedy Bass in 1948, utilizes a soft multituffed brush with bristles 0.007 inches in diameter. The bristles are placed at a 45-degree angle (See Fig. B-1) and directed into the gingival crevice. Short vibratory movements of the brush are performed to remove food material and bacterial film. On the linguals of the anterior teeth, the brush is turned to a vertical position (Bass 1948, 1954; Ray 2005). See also modified Bass toothbrushing technique.

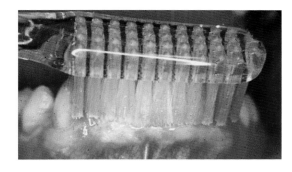

Fig. B-1

Bell Toothbrushing Technique—This technique of toothbrushing is also known as the physiologic technique, first described by T. Sidney Smith in 1940. It was highly advocated by Dickson Gabriel Bell in 1948 and today carries his name. Both Bell and Smith were from San Francisco, and this technique of toothbrushing was very popular in the West (Smith 1940; Bell 1948). See also physiologic toothbrushing technique.

Bennett Movement—A term used in the study of mandibular movement, referring to the lateral translation or side shift of the working condyle during lateral excursions of the mandible (Bennett 1908).

Berliner Epithelial Scalpel—In 1950 Abraham Berliner devised a self-limiting "epithelial scalpel" that effectively removed the epithelial lining and attachment in periodontal pockets, leading toward "new attachment." It successfully "peeled" out the epithelial lining and attachment, thus eliminating the tendency for shredding that occurs with conventional curettes during curettage (Berliner 1950). The ineffectiveness of the Berliner scalpel was studied in 1954 (Wertheimer 1954).

Bevelled Flap—This procedure, as defined by Nathan Friedman, is a thinning of the palatal flap in order to make it follow the osseous contour for adaptation to the alveolar crest. This distinguishes it from the apically repositioned flap of Friedman, because the palatal flap cannot be positioned apically (Friedman 1962a).

Bicuspidization—Treatment of the two sections of a bisected mandibular molar as premolars, mimicking their contour in the final prosthesis as if they were premolars (Augsburger 1976). The following requirements must be met for this technique to succeed: (1) adequate bone support to stabilize the remaining segments, (2) no severe fluting of the distal part of the mesial root and mesial part of the distal root, and (3) adequate separation of the mesial and distal roots to create an embrasure for adequate hygiene (Farshchian

and Kaiser 1988). See also bisectioning, root separation.

Bifurcation—The normal anatomic division of the roots of teeth into two parts. It should not be confused with the pathologic phenomenon of "bifurcation invasion" or "bifurcation involvement," where loss of periodontal attachment has occurred between the roots (ADA 1950; AAP 2001a). See also bifurcation invasion, bifurcation involvement.

Bifurcation Invasion—Also known as *bifurcation involvement*, this is the extension of pulpitis or periodontitis into a bifurcation (AAP 2001a). See also bifurcation, bifurcation involvement.

Bifurcation Involvement—An interradicular periodontal lesion (loss of attachment) between two roots of a multirooted tooth (See Fig. V-1a) (Glickman 1950a). See also bifurcation, bifurcation invasion.

Bifurcational Ridges—First described in 1958 by Everett and coworkers, these are distinct ridges or elevations within the bifurcation of mandibular first molars (See Fig. B-2). They originate from the mesial surface of the distal root, run across the bifurcation, and end high up on the mesial root, where they blend into the distal surface of the mesial root. They include the intermediate ridge, which consists mainly of cementum with only slight dentin, and the external or buccal and lingual ridges, which consist primarily of dentin with a thin covering of cementum (Everett et al, 1958).

Bilaminar Graft—This periodontal plastic surgery procedure, used for covering exposed root cementum in mucogingival defects, consists of overlying a free connective tissue graft with adjacent papillae over the root surface. Such "sandwiching" of flaps is done to ensure plasmatic circulation and a predictable outcome in covering roots with keratinized gingiva. The adjacent papillae (i.e., pedicles) may be either full- or partial-thickness grafts (Nelson 1987; Harris 1992). See also oral plastic surgery, periodontal plastic surgery, subpedicle connective tissue graft.

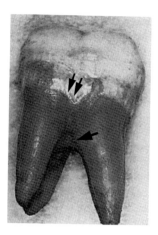

Fig. B-2: Single arrow, bifurcational ridge; Double arrow, cervical enamel projection (With permission from Elsevier Publishing)

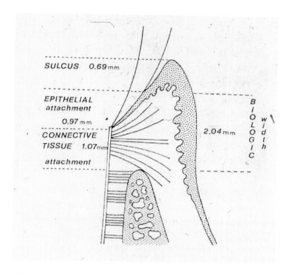

Fig. B-3

Biofilms—Within complex ecosystems, layers of bacteria reside on the surface of the mucosal epithelia of the oral cavity, respiratory tract, esophagus, GI tract, and urinary tract. Such matrices of bacterial populations are closely adherent to each other, protected by a shaped matrix or glycocalyx, and are highly interconnected with one another and/or to surfaces or interfaces (Cohen and Slavkin 2000; Socransky and Haffajee 2002).

Biointegration—An osseointegration in which a direct biochemical bone-to-implant interface occurs, which is confirmed at the electron microscopic level. This type of integration is associated with "bioactive" materials such as calcium phosphate, ceramic, or hydroxyapatite. It is independent of any mechanical "interlocking" mechanism (Meffert et al. 1987). See also fibroosseous integration, functional ankylosis, osseointegration.

Biological Width—The dimension from the crest of alveolar bone to the base of the sulcus, which includes the combined width of the connective tissue and epithelial attachment, i.e., the junctional epithelium (See Fig. B-3). This term was coined by Dr. D. Walter Cohen on June 3, 1962, in a lecture

at Walter Reed Army Medical Center, during a discussion on the periodontal preparation of the mouth for restorative dentistry (Ingber et al. 1977). This dimension was measured at 2.04 mm in a publication by Gargiulo and colleagues (Gargiulo et al. 1961). However, several authors have stated that the biological width should include the crevicular depth for a minimum of 2.7 to 3 mm (Nevins and Skurow 1984; Becker et al. 1998).

Bisectioning—The surgical splitting of a molar into two separate roots and their associated crown components. This usually applies to mandibular molars but can also apply to a maxillary molar where one root has been hemisectioned and the remaining roots and crowns of the teeth are split into two roots and their associated crown portions (Newell 1991). See also bicuspidization, root separation.

Blowout—A clinical situation in which rapid and extensive bone destruction occurs in a furcation following a minor osteoplasty while managing an incipient furcation involvement. It usually occurs in a molar having a short root trunk (Ochsenbein 1986). See also root trunk.

Blunt Dissection—The elevation of a full-thickness or mucoperiosteal flap from the necks of the teeth and underlying alveolar bone during periodontal surgery (Ammons and Smith 1976). See also full thickness flap, mucoperiosteal flap.

Bonded-Bracket Index (BBI)—An index devised to compare the accumulation of plaque on bonded versus banded teeth using the Quigley-Hein method. With the use of a disclosing solution, it exhibits a scale from 0 (no plaque on bracket or tooth surface) to 5 (plaque present on bracket and tooth completely covering the entire clinical crown) (Ciancio et al. 1985). See also Quigley-Hein plaque index.

Bone Blending—The mixing and blending of cancellous and cortical bone spicules in a sterile capsule and pestle, the type normally used for amalgam trituration, to produce a homogeneous mass. The bone is obtained from extraction sites, exostosis, tori, or edentulous ridges (Diem et al. 1972). This mixture is triturated for 60 seconds to obtain a particle size of 210 × 105 μ (Zaner and Yukna 1984). This technique is a modification of the osseous coagulum approach of R. Earl Robinson (Robinson 1969). See also osseous coagulum, osseous filtration.

Bone Factor—This expression, coined in 1944 by Irving Glickman, attempts to explain the systemic regulatory influence upon alveolar bone. That is, the response of alveolar bone to bone-destructive influences is subject to the patient's systemic background. Patients with a "positive" bone factor were considered resistant to periodontitis, whereas those with a "negative" bone factor were viewed as being susceptible to periodontitis (Glickman 1944, 1949; Glickman et al. 1944).

Bone Morphogenetic Protein (BMP)—Bone-inductive proteins (composed of acidic polypeptides) located in the cortical bone matrix and exposed when demineralized with 0.6N hydrochloric acid (Urist and Strates 1971). The amount of bone morphogenetic protein produced from 1 kg of fresh bone is about 1 mg (Urist et al. 1983). See also demineralized freeze-dried bone allograft (DFDBA), osteoinduction.

Bone Powder—A term coined by R. Earl Robinson for bone chips recovered during osseous surgery to be used in the repair of osseous defects. However, Walter Donnenfeld suggested the term *osseous coagulum* instead, and it has taken precedence in bone grafting studies (Dello Russo 1995) *Bone powder* also appears in the older literature in connection with heterogenous bone graft studies (Beube and Silvers 1934). See also osseous coagulum.

Bone Quality Classification—A system of describing the quality of bone according to the ratio of compact (cortical) to trabecular (spongy) bone. It was first presented in 1985 by U. Lekholm and G.A. Zarb in four categories: (1) almost all homogenous compact bone, (2) a thick layer of compact bone surrounding a core of dense trabecular bone, (3) a thin layer of cortical bone surrounding a core of dense trabecular bone of favorable strength, and (4) a thin layer of cortical bone surrounding a core of low-density trabecular bone (Lekholm and Zarb 1985). Carl E. Misch classified bone quality as (1) dense compacta, (2) porous compacta/coarse trabecular, (3) porous compacta/coarse-fine trabecular, and (4) fine trabecular (Misch 1988) Misch later used the term *bone density classification* and applied the symbols D1, D2, D3, and D4 to the four types of bone, respectively (See Fig. B-4) (Misch 1990, 1999, 2005).

Bone Sounding—A way of directing a periodontal probe into anesthetized soft tissue horizontally and vertically until it strikes the underlying alveolar bone (See Fig. B-5). The probe is moved in millimeter increments so as to determine the level and contour of the bone (see Figs. P-7b, T-4) (Easley 1967). See also transgingival probing.

Bone Swaging—This technique of autogenous bone grafting consisted of fracturing the bone without severing it completely

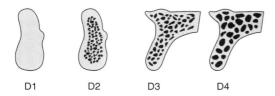

Fig. B-4: (With permission from Elsevier Publishing)

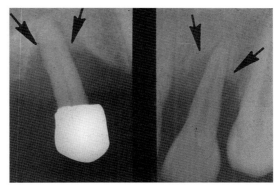

Fig. B-6: Arrow, bony defects

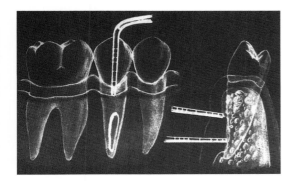

Fig. B-5: (With permission from the American Dental Association)

from its blood supply while it is moved into an osseous defect. It was used primarily in fracturing bone from edentulous areas into bony defects and treating bifurcation involvements or three-wall troughs (see Fig. C-6) (Ewen 1965). See also contiguous autogenous transplant.

Bony Defect—Also known as an *osseous defect*, refers to any pathologic aberration or deviation from normal within the alveolar supporting bone (See Fig. B-6). Numerous publications have illustrated and discussed these aberrations (Saari et al. 1968; Larato 1970a, 1970b, 1970c; Easley 1967; AAP 2001a). See also osseous defect.

Bridging—The periodontal surgical healing phenomenon where a soft tissue graft "takes" over an avascular area. It is the result of the development of collateral circulation from the vascular areas of the recipient bed and may originate from either epithelial or connective tissue. It may

occur also in lateral sliding flaps, subepithelial connective tissue grafts, or other surgical procedures where root coverage is planned or accomplished (Sullivan and Atkins 1968). See also take.

Bruxism—The clenching and/or grinding of the teeth when not masticating or swallowing (Posselt and Wolff 1963). Sigurd Ramfjord and colleagues have defined bruxism as nonfunctional gnashing and grinding of the teeth in eccentric excursions. They further describe "centric" bruxism as **clenching** and "eccentric" bruxism as **bruxism** (Ramfjord and Ash 1966). Bertrand S. Frohman, a physician, was one of the earliest writers to use this term (Frohman 1931). See also bruxomania, clenching, parafunction.

Bruxomania—In the early literature, this term referred to the gritting of teeth, as observed in patients who were afflicted with lesions in the central nervous system such as meningitis, paralysis, spasmodic hemiplegia, dementia, epilepsy, chorea, and so on (Marie and Pietkiewicz 1907). This was later referred to as bruxism by Bertrand S. Frohman (Frohman 1931). See also bruxism, Karolyi effect.

BULL Rule—A rather common term used in teaching the rules of selective grinding of posterior teeth in lateral excursions and position. This expression refers to grinding the **buccal** aspect of the **upper** and the **lingual** aspect of the **lower** cusps of posterior teeth. With this approach, there is little danger of disturbing centric stops, which are normally the lower buccal and upper lingual cusps (Schuyler 1935, 1947; Bjorndahl 1958). See also MUDL rule.

Bundle Bone—This is the compact bone lining the tooth socket, having many Sharpey's fibers imbedded in it (Weinmann and Sicher 1955). G. Stein and J.P. Weinmann have said that it is the alveolar bone on the side from which the teeth are moving and is rich in Sharpey's fibers; they called this bone *Bundelknochen* (Stein and Weinmann 1925). See also lamellar bone, woven bone.

Buttressing Bone—Bone formative activity that occurs in the repair of trauma from occlusion. It may occur **centrally,** along the endosteal surfaces of the trabeculae, and does not alter the morphology of the bone. When it occurs **peripherally,** on the external surface, it may produce bulbous contours to the buccal or lingual plate as a pronounced ridge at the cervical margin. (Glickman 1965).

![C](image of letter C)

Calciphylaxis—Dr. Hans Selye defined this term as a condition of induced systemic hypersensitivity in which tissues respond to appropriate challenging agents with a precipitous local calcification (Selye 1964). The administration of various calcifying factors, such as vitamin D, parathyroid hormone, or dihydrotachysterol (DHT) has been shown to produce calciphylaxis (Glickman et al. 1965).

Calculus (Attachment)—In September 1952 at the Annual Meeting of the American Academy of Periodontology in St. Louis, Helmut A. Zander presented his four methods of calculus attachment to root cementum. They are (1) attachment by means of the secondary cuticle, (2) attachment to the microscopic irregularities of the cementum surface, (3) attachment by penetration of microorganisms making up the matrix into the cementum, and (4) attachment into areas of cementum resorption (See Fig. C-1) (Zander 1953). Bernard S. Moskow presented another method of calculus attachment through cemental fragmentation from dentin at the cementoenamel junction. Calculus deposition occurs between dentin and cementum (separation) when the latter is fragmented from the underlying dentin surface (Moskow 1969).

Calculus (Dental)—Dental calculus may be defined as a hard concretion that forms on teeth or dental prostheses through calcifi-

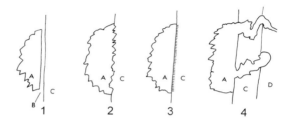

Fig. C-1: A, calculus, B, secondary cuticle; C, cementum; D, dentin (With permission from Elsevier Publishing)

cation of bacterial plaque (AAP 2001a). Historically, calculus has been typed as follows: (1) **salivary** (from saliva), (2) **serumal** (lodged in the subgingival space upon the enamel or cementum or both (from serum), and (3) **pus pocket** (deposited on roots of teeth where the periodontal attachment has been lost) (Black 1911). See also subgingival calculus, supragingival calculus, tartar, tooth accumulated material (TAM).

Calculus Surface Index (CSI)—This periodontal index measures supra- and/or subgingival calculus on four mandibular incisors. The four surfaces (two proximal, one labial, and one lingual) of each tooth are explored for the presence of calculus. A number is assigned to each tooth (0 to 4), corresponding to the number of surfaces with calculus. The total number of calculus-covered surfaces of all four teeth is referred to as the calculus surface index (Ennever et al. 1961).

Cellular Cementum—That portion of the cementum that contains cementocytes; it is found primarily in the apical third of the root (Goldman 1957; Aisenberg 1952). See also acellular cementum, altered cementum, cementum, intermediate cementum, osteocementum.

Cementoenamel Junction (CEJ)—The area of union between the cementum and enamel at the cervical region of the tooth (See Fig. C-2). The CEJ may have three types of relationships: (A) cementum and enamel do not touch (5 to 10% of the time), (B) cementum and enamel meet end to end (30% of the time), and (C) cementum overlaps a small portion of enamel (60 to 65% of the time) (Noyes et al, 1938). See also amelocemental junction.

Cementopathia—In 1946, Bernhard Gottleib changed his term *diffuse alveolar atrophy* to *cementopathia*, which explained the cemental changes occurring beneath the marginal tissue causing the wandering and loosening of teeth (Gottleib 1946). Basically, Gottleib saw an abnormality in or lack of cementum deposition as causing this periodontal pathosis. Recently, investigators have reconsidered this phenomenon as an initiating cause in early-onset periodontitis or aggressive periodontitis (Page and Baab 1985) See also diffuse alveolar atrophy.

Cementum—This portion of the attachment apparatus is mineralized connective tissue, consisting of 45 to 50% inorganic and 50 to 55% organic material, which covers the root surface of the tooth. It provides a surface area for the attachment of Sharpey's fibers of the periodontal ligament and some collagen fibers of the gingiva (Kerr 1961; Hassell 1993). Several varieties of cementum have been described beyond the classical acellular or primary cementum and cellular or secondary cementum (Ten Cate et al. 1997). Acellular cementum has been further shown to be acellular afibrillar, acellular extrinsic fiber, and

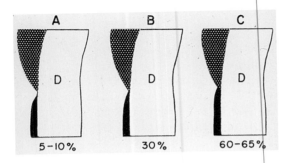

Fig. C-2

acellular intrinsic fiber cementum. Cellular cementum, likewise, has been shown to be cellular fiber and cellular mixed stratified cementum. The latter is a mixture of cellular intrinsic fiber and acellular extrinsic cementum (Bosshardt and Selvig 1997). See also acellular cementum, altered cementum, attachment apparatus, cellular cementum, intermediate cementum.

Centric Occlusion (CO)—According to the Academy of Prosthodontics, centric occlusion is the occluding of opposing teeth when the mandible is in centric relation; this may or may not coincide with the maximum intercuspation position (AP 1994). On the other hand, the American Academy of Periodontology defines it as the maximum intercuspation or contact of the opposing arches (AAP 2001a). Synonyms are *maximum intercuspation, habitual position, acquired position*, and *intercuspal contact*; all are tooth-guided. See also centric relation (CR), clenching, freeway space, maximum intercuspation, postural position, retruded contact (RC).

Centric Relation (CR)—The terminal hinge relationship of the mandible, which is reproducible and can be recorded with accuracy (Posselt 1968). It has also been explained as the most retruded physiologic relation of the mandible to the maxilla from which lateral movement can be made (AAP 2001a). Other authors have described it as the most retruded, unstrained position of the condyles in the glenoid fossae from which lateral excursions can be made (Pugh and Smerke 1969). See also centric occlusion, retruded contact (RC).

Cervical Enamel Projection (CEP)—This anatomic variant is a dipping of the enamel from the cementoenamel junction (CEJ) apically toward the furcation area of molars; it is covered by junctional epithelium rather than connective tissue (Swan and Hurt 1976). Donald H. Masters and Sam W. Hoskins, Jr., first named and classified the CEJs into three grades: grade I, a distinct change in CEJ attitude with enamel projecting toward the bifurcation (See Fig. C-3a); grade II, the enamel projection approaches the furcation but does not come into contact with it; and grade III, the enamel projection extends into the furcation proper (See Fig. C-3b) (Masters and Hoskins 1964). If present, it occurs in the "flute" portion of the furcation. See also enamel pearl, flute, radicular enamel.

Cervical Plaque Index (CPI)—A measuring system to record the accumulation of cervical plaque was reported in 1976, grading six surfaces of each tooth (i.e., mesial buccal, buccal, distal buccal, distal lingual, lingual, and mesial lingual). The degree of plaque accumulation is measured as follows: grade 0, no cervical plaque; grade 1, up to 1 mm of thin cervical plaque; grade 2, over 1 mm of thin cervical plaque; grade 3, up to 1 mm of thick cervical plaque; and grade 4, over 1 mm of thick cervical plaque (Schmid et al. 1976).

Charters Toothbrushing Technique—The Charters approach to toothbrushing is primarily designed to stimulate the interdental gingiva through vibratory motions with the sides of the bristles. The brush head is placed so the bristle ends are directed toward the occlusal/incisal edges, being careful not to pierce the gingival tissue. Emphasis is placed on increasing the circulation through vibratory motions, thus forcing out toxic products (Ray 2005). This technique was first described in 1819 by Leonard Koecker, a German-born den-

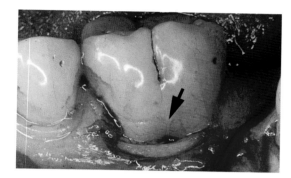

Fig. C-3a: Arrow, grade I CEP

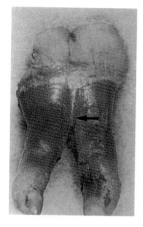

Fig. C-3b: Arrow, grade III CEP (With permission from Elsevier Publishing)

tist, who practiced in Baltimore, Maryland. However, it was William J. Charters, of Des Moines, Iowa, who endorsed and documented this technique in 1928 and 1932, describing his technique, purpose, and goals in achieving a cleaner mouth (Charters 1928, 1932) This technique became popular in the Midwest because of Dr. Charters' home in Iowa. To promote his ideas of preventing gum disease, Charters established the Des Moines Toothbrush Clinic. (Held 1989). See also toothbrushing technique.

Chronic Desquamative Gingivitis (CDG)—This disease, also known as desquamative gingivitis, is a clinical syndrome consisting of gingival changes and associated symptoms that may be a specific disease entity or a manifestation of other diseases (See Fig. D-3) (Glickman and Smulow 1964). See also desquamative gingivitis, gingivosis.

Cinguloradicular Groove—Also known as the palatogingival groove. As with the other synonyms for this developmental anomaly of the maxillary incisor teeth, the groove, if it extends onto the root, serves as a reservoir for plaque and calculus, leading to the development of localized periodontitis (Assaf and Roller 1992). See also distolingual groove, palatal groove, palatogingival groove, palatoradicular groove, radicular lingual groove.

Circular Fiber Group—These connective tissue fibers, being part of the gingival fiber group, lie just apical to the gingival epithelium and completely encircle the tooth, providing tonus, support, and contour to the free gingival (See Fig. C-4a,b). They occupy a large part of the available space between the alveolar crest and gingival margin. Sumter S. Arnim and David A. Hagerman first described this fiber group (Arnim and Hagerman 1953) See also gingival fiber group, ligamentum circulare dentis.

Circular Toothbrushing Technique—This method of toothbrushing is also known as the Fones toothbrushing technique (Ray 2005). See also Fones toothbrushing technique, toothbrushing technique.

Circumferential Defect—A type of infrabony defect whose four osseous walls are the buccal, lingual, mesial, and distal (Goldman and Cohen 1958). See also infrabony defect, osseous defect.

Circumferential Supracrestal Fiberotomy (CSF)—This surgical procedure is also known as fiberotomy. CSF is a more specific term because it includes not only transection of the gingival fibers but also that of the transseptal fibers. The surgical blade is placed 2 to 3 mm apical to the crest of the alveolar bone to alleviate re-

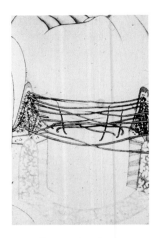

Fig. C-4a: Facial view (With permission from the American Dental Association)

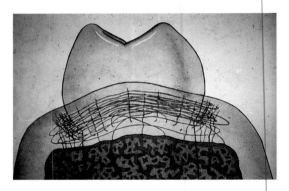

Fig. C-4b: Interproximal view (With permission from the American Dental Association.)

lapse of orthodontically rotated teeth. This term was coined by P.M. Campbell, J.W. Moore, and J.L. Matthews (Campbell et al. 1975). See also fiberotomy, supracrestal fiberotomy.

Circumferential Suture—In this suturing method, the suture encircles the tooth when only one flap (buccal or lingual) is involved and when the tissue is suspended at a desired level rather than being pulled taut as far as possible (Morris 1965a). See also suture.

Citric Acid—A tricarboxylic acid used as a root biomodifier when placed in a near-saturated solution at a pH of 1.0 to 1.4 (See Fig. R-4). It is claimed to aid in the detoxification and cleansing of diseased root surfaces and exposing intrinsic collagen fibers in new attachment procedures (AAP 2001a). Extensive reviews of citric acid use in root biomodification have been published (Fialkoff and Fry 1982; Holden and Smith 1983). See also root biomodification.

Clark's Rule—In 1910, C.F. Clark introduced the parallax method for identifying the location and position of impacted teeth, especially maxillary canines (Fig. C-5a,b,c). If the cuspid moves in the same direction as the tube head when two periapical films are taken in the same horizontal plane for comparison (one film taken at a more distal position), then the cuspid is in a palatal position. If the cuspid moves in the opposite direction, it is in the facial position. If there is little discernible movement radiographically, the cuspid is in a relatively normal position in the alveolar ridge. The acronym **slob** may be used in recalling the principle of tube shift: **s**ame, **l**ingual, **o**pposite, **b**uccal (i.e., **same** direction of movement of the image of the impacted tooth as the tube moves, then the tooth is **lingual**; **opposite** direction of movement to the tube, then the tooth is **buccal**) (Clark 1910; Wise 1981; Jacobs 1999).

Clenching—Clenching, according to Sigurd P. Ramfjord and Major M. Ash, is defined as centric bruxism or tooth grinding in centric occlusion (Ramfjord and Ash 1966). See also bruxism, centric occlusion, parafunction.

Closed Crevicular Curettage—This term refers to performing a soft tissue curettage rather than a flap procedure in treating periodontal pockets. According to Ralph Pollack, this approach has several advantages. It may be used (1) for initial preparation to obtain predictable soft tissue shrinkage, (2) when surgery is contraindicated for health or medical reasons, (3) when emotional patients cannot tolerate

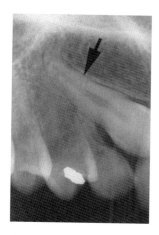

Fig. C-5a: Arrow, impacted canine

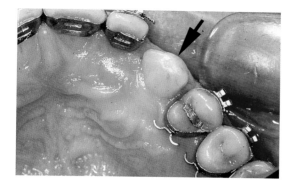

Fig. C-5b: Arrow, retained deciduous canine

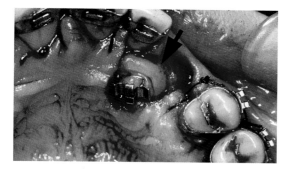

Fig. C-5c: Arrow, exposed canine; removal of deciduous canine

definitive surgery, and (4) when esthetic concerns are a consideration (Pollack 1984). See also closed curettage, curettage, subgingival curettage.

Closed Curettage—This refers to the debridement of deep periodontal pockets (scaling, root planing, and soft tissue curettage) where access to root surfaces is poor (See Fig. S-7a,b). This is in contrast to performing the same procedure after flap elevation. Sigurd P. Ramfjord called this procedure a "blind curettage" (Ramfjord 1980; AAP 2001a). See also closed crevicular curettage, curettage, subgingival curettage.

Codestructive Factor—A term coined by Irving Glickman during his studies of the interaction between inflammatory periodontal disease and trauma from occlusion. The codestructive factor consists of the **zone of irritation** (bounded by the marginal gingiva and transseptal fibers) and the **zone of codestruction** (which includes the periodontal ligament, alveolar bone, and cementum). It is known that trauma from occlusion has no effect on inflamed gingiva or the zone of irritation (Goldman 1956); however, when inflammation progresses to the supporting structures of the tooth or to the zone of codestruction, trauma from occlusion results in further spread and destruction of the periodontal attachment. These two zones make up the codestructive factor (Glickman 1963).

Col—The shape or contour, in a buccal-lingual direction, between the buccal and lingual papillae when the teeth are in contact (Cohen 1959). The American Academy of Periodontology has defined it as a valley-like depression of the interdental gingiva that connects facial and lingual papillae that conforms to the shape of the interproximal contact area (AAP 2001a). The term is borrowed from mountaineering, where it is used to describe a ridge-shaped depression adjoining two adjacent peaks (Fish 1961). See also interdental col, interdental papilla.

Community Periodontal Index of Treatment Needs (CPITN)—An index developed by the World Health Organization in 1978 to measure the periodontal treatment needs of a population. It was based on a clinical examination developed by Jukka and Anja Ainamo and a screening system developed by Timothy O'Leary and J.R. Johansen, P. Gjermo, and H.T. Bellini (Ainamo and Ainamo 1978; O'Leary 1967; Johansen et al. 1973). The dentition is divided into sextants and every tooth in each sextant is probed with a WHO or PSR probe for bleeding, calculus, and depth. The index is derived by assigning the worst condition (code 0 to 4) around any single tooth in each sextant. The codes are as follows: 0, no signs of disease; 1, gingival bleeding on gentle probing; 2, supra- or subgingival calculus; 3, pathologic pockets of 4 to 5.5 mm; and 4, pathologic pockets of 6 mm or more. The description and methodology for using the CPITN were first given by Jukka Ainamo, David Barmes, George Beagrie, Terry Cutress, Jean Martin, and Jennifer Sardo-Infirri (Ainamo et al. 1982). See also periodontal screening and recording (PSR) probe.

Complete Denudation—A term in mucogingival surgery coined by Henry M. Goldman, Saul Schluger, Lewis J. Fox, and D. Walter Cohen for the now obsolete term "pushback" procedure (Goldman et al. 1964). See also pushback.

Composite Graft—A hard tissue graft utilized to augment periodontal or osseous defects or for sinus augmentation, etc. It consists of more than one graft material (Valentini and Abensur 1997).

Composite Index—An index with both reversible and irreversible components. Examples are (1) periodontal index, (2) periodontal disease index, and (3) gingival–bone count index (AAP 1996a, 2005a). See also index, irreversible index, reversible index.

Confirm Bleeding Day Index—This index is positive only when the probed area, upon

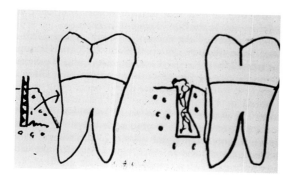

Fig. C-6: (With permission from Elsevier Publishing)

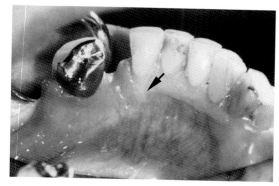

Fig. C-7a: Arrow, gingival recession

provocation 48 to 72 hours after initially probed, bleeds a second time (Watts et al. 1979).

Contiguous Autogenous Transplant—A technique of bone augmentation similar to "bone swaging"; however, the osseous graft is not completely detached from the donor site but is moved against the tooth, similar to a greenstick fracture (See Fig. C-6). According to the authors, the bone is repositioned, not "swaged," since the latter term refers to the remodeling of metallic objects. A contiguous autogenous transplant is indicated for infrabony pockets with one osseous wall (Ross et al. 1966). Histologic assessment has also been reported (Zubery et al. 1993). See also bone swaging.

Contiguous Pedicle Graft—A term coined by Herman Corn in 1964 for his edentulous area pedicle graft procedure (See Fig. C-7a,b,c) (Corn 1964). See also edentulous area pedicle graft, lateral repositioned flap, sliding flap.

Contiguous Soft Tissue Autograft—A term coined by D. Walter Cohen to refer to the repositioning of existing gingiva to create more gingiva on a recipient tooth. The word contiguous implies that a connection exists between the flap or graft's donor site with the recipient site by a soft tissue pedicle. Synonyms of this term include the following: (1) laterally positioned flap, (2) oblique rotated flap, (3)

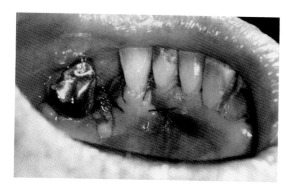

Fig. C-7b: Pedicle graft sutured

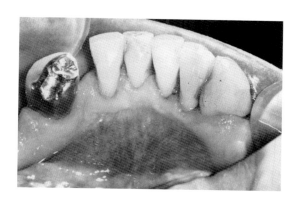

Fig. C-7c: Postoperative results

double papillae flap, (4) coronally positioned flap, and (5) apically positioned flap (Cohen 1969).

Continuous Sling Periosteal Suture—This type of suturing is utilized in the apical positioning of a partial-thickness flap when an attempt is being made to increase the zone of attached gingiva. The continuous sling suture passes through the periosteum in such a manner as to "hold" the flap in an apical position (Douglas 1976). See also interrupted periosteal suture, suture.

Continuous Sling Suture—This type of suture is employed in closing the facial and palatal (lingual) flaps independent of each other. The clinician is able to "sling" the buccal or facial flap apically to a desired position and yet draw the prescalloped palatal flap tightly around the necks of the teeth (Dahlberg 1969). See also sling suture, suture.

Continuous Suture—This suturing technique is utilized in closing both the buccal and lingual flaps simultaneously when there is little discrepancy between the facial and lingual osseous levels (Rosner 1977). See also suture.

Coronal Flap Positioning—The placement of a flap coronally, beyond its original presurgical position, to facilitate the healing of intrabony defects or furcation defects or in the course of other types of guided tissue regenerative procedures. The flap retention on the crown is achieved through placement of brackets, adhesives, or other individualized suturing techniques (Pontoriero et al. 1988). See also coronally advanced flap, coronally displaced flap, coronally positioned flap.

Coronal Migration—A synonym for creeping attachment, the physiologic migration of the epithelial attachment coronally following various surgical procedures. This expression was used to describe "coronal migration" of the gingival margin following the frenectomy procedure (Waltzer and Halik 1954). See also creeping attachment, physiologic regeneration, secondary root coverage.

Coronally Advanced Flap—Also known as coronal flap positioning (Francetti et al.

2000). See also coronal flap positioning, coronally displaced flap, coronally positioned flap.

Coronally Displaced Flap—Also known as coronal flap positioning. Following two vertical incisions, the flap is sutured coronally by passing the suture through a previously placed orthodontic plastic tube or button (Gantes and Garrett 1991). See also coronal flap positioning, coronally advanced flap, coronally positioned flap.

Coronally Positioned Flap—Also known as coronal flap positioning. This surgical procedure was introduced in 1926; its use has frequently been reported in the current periodontal literature (Norberg 1926; Garrett et al. 1994). See also coronal flap positioning, coronally advanced flap, coronally displaced flap.

Coronally Positioned Palatal Sliding Flap—A periodontal surgical flap devised to cover implants inserted in compromised positions when augmented with barrier membranes. Following elevation of a palatal mucoperiosteal flap, a series of incisions are made in the flap, allowing movement of the outer surface of the palatal flap coronally. This "sliding" flap will cover the barrier and approximate the implant, eventually being sutured to the buccal flap. This procedure may accomplish ridge augmentation as well as increasing the zone of keratinized gingiva adjacent to the implant. It may be indicated in a variety of periodontal surgical procedures, especially GTR and implant surgery (Tinti et al. 1995).

Coronally Repositioned Flap—A surgical procedure performed in the management and treatment of gingival recession. The flap is "repositioned" to its original presurgical position for improvement of esthetics, management of symptoms, and aid in health/function (Bernimoulin et al. 1975). This periodontal plastic procedure may be used alone (Guinard and Caffesse 1978) or in combination with a free soft tissue autograft (Caffesse and Guinard

1978). See also incisal repositioning flap, semilunar coronally repositioned flap.

Coronectomy—A term introduced in 1989 by Gerald M. Bowers and colleagues in their histologic study of the new attachment of periodontally involved teeth. It made reference to the process of submerging vital roots by the removal of the tooth's crown (Bowers et al. 1989).

Corrosion—The chemical or electrochemical dissolution of tooth surfaces by either endogenous or exogenous sources. Endogenous sources may include gastric acids due to bulimia nervosa or gastroesophageal reflux disease (GERD) (Grippo et al. 2004) or gingival crevicular fluid flow, as once suggested by Bodecker (Bodecker 1945). Exogenous sources include acidic food and/or beverages consumed in excess (See Fig. C-8a,b,c). Excessive dissolution of tooth structure has also been reported following a health-conscious patient's habitual chewing of 500-mg tablets of vitamin C (Ciancio 2004). It has been proposed that the term corrosion supplant the term erosion in the dental lexicon (Grippo et al. 2004). See also abfraction, abrasion, attrition, erosion.

Corticotomy—Also known as cortical osteotomy, this is a partial osteotomy, involving only the cortical plate, designed to weaken the resistance of the bone to the application of force. Such a procedure is routinely performed prior to distraction osteogenesis for elongation of the mandible or maxilla (Daskalogiannakis 2000). See also distraction osteogenesis.

Cosmetic Periodontal Surgery—Esthetic or cosmetic periodontal surgery has taken on an entirely new meaning since the early days of managing mucogingival defects, especially when they occur to the maxillary anterior gingiva. These problems may be related to (1) excessive gingival display with insufficient clinical crown length (See Fig. C-9a,b), (2) asymmetry of gingival margins, (3) improper relationship of gingival margins, (4) flat marginal contour, (5) localized marginal tissue re-

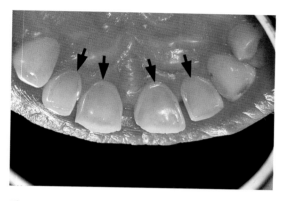

Fig. C-8a: Arrows, corrosion due to lemon sucking

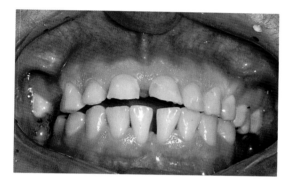

Fig. C-8b: Loss of tooth enamel due to lemon sucking

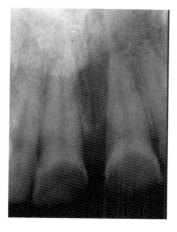

Fig. C-8c: Radiographic image of enamel loss

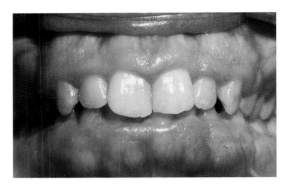

Fig. C-9a: Pretreatment (With permission from the Indiana Dental Association)

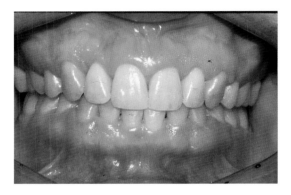

Fig. C-9b: Seven months posttreatment (With permission from the Indiana Dental Association)

cession, and (6) localized alveolar ridge deficiency (Allen 1988). See also mucogingival surgery, periodontal plastic surgery.

Costen Syndrome—This eponym, named after James B. Costen, an American otolaryngologist, was the first attempt to describe completely the framework of the etiology, pathogenesis, and treatment of the myofascial pain dysfunction syndrome. This syndrome, as stated by Costen, was explained as compression placed on the eustachian tube from the upward pressure of the condylar head through the tympanic plate and finally against the temporal and chorda tympani nerves (Sperber and Buckingham 2000).

According to Costen, this syndrome of ear and sinus symptoms is frequently seen in edentulous patients or those with marked overbite and manifests itself by impaired hearing, buzzing, snapping, pain, headaches, and a burning sensation in the throat (Costen 1934). See also myofascial pain dysfunction syndrome (MPD), temporomandibular disorders (TMD).

Cracked-Tooth Syndrome—This syndrome, which occurs most frequently to the mandibular second molars, may be diagnosed by (1) discomfort in chewing, (2) unexplained sensitivity to cold, and (3) severe pain in the absence of dental caries (Cameron 1976). In addition to pulpal problems associated with the cracked-tooth syndrome, periodontal pockets have also been shown to occur along the line of fracture (Hiatt 1973).

Crane-Kaplan Technique—This surgical approach to treating pyorrhea alveolaris, introduced in 1931, is a conservative technique for eliminating all unsupported gingival tissue (pockets) with minimal osseous reduction. After the establishment of bleeding points and subsequent tissue removal by following the points, the complete labial and lingual gingival flap of tissue is removed. The teeth are then thoroughly scaled, all unsupported tissue removed, and the underlying bone beveled. Once the hemorrhage is controlled, a cement pack is placed for protection and tissue healing. The establishment of normal periodontal relationships usually occurs in 1 to 3 months, with the end result closely resembling normal recession (Crane and Kaplan 1931; Kaplan and Milobsky 1951).

Crater Defect—The crater is a two-walled infrabony pocket located interdentally and bounded by buccal and lingual walls (Goldman and Cohen 1958). It is the most common infrabony pocket found in patients with periodontitis (Saari et al. 1968). Clifford Ochsenbein and Harry Bohannan have further classified craters by their depth and the thickness of their walls, as follows: class I, 2- to 3-mm osseous concavities with relatively thick buccal and lingual walls; class II, 4- to 5-mm osseous concavities with wide orifices and thinned walls; Class III, 6- to 7-mm osseous concavities with a sharp drop of the crater wall from the margins to a broad flat bone; and class IV, the least common, various depths with extremely thin buccal and lingual walls (Ochsenbein and Bohannan 1964). See also infrabony defect, interdental crater, interproximal crater.

Creeping Attachment—This phenomenon involves the postoperative migration of the gingival margin in a coronal direction over portions of a previously denuded root. Such migration is often seen to continue for long periods postoperatively until a consistent marginal level is reached. The gingival tissue is attached firmly to the root and positive exploration by a probe does not reveal any clinical sulcular depth. This phenomenon is a clinical observation that cannot be substantiated scientifically. It cannot be predicted on a routine clinical basis (Goldman et al. 1964). It has been described as a result of (1) progressive movement of the attachment apparatus or (2) a neoformation of attached gingiva and periodontal fibers on the denuded root surface (Matter and Cimasoni 1976). See also coronal migration, physiologic regeneration, secondary root coverage.

Crestal Incision—This type of incision during periodontal surgery aims to direct the tip of the Bard Parker scalpel at the **crest** of the alveolar process. It is most frequently utilized in the elevation of a full-thickness mucoperiosteal flap (Litch et al. 1984). See also subcrestal incision, sulcular incision.

Crestal Lamina Dura—The radiographic white line observed at the crest of the alveolar bone in properly angulated and processed dental radiographs. It is often assessed by clinicians in judging periodontal health, but caution must be exercised when using the integrity of the crestal lamina dura as an indicator for either peri-

odontal health or the need for treatment (Rams et al. 1994). See also lamina dura.

Crevicular Epithelium—(see Fig. J-1) Also known as sulcular epithelium, this refers to the nonkeratinized epithelium lining the gingival crevice (Bral and Stahl 1977). See also sulcular epithelium.

Crevicular Incision—Also known as a sulcular incision, this is one of several incisions utilized during flap surgery when the tip of the Bard Parker scalpel is inserted into the gingival crevice (pocket) for flap elevation or in the process of removing inflamed sulcular tissue (Johnson, RH 1976). See also sulcular incision.

Cribriform Plate—The inner wall of the tooth socket, which is perforated by many openings, being sieve-like in appearance in dry skull specimens. These openings carry the nerves and blood vessels into the periodontal ligament (Orban 1957). See also alveolar bone proper, lamina dura.

Critical Mass of Alveolar Bone Support—That remaining level of alveolar bone support, although reduced, which will permit tooth mobility to be reversed. It allows for physiologic adaptive changes to occur that mediate reparative and regenerative processes and thus reduce or eliminate tooth mobility (Perlitsh 1980).

Critical Probing Depth (CPD)—The initial probing depth value below which loss of attachment occurred as a result of treatment and above which gain of attachment resulted (Lindhe et al. 1982).

Crown Lengthening—A surgical procedure designed to increase the extent of supragingival tooth structure for restorative or esthetic purposes (See Fig. C-9a,b). It is achieved by apically positioning the gingival margin, removing supporting bone, or both. This may also be accomplished by orthodontic tooth movement (Allen 1993a; Wagenberg et al. 1989; Becker et al. 1998; Wagenberg 1998; AAP 2001a; Hildebrand 2003). See also forced eruption, tooth lengthening, vertical extrusion.

Cryosurgery—One form of "cryotherapy," or the destruction of tissue by extreme cold, usually by the use of liquid nitrogen or carbon dioxide (See Fig. C-10a,b) (AAP 2001a). Its first use in dentistry was to treat malignant and benign lesions of the oral cavity (Gage et al. 1965; Emmings et al. 1967); thereafter its suitability in treating periodontal disease was shown by Ronald Odrich and Charles Kelman in 1967 (Odrich and Kelman 1967).

Curettage—A surgical technique in dentistry designed to remove, by debridement, the inner aspect of the diseased gingival wall, including the ulcerative and hyperplastic gingival epithelium and the contiguous zone of damaged connective tissue downward and outward to the firm and intact aspect of the gingival corium, thus converting diseased tissue to a surgical wound (Kon et al. 1969; Pollack 1984). The current statement on gingival curettage from the American Academy of Periodontology has been published (AAP 2002a). See also closed curettage, closed crevicular curettage, root curettage, subgingival curettage.

Curtain Technique—A surgical flap technique designed to permit conservation of the maxillary anterior esthetics as well as to preserve phonetics. During the procedure, the triangular piece of labial papilla that remains is referred to as the **curtain,** and its preparation as such represents the entire extent of the labial surgery. It retains its vital connection with the intact labial attached gingiva (Frisch et al. 1967). This technique has received more attention lately and its esthetic preservation is described and illustrated by presenting several completed cases; its author has called it the *modified resective technique,* or MRT (Lie 1992).

Curve of Spee—As used in the study of mastication, this is the anteroposterior curve of occlusion, which is concave upward. It was named after the German embryologist, Ferdinand Graf von Spee and was described by him in 1890 (Spee 1890; Sperber and Buckingham 2000). A literal translation of Spee's initial statement is as

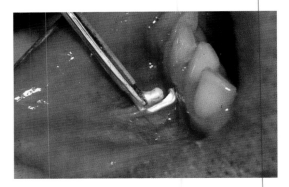

Fig. C-10a: Cryosurgery probe placed on frenum

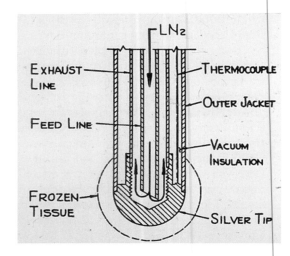

Fig. C-10b: Schematic diagram of liquid nitrogen cryosurgery probe

follows: "If a curved line be drawn touching the summits of the buccal cusps of the upper or lower teeth from first bicuspid to third molar, it will more or less accurately correspond to the arc of a circle with its convexity downward. This curve varies in different individuals. If, in a skull with typical dentin, it is considered in a projection of the jaw upon the vertical sagittal plane, it touches the anterior face of the articular surface of the condyle. This is the most ideal form. In the case of man, the center of the curve lies behind the crista lacrymalis posterior and on the line bisecting the horizontal plane passing through the orbit" (Nagao 1919).

Cuspid Rise—In the study of occlusion during lateral movement of the mandible, disarticulation of the dentition by opposing cuspids. This prevents trauma to the temporomandibular articulation and the periodontium (D'Amico 1958, 1959). *Synonyms are cuspid guidance and cuspid protected occlusion* (AAP 2001a).

Cutback Incision—As used during periodontal surgery, this incision is placed in the alveolar mucosa so as to relieve flap tension, enabling the flap to move more freely around its base. The cutback incision is placed in the direction to which the flap (pedicle) is to be moved (Corn 1964).

Cyanoacrylates—In the 1960s, Surindar N. Bhaskar studied the ability of certain chemical substances to adhere to and cement moist, living tissue. These chemical substances, known as cyanoacrylates, were found to be beneficial in protecting both orofacial wounds and selected periodontal wounds following surgery. They eliminated the need for sutures, provided homeostasis, and were biodegradable in 7 to 10 days. The two cyanoacrylates that proved acceptable to living tissues were the butyl and isobutyl types (Bhaskar et al. 1966; McGraw and Caffesse 1978). See also periodontal dressing, suture.

Cyclic Neutropenia—A decrease or lack of circulating neutrophils (white blood cells), occurring every 3 to 4 weeks. Its clinical and radiographic appearance periodontally closely resembles that of an "aggressive" periodontitis (Cohen and Morris 1961; Scully et al. 1982). The neutrophil count should be less than 500/mm for 3 to 5 days during each of at least three successive cycles in order to make this diagnosis. Fortunately, the symptoms related to cyclic neutropenia seem to diminish after the second decade of life despite the fact that the cycling of the neutrophils continues. (Neville et al. 2002).

Cytokines—A group of bioactive polypeptides produced by a wide variety of cells that mediate a variety of metabolic and immunologic functions (Van Dyke et al. 1993). Another source has described them as a large group of proteins made by cells capable of regulating a wide variety of cellular functions (AAP 2001a). See also growth and differentiation factors.

D

Decalcified Freeze Dried Bone Allograft (DFDBA)—Also known as *demineralized* freeze-dried bone allograft (Mellonig 1998), DFDBA fulfills four important functions in periodontal regenerative surgery: (1) osteoinductivity, (2) osteoconductivity, (3) space making, and (4) clot stabilization (Reddie 1987). See also allograft, demineralized freeze-dried bone allograft (DFDBA).

Decayed, Missing, Filled Index (DMF)—This irreversible index provides information as to the prevalence and incidence of dental caries and their sequelae. The "D" represents open cavities or decay, the "M" refers to missing teeth or those designated for removal, and "F" indicates filled cavities. The index was developed by H. Trendley Dean and further elaborated upon in 1938 by H. Klein, C.E. Palmer, and J.W. Knutsen (Klein et al. 1938). See also irreversible index.

Decortication—This term refers to the removal of dense or sclerotic bone in an intrabony pocket via multiple intramarrow penetrations or perforations, thus providing for a greater vascularized surface that is more osteogenic for periodontal regeneration (Nabers and O'Leary 1965, 1967; AAP 2001a; Cohen 1989).

Deepithelized Connective Tissue Pedicle Graft—In the interest of augmentation of residual ridges for prosthetics, a technique for ridge augmentation was introduced in 1980 by placing a connective tissue pedicle graft labially to an edentulous area in order to create the desired esthetic result (Abrams 1980) David Garber and Edwin Rosenberg modified this technique by suturing a combined epithelial and connective tissue graft, removed from the tuberosity, onto the deepithelized ridge (Garber and Rosenberg 1981). See also ridge augmentation.

Dehiscence—The absence of alveolar cortical plate sometimes exceeding more than half of the root length and often resulting in a denuded root surface (See Fig. D-1a,b) (Elliott and Bowers 1963; Larato 1970d) When a dehiscence has resulted in severe loss of the alveolar cortical plate, it has been called a class III fenestration (See Fig F-6a,b for a postoperative view) (Stahl et al. 1963). See also fenestration.

Delayed Passive Eruption—A dentogingival relationship in which the margin of the gingiva is positioned incisally/occlusally on the anatomic crown in adulthood and does not approximate the cementoenamel junction (Volchansky and Cleaton Jones 1976). It has been further classified according to (1) gingival/anatomic crown relationships and (2) alveolar crest/CEJ relationships with associated types and subgroups. (Coslet et al. 1977) A more current overview of de-

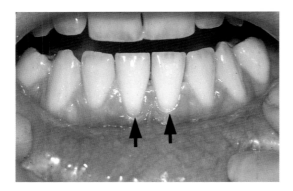

Fig. D-1a: Arrow, facial dehiscences

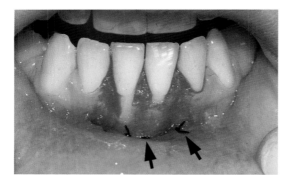

Fig. D-1b: Hidden dehiscences, surgically exposed; arrows, sutures (With permission from the American Academy of Periodontology)

layed passive eruption has been presented (Weinberg and Eskow 2000a). See also altered passive eruption, passive eruption.

Demineralized Freeze-Dried Bone Allograft (DFDBA)—A bone graft with an identified bone morphogenetic protein (BMP) that is capable of osteogenic induction by inducing primordial cells to differentiate into osteoblasts even when implanted in tissues that would otherwise not form bone (Urist 1965). Also known as a decalcified freeze-dried bone allograft (Mellonig 1998). A status report on the use of bone allografts in periodontal regeneration is available (AAP 2001b). See also allograft, decalcified freeze-dried bone allograft (DFDBA).

Dental Health Center (DHC) Index—An index that measures gingival inflammation and the propensity for loss of attachment by assessing the degree of gingivitis, loss of attachment, and supra- and subgingival dental calculus around eight teeth. These teeth include all the permanent first molars, the upper right central incisor, the upper left first bicuspid, the lower left central incisor, and the lower right first bicuspid (Suomi et al. 1969).

Dentogingival Complex—The dentogingival complex comprises three components: (1) the connective tissue fibrous attachment, (2) the junctional epithelium or epithelial attachment, and (3) the gingival sulcus (Kois 1994). It is also known as the dentogingival unit. See also dentogingival unit.

Dentogingival Fiber Group—This group of collagenous fibers runs from the supra-alveolar cementum, beneath the junctional epithelium, and outward in a flaring fashion into three distinct groups: (1) group A, into the free gingiva; (2) group B, into the attached gingiva; and (3) group C, into the periosteum (See Fig. D-2) (Orban 1957). See also gingival fiber group.

Dentogingival Junction—According to Harry Sicher, this is the functional unit of the periodontium composed of the connective tissue attachment of the gingiva and the epithelial attachment (Sicher 1959). The first detailed description of the "physiologic" dentogingival junction was by Anthony W. Gargiulo, Frank M. Wentz, and Balint Orban, who described in detail the measured anatomic relationships of the dentogingival junction (Gargiulo et al. 1961).

Dentogingival Unit—Also known as the dentogingival complex (Listgarten MA 1970). See also dentogingival complex.

Dentoperiosteal Fiber Group—This group of collagenous fibers, part of the gingival fiber group, extends from the lateral (outer) surfaces of the alveolar bone to the root cementum. They function to anchor the tooth to the bone (Orban 1957). See also gingival fiber group.

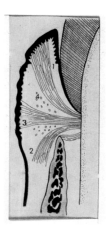

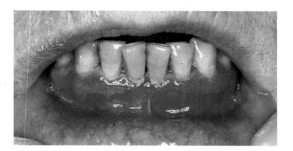

Fig. D-3

Fig. D-2: 1, free gingival fiber group A; 2, periosteal fiber group C; 3, attached gingival fiber group B; 4, circular fiber group (cross-sectional view)

Denudation—This term refers to the baring or exposure of the alveolar process during periodontal surgery. It was a popular and major technique in the management of mucogingival defects in the "pushback" procedure (Friedman 1957). R. Earl Robinson introduced bone denudation as his second incision in the periosteal fenestration technique (Robinson 1961), and Herman Corn bared the bone in vestibular deepening during the periosteal separation procedure (Corn 1962). See also periosteal fenestration; periosteal separation; pushback procedure.

Desquamative Gingivitis—A nonspecific term denoting chronic, diffuse inflammation of the gingiva with sloughing of the surface (See Fig. D-3) (AAP 2001a). It can be found in several mucosal diseases such as erosive lichen planus, benign mucous membrane pemphigoid, bulbous pemphigoid, and pemphigus vulgaris. It was first described by J. Tomes and G. Tomes in 1894 and later elaborated by H. Prinz, who called it chronic desquamative gingivitis. He defined it as a chronic diffuse inflammation of the marginal gum tissue characterized by desquamation of the epithelium of the papilla, deep bluish red-

ness of the underlying connective tissue, readily bleeds upon irritation and rarely affects the palatal region (Prinz 1932). See also chronic desquamative gingivitis (CDG), gingivosis.

Dieback—Coined by Kevin G. Murphy, this expression denotes the sloughing or necrosis of the gingival flap when guided tissue regeneration procedures are performed. It is due to the deprived blood supply to the gingiva when a nonresorbable barrier is used (Murphy 1995a, 1995b).

Diffuse Alveolar Atrophy—Severe alveolar bone resorption with loss of periodontal ligament fiber orientation but without gingival alterations. It was first described by Bernhard Gottleib in 1920, when he noticed wandering and loosening of teeth as an early periodontal symptom, with pocket formation and suppuration coming later (Gottleib 1920, 1928). In 1946, he changed this term to *cementopathia* (Gottleib 1946). See also cementopathia, juvenile periodontitis, periodontosis.

Digital Subtraction Radiography—See also subtraction radiography, digital.

Disclosing Agent—A disclosing agent, as defined by Murray Raybin, is a solution that, when applied to teeth, makes roughness and foreign matter on the teeth visible by staining (See Fig. D-4a,b). "Foreign matter" here includes mucinous plaques, calculus and materia alba/food debris, bacteria and their products, and dead tissue elements (Raybin 1943, 1945) Sumter

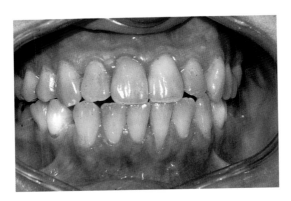

Fig. D-4a: Before plaque disclosure

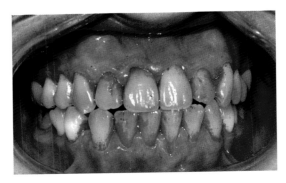

Fig. D-4b: Plaque disclosed

S. Arnim popularized the use of disclosing agents as routine adjuncts to oral hygiene by introducing erythrosin FDC Red Dye #3 to dentistry (Arnim 1963). The important role of disclosing agents in educating patients in oral physiotherapy is frequently stressed in the literature (Tan AES 1981).

Displaced Flap—The displaced flaps, included in both the "pushback" and "pouch" procedures, no longer have a role in periodontal therapy. They were used in the early days of mucogingival surgery in attempts to deepen the vestibular fornix and create a wider zone of attached gingiva. These procedures marked the beginning of the era of mucogingival surgery (Gargiulo 1969). See also gingival extension, pouch procedure, pushback procedure.

Distal Wedge—The distal wedge procedure was introduced to periodontics by R. Earl Robinson; it is designed to manage periodontal pockets on a terminal tooth in either the retromolar or tuberosity areas. The incision outline may be either triangular, square, or linear. Robinson initially presented it before the Western Society of Periodontology in Palm Springs, California, in November 1963 (Robinson 1966). See also modified distal wedge, proximal wedge.

Distolingual Groove—Also known as the palatogingival groove. This tooth anomaly or variation in anatomy is akin to the dens in dente, often found in the same location on the maxillary lateral incisors (Everett and Kramer 1972). See also cinguloradicular groove, palatal groove, palatogingival groove, palatoradicular groove, radicular lingual groove.

Distraction Osteogenesis—This surgical technique lengthens long bones of the extremities by gradual distraction of a fracture callus; it is associated with its developer, the Russian orthopedic surgeon Gavriel A. Ilizarov (Ilizarov 1988). It is also used in the craniofacial area for the correction of bone defects in the skull and the treatment of vertical deficiencies in the maxilla or mandible prior to implant placement. It involves a corticotomy followed by gradual distraction of the segments, with formation of new bone (regenerate bone) between them. The distraction can be performed by an external or an intraoral device containing some type of screw that can be wound gradually, in a manner similar to rapid maxillary expansion (Daskalogiannakis 2000; McAllister and Gaffaney 2003). See also corticotomy.

Double-Flap Procedure—A surgical procedure devised in 1960 by Clifford Ochsenbein to treat periodontal pockets in the mandibular arch when they traverse a narrow band of attached gingiva in the presence of a shallow vestibular fornix. It provides the means of gaining access to and correcting the bony lesion while maintaining a tissue cover over all bone not immediately involved in the resection (Ochsenbein 1960, 1963).

Double Papillae Repositioned Flap—A plastic and reconstructive surgical approach to restoring lost gingiva where recession has occurred on the labial or lingual gingiva, when there is no loss of the interdental papillae on either side of the denuded area. The advantages of the double papillae flap over the laterally positioned flap are (1) minimal exposure of underlying periodontium at the interdental donor sites, (2) reduction of tension and pull on the repositioned flap, and (3) a greater amount of gingiva in the interdental locations than on the adjacent labial or buccal surfaces (Cohen and Ross 1968; Ross et al. 1986). See also interdental papillae graft.

Early-Onset Periodontitis—A group of dissimilar destructive periodontal diseases that affect very young patients. They are prepubertal periodontitis, juvenile periodontitis, and rapidly progressive periodontitis (AAP 1989; Albander et al. 1997). See also aggressive periodontitis, generalized juvenile periodontitis (GJP), juvenile periodontitis, localized juvenile periodontitis (LJP), pre-pubertal periodontitis, rapidly progressive periodontitis (RPP).

Eastman Interdental Bleeding Index (EIBI)—Also known as the Interdental Bleeding Index (IBI). This is a clinical evaluation of gingival health based on the bleeding tendency following stimulation with wooden interdental cleaners (Caton et al. 1989). See also interdental bleeding index (IBI).

Edentulous Area Pedicle Graft—This plastic surgery technique applies to those situations where teeth adjoining edentulous areas exhibit the following: (1) pockets involving the mucogingival junction, (2) an absence or near absence of functional gingiva on the radicular surface, and (3) the presence of a related shallow vestibular fornix or frenum involvement (See Fig. E-1a,b,c,d). The success of this pedicle graft is dependent on (1) a suitable surgical design, (2) preparation of the pedicle at the donor site, (3) preparation of the recipient site, and (4) proper atraumatic surgical technique in the graft transplanta-tion (Corn 1964). See also contiguous pedicle graft, lateral repositional flap.

Edlan-Mejchar Technique—A plastic surgical periodontal procedure used for deepening the vestibular trough in the mandibular anterior region. This approach is most applicable where there are no pockets and little to no gingival tissue to make apical positioning practical (Edlan and Mejchar 1963). Long-term studies have shown this procedure to be predictable and to maintain the established vestibular depth over a 5-year period; however, the operation is technically difficult (Bergenholtz and Hugoson 1973).

Elaunin Fibers—Immature elastic fibers of human gingiva located in the middle layer of human gingival connective tissue. The upper layer contains oxytalan fibers and the lower layer consists of elastic fibers. These three layers (upper, middle, and lower) represent the consecutive stages of elastogenesis (Chavrier 1990). See also oxytalan fiber.

Electrocoagulation—The most commonly used electrosurgical procedure in dentistry, utilizing a biterminal technique with a partially rectified or fully modified rectified current (See Fig. E-2). It requires a damped or interrupted wave train, which prevents or controls hemorrhage. The coagulation electrodes are much bulkier than those used in electrosection

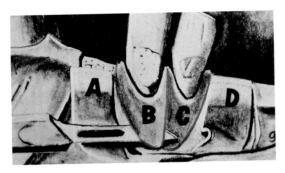

Fig. E-1a: B,C, tissue to be removed; A,D, tissue to reposition over area B,C (With permission from the American Academy of Periodontology)

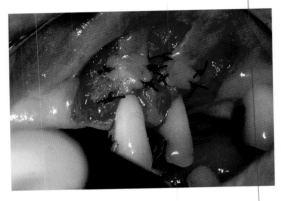

Fig. E-1c: Pedicle grafts repositioned

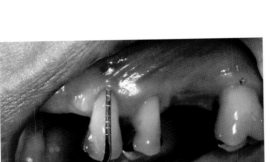

Fig. E-1b: Presurgical site

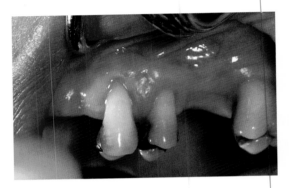

Fig. E-1d: Healing after 3 months

and have a shape of either a ball, bar, or cone (Flocken 1980; Azzi 1981). See also electrosurgery.

Electrodesiccation—A monoterminal electrosurgical technique that has little or no application in dentistry. It uses a dehydrating current and is the most dangerous electrosurgical technique. The active electrode is inserted in situ to coagulate a mass of tissue, being useful in dermatology, cancer surgery, and the treatment of cancerous hemangiomas. The operator has no control over the amount of tissue destroyed (Flocken 1980, Azzi 1981). See also electrosurgery.

Electrofulguration—This monoterminal electrosurgical technique is seldom used in dentistry. The active electrode is held slightly out of tissue contact and moved over the tissue, spraying sparks to produce a hard crust or scab, as from a burn (i.e., an eschar) (Flocken 1980; Azzi 1981). See also electrosurgery.

Electromyography—The study of electrical activity in muscle. Every time a muscle contracts, a minute fraction of the total energy liberated appears as electrical energy. This electrical activity is recorded by strategically placed electrodes over muscle groups and printed out on special graph paper. Researchers or electromyographers are then able to investigate the behavior of skeletal muscle (i.e., muscles of mastication) in humans under known or controlled conditions (Pruzansky 1960).

Electrosection—A biterminal technique of electrosurgery commonly used in den-

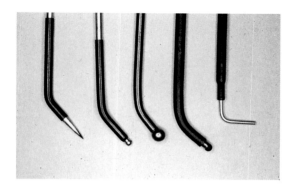

Fig. E-2: Electrocoagulation electrodes

tistry, requiring an undamped or continuous wave train. The procedures performed include (1) incisions and excisions and (2) planing. Incisions and excisions are performed by single-wire active electrodes that can be bent or adapted for any type of cutting procedure. Planing of tissue can be accomplished by selection of an appropriate loop electrode (Flocken 1980; Azzi 1981). See also electrosurgery.

Electrosurgery—The division of tissue by a high-frequency current, ranging from 1.5 to 7.5 million cycles per second, applied locally with a metal instrument or needles (AAP 2001a). Electrosurgical techniques may be either monopolar or bipolar. The monopolar method involves the cutting of tissue by means of an advancing spark with the patient grounded and in the electrical loop: it causes sparking, current spread, and thermal damage to the tissue, with delayed healing. The bipolar method involves the cutting of tissue without sparking or charring. It is not based on vaporization or an advancing spark but rather on molecular resonance. It both cuts and coagulates (Shuman 2001). The science and clinical applications of electrosurgery in both restorative dentistry and periodontics have been reviewed (Flocken 1980; Azzi 1981). See also electrocoagulation, electrodesiccation, electrofulguration, electrosection.

Enamel Matrix Derivative—Proteinaceous materials composed principally of amelogenins and related proteins derived from porcine tooth buds. The enamel matrix proteins (derivatives) are important for the development of acellular cementum, periodontal ligament, and alveolar bone (Mellonig 1999). See also amelogenins, enamel matrix proteins.

Enamel Matrix Proteins—These are thought to be synthesized by the cells of the epithelial root sheath; they play a fundamental role in the formation of acellular cementum. A dominating constituent of the enamel matrix protein is amelogenin, a hydrophobic, low-molecular-weight protein (Hammarstrom 1997, Hammarstrom et al. 1997). See also amelogenins, enamel matrix derivative.

Enamel Pearl—Isolated islands of large spheroidal ectopic enamel, rather than extensions of coronal enamel, formed apical to the cementoenamel junction on the root surface (See Fig. E-3a,b). The later cervical enamel projections are found on the lateral surface of the roots or furcations of molars (See Fig. C-3a,b) (Moskow and Canut 1990). See also cervical enamel projections (CEP), radicular enamel.

Endodontic-Periodontal Lesion—This lesion is characterized by a deep, localized periodontal pocket emanating from infected pulpal tissue. After a thorough examination, definitive treatment and cure is obtained by endodontic treatment (Solomon et al, 1995) See also retrograde periodontitis.

Envelope Flap—A periodontal flap with no vertical or releasing incisions (Dello Russo 1998). It is created by an inverse bevel incision and then freed from the remaining gingival margin and positioned according to the requirements of the area. It cannot be moved obliquely or laterally to a different position (Barrington 1973). See also relaxed flap.

Envelope Of Motion—The capacity of the mandible to move in all three planes in space, including the postural position, the

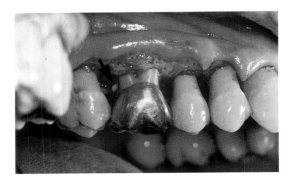

Fig. E-3a: Arrow, enamel pearl

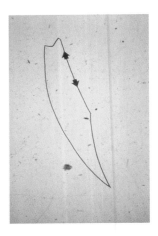

Fig. E-4

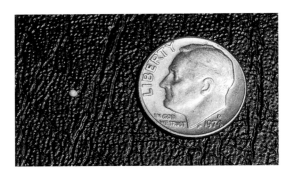

Fig. E-3b: Enamel pearl sized to coin

intercuspal position, the retruded position, and the position of maximum opening (See Fig. E-4). Ulf Posselt traced the path of the mandibular incisor teeth in the median plane throughout the range of mandibular movement and identified the relative location of these positions. The diagrammatic representation of all these mandibular border movements in a sagittal plane is known as the envelope of motion (Posselt 1968).

Envelope Technique—An innovative approach for covering localized areas of root exposure with a free connective tissue graft harvested from the depth of the hard palate. The graft is placed into an "envelope" on the recipient tooth previously created by partial-thickness dissection of tissues surrounding the defect. In this procedure, both sides of the graft are in inti-

mate contact with vital tissues (Raetzke 1985). See also Raetzke's pouch.

Epidemiology—The science concerned with the factors and conditions determining the occurrence and distribution of health, disease, defects, disability, and death among groups of individuals. The principal distinction between epidemiology and clinical practice is that the epidemiologist observes groups of individuals and his or her observations pertain to the whole group, both the affected and the unaffected, whereas a clinician is concerned with the individual patient (AAP 1996a, 2005a). One of the first attempts to categorize the severity of "periodontal" infection in a dental population, using merely a questionnaire and radiographic evidence, was undertaken in 1918 (Black 1918). See also incidence, prevalence.

Epithel Ansatz—The German term for epithelial attachment. (Gottlieb 1921). See also epithelial attachment.

Epithelial Attachment—The "organic" connection between the gingival epithelium and the tooth substance, discovered by Bernhard Gottlieb in 1921 (See Fig. J-1) (Gottlieb 1921). It comprises nonkeratinizing cells in one or more layers adhering to the tooth surface at the base of the gingival crevice (AAP 2001a). The attaching medium of the epithelial cells to the tooth surface is a product of the epithelial cells themselves (Stallard et al. 1965). Today, the epithelial attachment is called the "junctional epithelium" (AAP 2001a). See also junctional epithelium.

Epithelial Cuff—The gingival epithelium, which Jens Waerhaug suggested was in contact with the tooth structure but not really attached to it. According to Waerhaug, the bottom of the pocket is consistently reported to be situated at the cemento-enamel junction, with a capillary space between the gingiva and the tooth (Waerhaug 1952). As early as 1920, Arthur D. Black theorized that an epithelial cuff existed and "adjusted" to the enamel surface with no organic connection to it (Black 1920). See also attached epithelial cuff.

Epithelial Rests of Malassez—During tooth development, as cementum is deposited on dentin, the Hertwig epithelial root sheath disintegrates, resulting in deposition of epithelial cells within the periodontal ligament. These epithelial rests of Malassez, as they are now called, are isolated as either clusters of cells or interlocking strands near the cementum, decreasing in prevalence with increasing age (Orban 1952). They were named after the French physiologist Louis Charles Malassez, who described them in 1885 (Malassez 1885). The French anatomist Antonine Serres was likely the first to describe these rests; he called them "glandulae tartarica," believing them to be a possible source of dental calculus (Serres 1817). The rests of Malassez and Serres glands as eponyms were discussed by Sperber and Buckingham in 2000. See also Hertwig epithelial root sheath.

Erosion—An apparent chemical dissolution of enamel and dentin, unrelated to caries, causing a cavity that has a hard, smooth base (AAP 2001a). Its history in the dental literature can be traced back almost 100 years (Miller 1907). According to J.O. Grippo, M. Simring, and S. Schreiner, the term erosion should be deleted from the dental lexicon and supplanted by the term corrosion, to denote the chemical dissolution of teeth (Grippo et al. 2004). See also abfraction, abrasion, corrosion.

Established Periodontitis—A clinical entity based on the following: (1) clinical attachment level of ≥ 6 mm in two or more teeth and (2) one or more sites with probing depths of ≥ 5 mm. This expression may be useful in focusing on the subset of the population that may be at greatest risk for periodontal breakdown (Machtei et al. 1992).

Esthetic Zone—The area incorporated by the perimeter of the lips. The relationship of the three components involved in the smile—the teeth, the lips, and the gingiva—determines whether a particular smile has a high, medium, or low lip line. These components, in turn, determine subjectively whether or not a smile is attractive (Saadoun 1997).

Everett-Fixot Grid—This diagnostic x-ray grid, consisting of embedded wires in a piece of Plexiglass, is helpful for comparing bone levels in radiographs taken at various times under similar conditions (See Fig. E-5a,b,c,d,e). It is placed between the object to be studied and the dental film. The calibrated grid is divided into millimeters, running both horizontally and vertically, with every fifth millimeter accentuated by a heavier line for easier reading (Everett and Fixott 1963).

Evidence-Based Periodontal Treatment—The gathering of unbiased data (evidence) by investigators using specific rules of evidence to quantify therapeutic recommendations. The three steps used in gathering clinical information from the literature are (1) search, (2) evaluate, and (3) rank. This gathered information (i.e., evidence) can then be used to formulate new decision pathways in practice and treatment (McGuire and Newman 1995). A summary of the 1996 World Workshop in Periodontics, reporting on evidence-based periodontal therapy, was published in 1997 (Jeffcoat et al. 1997).

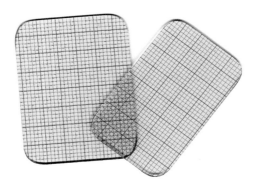

Fig. E-5a: Grids sized for no. 1 and 2 radiographic film

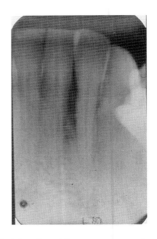

Fig. E-5d: No. 1 grid on preoperative GTR anterior film

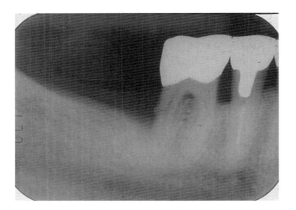

Fig. E-5b: No. 2 grid on preoperative GTR molar film

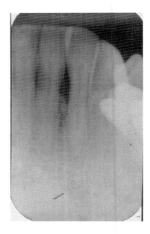

Fig. E-5e: No. 1 grid on postoperative GTR anterior film

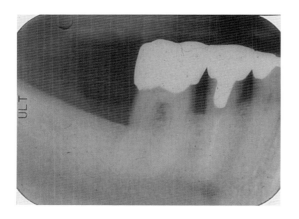

Fig. E-5c: No. 2 grid on postoperative GTR molar film

Excisional New Attachment Procedure (ENAP)—An approach to reestablishing periodontal attachment and reducing pocket depths (See Fig. E-6). It is attempted by surgically removing sulcular and junctional epithelium, the transseptal and gingival crest fibers, root calculus, and involved cementum, through an internal beveled incision without detachment of the mucogingival complex. Commonly called the ENAP, it was first presented and

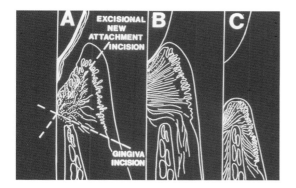

Fig. E-6: A, incisions for E-NAP and gingivectomy (GV); B, postoperative tissue height with E-NAP; C, postoperative tissue height with GV

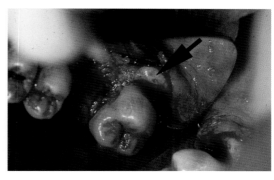

Fig. E-7c: Arrow, preoperative palatal exostosis (type C)

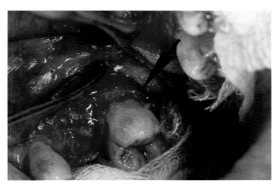

Fig. E-7d: Arrow, postoperative palatal exostosis removed (type C)

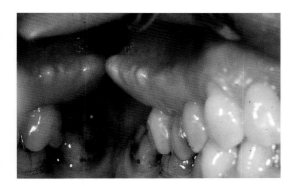

Fig. E-7a: Buccal exostosis (With permission from the Indiana Dental Association)

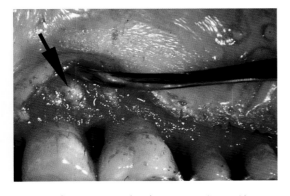

Fig. E-7b: Arrow, palatal exostosis (type A)

evaluated experimentally and clinically in 1976 (Yukna et al. 1976; Yukna 1976). See also internal bevel incision.

Exostosis—A benign bony growth projecting outward from the surface of a bone (See Fig. E-7a,b,c,d) (AAP 2001a). Exostoses are frequently uncovered upon the elevation of posterior flaps during periodontal surgery. They have been classified into five types: type A, small nodules of bone; type B, large nodules of bone; type C, a sharp ridge of bone; type D, spike-like projections of bone; and type E, combinations of A, B, C, and D (Larato 1972). Exostoses may also occur along the buccal aspect of the mandibular and maxillary alveolar ridge (Neville et al. 2002). See also Fig. C-9a under the term crown lengthening. The significance of these exostoses in the planning of periodontal surgery has been emphasized (Nery et al. 1977). See also torus.

Extent and Severity Index (ESI)—An index measuring both the number of sites exceeding a certain threshold (extent) and the mean level of attachment (a measure of severity). The ESI uses estimates of attachment level from probing measurements of 14 sites in one maxillary quadrant and 14 sites in the contralateral mandibular quadrant (Carlos et al. 1986).

External Bevel Gingivectomy—Also known as the gingivectomy procedure, it is a method of eliminating excessive pocket depth and exposing additional coronal tooth structure. It is performed when there is more than adequate width of attached gingiva and no bone involvement (Yuodelis and Smith 1976). See also gingivectomy, internal bevel gingivectomy.

Extrasulcular Incision—The incision placement during periodontal flap surgery at some point between the gingival margin and the mucogingival junction. It is determined by the depth of the pocket relative to the amount of attached gingiva (Dello Russo 1998). See also subsulcular incision.

F

Facial Radicular Groove—Refers to a facial anomaly in a maxillary central incisor that extends coronally and apically to the cementoenamel junction. This developmental groove forms a nidus for plaque and calculus formation, encouraging the development of periodontitis (Kozlovsky et al. 1988). See also labiogingival notch.

Factitial Gingival Traumatism—An unusual self-mutilation habit involving the gingival/periodontal structures that results in localized gingival destruction (See Fig. F-1a,b) (Hasler and Schultz 1968). The word *factitious* applies to a state or situation produced by other than natural means, as in the case of self-inflicted trauma (AAP 2001a). This term has been further subdivided into three classifications: type A, injuries superimposed on a preexisting condition (e.g., herpetic lesions, localized infection); type B, injuries secondary to other established lesions (e.g., finger sucking or nail biting); and type C, injuries of unknown and/or complex etiology (e.g., psychological problems) (Stewart and Kernohan 1972).

Fenestration—This term is derived from the Latin word fenestra, meaning "window." In periodontology, it has been described as a window-like aperture or opening, such as may be found in the alveolar bone over the root of a tooth (AAP 2001a). It has also been classified as a defect in the cortical plate of bone that exposes the facial or

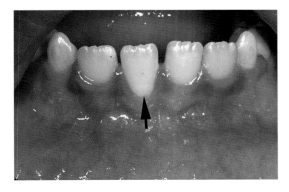

Fig. F-1a: Arrow, localized gingival recession

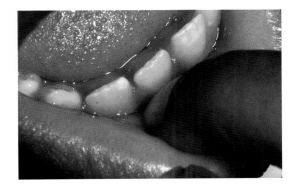

Fig. F-1b: Self-inflicted injury from fingernail habit

lingual root surfaces (Elliott et al. 1963; Larato 1970d). In 1963, S.S. Stahl et al. graded fenestrations into three categories:

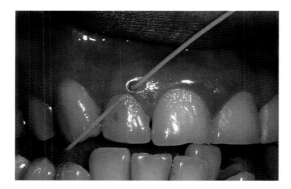

Fig. F-2a: Gingival fenestration

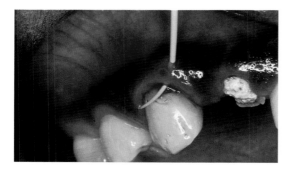

Fig. F-2b: Gingival fenestration

stage 1 is the smallest opening seen with the naked eye, stage 2 is an opening between stages 1 and 3, and stage 3 occurs when the loss of buccal vertical bone extends into the alveolar crest (Stahl et al. 1963). Stage 3 may also be referred to as a dehiscence. Although fenestrations are often thought of as osseous defects, they have also occurred in the gingiva, where they are called gingival fenestrations (See Fig. F-2a,b) (Lane 1977). See also dehiscence.

Festooning—Also known as vertical grooving of the osseous tissue, a procedure performed during osteoplasty (Ochsenbein 1958). See also vertical grooving.

Fiberotomy—Also known as gingival fiberotomy, this is a circumferential crevicular incision through all gingival and periodontal fibers coronal to the crest of the alveolar bone (AAP 2001a). Fiberotomy was introduced as a surgical technique in 1970 to reduce the rotational relapse of orthodontically repositioned teeth (Edwards 1970). Edwards's technique consisted of severing all fibrous attachments surrounding the tooth to a depth of approximately 2 to 3 mm below the alveolar crest. This technique has been shown to sever all supracrestal fibrous attachments to a rotated tooth. See also circumferential supracrestal fiberotomy (CSF), supracrestal fiberotomy.

Fibronectin—This term originates from two Latin words, *fibra* for fiber and *nectere* for link. It is a high-molecular-weight glycoprotein composed of two disulfide-linked polypeptides. Functional domains of the molecule have an affinity for cells and the extracellular matrix components found on cell surfaces, in connective tissues, in the blood, and in other body fluids (AAP 2001a). Fibronectin acts as a chemoattractant on fibroblasts and enhances the adherence of fibroblasts to root surfaces (Baum and Wright 1980). See also root biomodification.

Fibroosseous Integration—The interposition of healthy, dense collagenous tissue between a dental implant and bone (AAID 1986; Weiss 1986; AAP 2001a). See also biointegration, functional ankylosis, osseointegration.

Fixed Long Labial Mucosal Flap—This surgical procedure, introduced in 1963 by Henry M. Bohannon, is a combination of bilateral vertical incisions, an internal beveled incision, and a mucoperiosteal flap reflection by blunt dissection to the mucogingival junction. Sharp dissection is then resumed, leaving a curtain of periosteum covering all but 2 mm of exposed bone. The flap is sutured apically and a dressing is placed (Bohannon 1963a). This is specifically applicable in vestibular deepening in the mandibular anterior area, particularly when there is little or no attached gingiva. It is a modification of Friedman's apically repositioned flap (1962) and a refinement of Naber's repositioning of the attached gingiva (1954). This procedure is based on Bohannon's thesis entitled "Preliminary Investigation into the Results Obtained from the Vestibular Fornix Extension Operation" at the University of Pennsylvania in 1960. Additional papers from his studies included (1) complete denudation (1962a), (2) periosteal retention (1962b), and (3) vestibular incision (1963b).

Flossing Clefts—Comprised of linear or V-shaped marginal deformities of the interdental tissue, flossing clefts result from the improper use of dental floss (See Fig. F-3a,b). They are often observed in the posterior areas and will heal completely when an early diagnosis is made and the habit corrected (Hallmon et al. 1986; Gillette and Van House 1980).

Flute—That part of the tooth's furcation which is concave or grooved and is just coronal to the separation of the roots (Saadoun 1985). See also cervical enamel projection (CEP).

Fones Toothbrushing Technique—This technique is also known as the circular toothbrushing technique. With the teeth held together, the brush is placed parallel to the line of occlusion and moved in a rotary (circular) motion. The circular path of the brush should include all the gingiva up to the mucobuccal fold (Ray 2005). The objective is for the bristles to penetrate between the teeth and clean interproximally without using a crosswise motion against the teeth and gums (Fones 1915).

Food Impaction—The forceful wedging of food through occlusal pressure into the interproximal spaces (Hirschfeld 1930). In addition to the vertical impaction due to chewing pressure, it also includes the horizontal impaction by the forcing of food interproximally by tongue or cheek pressure (AAP 2001a). A study of the effect of food impaction on interproximal bony defects has been reported (Larato 1971).

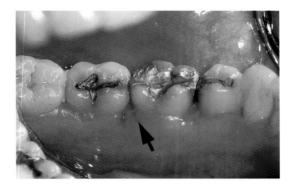

Fig. F-3a: Arrow, linear gingival deformity

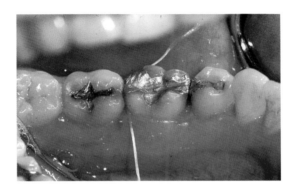

Fig. F-3b: Incorrect floss placement

Forced Eruption—Crown lengthening through orthodontics, which extrudes the tooth and, if needed, levels intrabony defects at the same time. This often eliminates the need for corrective periodontal therapy, thus preserving the patient's esthetics (Ingber 1974). See also crown lengthening, molar uprighting, vertical extrusion.

Free Gingiva—The free gingiva is that part of the gingiva, 0.5 to 1.5 mm wide, which surrounds the tooth like a collar and is not directly attached to the tooth surface (See Fig. F-4). It forms the outer wall of the gingival sulcus and extends from the bottom of the gingival sulcus to the coronal border of the gingiva, or its margin (Orban

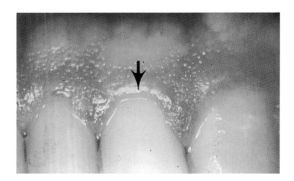

Fig. F-4: Arrow, free gingiva

1948a; AAP 2001a). See also marginal gingiva.

Free Gingival Graft—This expression, designating an autogenous gingival graft, is a misnomer. The usual donor site for an autogenous gingival graft is masticatory mucosa from the palate and not free gingiva. The free gingiva is a distinct anatomic entity of the gingival unit and is not used for grafting (Cohen 1969). See also free soft tissue autograft.

Free Gingival Groove—The free gingival groove is a shallow line or depression on the surface of the gingiva between the free and attached gingiva. It is the dividing line between these two parts of the gingiva and runs parallel to the margin of the gingiva at a distance of 0.5 to 1.5 mm. The free gingival groove is believed to arise from functional impacts on the movable free gingiva back on the attached and immovable zone (Orban 1948a). The frequency of the occurrence of the free gingival groove varies widely (AAP 2001a), and the groove does not necessarily correspond to the level of the bottom of the gingival crevice or pocket (Ramfjord and Kiester 1954). See also attached gingiva.

Free Masticatory Mucosal Graft—This term, designating a free soft tissue autograft, specifically mentions the source of the autograft; the gingiva and mucosa covering the hard palate (Pennel et al. 1969). See also free soft tissue autograft.

Free Mucosal Graft—As used by R. Earl Robinson for the free soft tissue autograft, this term is more specific than merely referring to "soft tissue" as the tissue type (See Fig. F-5a,b,c) (Robinson 1967). See also free soft tissue autograft.

Free Soft Tissue Autograft—This soft tissue grafting procedure is performed when the grafted tissue is completely detached from its donor area and relocated elsewhere in the same mouth (See Fig. F-6a,b and for a preoperative view See Fig. D-1a,b) (Cohen 1969). It was first introduced to periodontics in the Swedish literature by Hilding Bjorn, an oral surgeon (Bjorn 1963a, 1963b), and then was presented in the United States in 1964 before the Philadelphia Society of Periodontology (King and Pennell 1964; Allen and Cohen 2003). Its primary purpose is to (1) increase the zone of attached gingiva, (2) extend the vestibular fornix, (3) manage gingival recession, and (4) eliminate muscle or frenum pull (Sullivan and Adkins 1968). See also free gingival graft, free masticatory mucosal graft, free mucosal graft, soft tissue autograft.

Freedom in Centric—In the study of occlusion, this phrase refers to the anteroposterior movement of the mandible between "retruded contact," a ligament-guided position, and "centric occlusion," a tooth-guided position (Schuyler 1969). In only 10% of the population does the retruded contact position equal centric occlusion; the remaining 90% of people have a centric occlusion or intercuspal contact about 0.25 to 2.25 mm anterior to the retruded contact position. This is referred to as the freedom of movement in centric (Ramfjord and Ash 1966). See also centric occlusion (CO), long centric, retruded contact (RC).

Free-Way Space—In the study of occlusion, this term refers to the interocclusal distance between (tooth-guided) centric occlusion and (muscle-guided) postural position, or when the muscles of mastication are in equilibrium (AAP 2001a). This

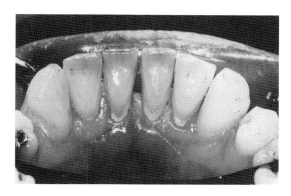

Fig. F-5a: Preoperative view

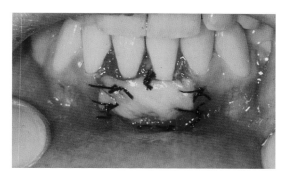

Fig. F-6a: Free soft tissue autograft

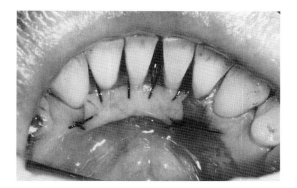

Fig. F-5b: Mucosal graft sutured

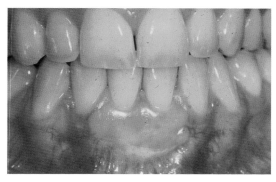

Fig. F-6b: Five years postoperatively

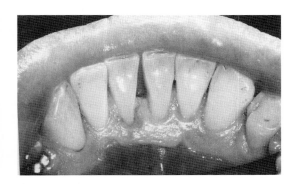

Fig. F-5c: Twelve months postoperatively

space or distance between the occlusal surfaces of the maxilla and mandible is between 2 and 4 mm. It is also called the interocclusal distance or clearance

(Posselt 1968). See also centric occlusion (CO), postural position.

Freeze-Dried Bone Allograft (FDBA)—This term refers to lyophilized (freeze-dried) bone allograft for the removal of organic/cellular elements (Mellonig 1981). It was first introduced as an osteoconductive agent for treating periodontal osseous defects (Mellonig et al. 1976); the methods for its preparation were described in 1980 (Mellonig 1980). The American Academy of Periodontology has published a position paper on tissue banking that includes an in depth review of FDBA (AAP 2001b). See also allograft.

Fremitus—This term refers to a palpable or visible movement of a tooth when subjected to occlusal forces (AAP 1996a and AAP 2001a).

Frenectomy—A surgical procedure to eliminate the retraction or movement of marginal gingiva or the interdental papilla by the action of the frenum (i.e., frenulum) by excising it (See Fig. F-7a,b) (AAP 2001a). Robert Gottsegan gives credit to Henry M. Goldman (Goldman 1953) for having been the first to develop a technique for correcting frenulum discrepancies (Gottsegan 1954). However, F. Helming has been credited for having been the first to sever the frenum and mucobuccal fold extension with surgical techniques in periodontics (Ramfjord and Costich 1968). See also frenulectomy, frenulumectomy, mucobuccal fold extension.

Frenotomy—The simple excisional release of the frenum from the apex of its insertion to its base and down to the alveolar process (Cohen 1989). It is derived from *frenum*, Latin for "curb" or "restraint" and *-tome*, Greek for "cutting"; in other words, it is the cutting of a frenulum, as seen in the release of ankyloglossia (AAP 2001a). See also frenulotomy.

Frenulectomy—Also known as frenectomy (Prichard 1972; AAP 2001a). See also frenectomy.

Frenulotomy—Also known as frenotomy. See also frenotomy.

Frenulumectomy—A procedure whereby a frenum is surgically removed by a horizontal incision, with the dissection of muscle fibers (Robinson 1956). According to R. Earl Robinson, this term was suggested as a synonym for *frenectomy* by Balint Orban during a 1956 Colorado Springs Seminar (Robinson 1957). See also frenectomy, mucobuccal fold extension.

Frenum—The frenum (frenulum) consists of variable amounts of loose connective tissue between two folds of mucous membrane (See Fig. F-7a). Muscles are never found in these folds and larger vessels are likewise absent (Sicher 1949). Isadore Hirschfeld was the first to draw attention to the frenum as an etiologic factor in peri-

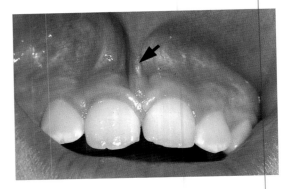

Fig. F-7a: Arrow, frenum

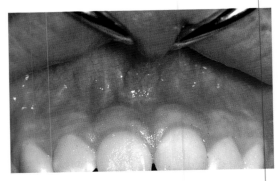

Fig. F-7b: Two weeks postoperatively

odontal disease (Hirschfeld 1939). The dispute over the existence of muscle fibers within the frenum has been persistent over the years (Noyes 1935; Gottsegan 1954).

Frontal Resorption—Physiologic resorption of alveolar bone on the periodontal ligament side in response to a light pressure on the teeth that has not caused necrosis of the periodontal ligament. It is an attempt to restore normal width to the periodontal ligament during tooth movement (Gottleib 1942). See also rear resorption.

Full Mouth Index—A system for measuring or recording a patient's entire periodontium or dentition for either epidemiologic or clinical purposes. An example would be Russell's Periodontal Index (Russell 1956). See also Periodontal Index (PI).

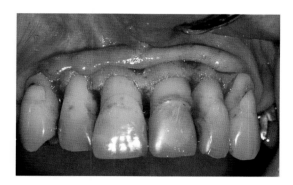

Fig. F-8

Full-Thickness Flap—During periodontal surgery, the gingiva, alveolar mucosa and periosteum may be elevated in one unit to produce this flap (See Fig. F-8). An inverse incision is made at the gingival margin and the blade inserted until the bony margin is contacted. The gingival tissue and periosteum are reflected in one piece, exposing the surface of the bone (Barrington 1973). See also blunt dissection, gingival mucoperiosteal flap, mucoperiosteal flap.

Functional Ankylosis—An ankylotic type of connection between bone and a hollow cylinder of a titanium implant flashed with titanium powder (rough surface). This implies an absence of an intervening layer of connective tissue as well as of relative movement between the implant and the socket (Schroeder et al. 1981). See also biointegration, fibroosseous integration, osseointegration.

Functional Repair—The formation of new alveolar bone, cementum, and periodontal ligament with regeneration of oral epithelium following periodontal treatment of a previously diseased root surface. It implies that there is no anatomic deformity (Staffileno et al. 1962). See also periodontal regeneration repair.

Furca—This term, Latin for "fork," refers to that portion of a multirooted tooth which lies between the roots. It extends (1) laterally to the same boundaries as the interradicular space, (2) apically to and includ-

ing the crest of the bifurcational ridges, and (3) coronally to and including the interradicular fluting (Heins and Canter 1968). See also bifurcational ridges, flute, furcation.

Furcaplasty—The reduction of the horizontal dimensions of a furcation by grinding away some tooth structure with steel burs or diamond points. It is usually combined with osteoplasty to reshape adjacent osseous defects and create a smooth confluence between bone and tooth. It is odontoplasty confined to the areas of furcations (Highfield 1978).

Furcation—The anatomic part of a multirooted tooth where the roots divide from the common root trunk into the bifurcation or trifurcation. It consists of three parts: the interradicular area, the flute, and the root roof (Saadoun 1985). Simply stated, it is the normal anatomic division of the roots of teeth into separate branches, as in the posterior teeth (ADA 1950), or it may be referred to as the anatomic area of a multirooted tooth where the roots diverge (AAP 2001a). See also bifurcation, flute, interradicular, root roof, root trunk, trifurcation.

Furcation Arrow—A small, triangular, radiolucent shadow across the mesial or distal roots of some maxillary molars associated with a proximal furcation involvement (See Fig. F-9). The apical base of the arrow

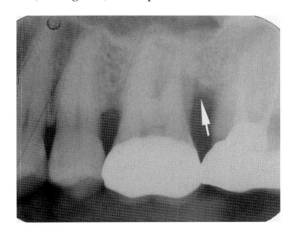

Fig. F-9: Arrow, furcation

is formed by the bone remaining in the furcation area. The classic presentation of the arrow would occur when the vertical component of bone loss was minimal. As the vertical component increases, the image broadens and becomes more diffuse (Hardekoph et al. 1987). See also furcation involvement.

Furcation Classification (Easley and Drennan)—A classification system based on the position (form and function) of the dentogingival junction, the periodontal ligament, and the bone within the furca. It is either class I (normal furca); class II (incipient or partially involved furca), further divided into types 1 and 2; or class III (completely involved furca), subsequently divided into types 1 and 2 (Easley and Drennan 1969). See also furcation involvement.

Furcation Classification (Eskow and Kapin)—A classification system designed to directly correlate with prognosis and treatment. It combines the horizontal system of Hamp, Nyman, and Lindhe (I, II, III) with a vertical interradicular destruction system (A, B, or C). The "A" is vertical destruction up to one-third of the total interradicular height, the "B" is vertical destruction reaching two-thirds of the interradicular height, and the "C" is interradicular osseous destruction into or beyond the apical third. The classification would then read IA, IB, IC; IIA, IIB, IIC; and IIIA, IIIB, IIIC (Eskow and Kapin 1984a, 1984b; Kapin and Eskow 1984a, 1984b). See also furcation classification (Hamp, Nyman, and Lindhe).

Furcation Classification (Fedi, Vernino, and Gray)—This system is similar to Glickman's 1953 classification with one modification: under the grade II classification, a degree I is recorded when there is > 1 mm but < 3 mm of horizontal bone loss in the furcation. Likewise, a degree II is noted when there is > 3 mm of horizontal bone loss but no through-and-through involvement (Fedi et al. 2000). See also furcation classification (Glickman).

Furcation Classification (Glickman)—Irving Glickman was the first to classify furcation invasion based on the degree of lateral periodontal destruction under the roof of the furcation. It reads: "*Grade I* is involvement of the periodontal membrane in the bifurcation or trifurcation without any gross or radiographic evidence of appreciable loss of alveolar bone. *Grade II* are cases where there is bone loss in one or more aspects of the bifurcation or trifurcation, but a portion of the alveolar bone and periodontal membrane remain intact. The intact periodontal structures permit partial penetration of a blunt probe into the bifurcation area but obstruct complete passage of a probe in the buccolingual or mesiodistal directions. *Grade III* are cases in which the alveolar bone has been destroyed to such a degree as to permit complete passage of a probe through the bifurcation or trifurcation in a buccolingual or mesiodistal direction. The bifurcation or trifurcation may be occluded by gingival tissue in this grade of involvement. *Grade IV* are cases in which the periodontium in relation to the bifurcation or trifurcation has been destroyed to such a degree as to create an open area through which a probe can be passed without difficulty. The bifurcation or trifurcation is exposed and clearly visible to clinical examination" (Glickman 1953).

Furcation Classification (Goldman and Cohen)—Terminology for interradicular involvement has been changed many times over the years, often confusing the student of periodontology with synonyms and new expressions for commonly accepted nomenclature. One example has been Goldman and Cohen's description for Glickman's grade I, grade II, grade III, and grade IV furcation classification to incipient (grade I), cul-de-sac (grade II), and through-and-through (grade III) (Goldman and Cohen 1968).

Furcation Classification (Hamp, Nyman, and Lindhe)—The amount of furcation involvement, denoted with Roman numerals in this classification, is measured by severity in millimeters. They are grade I, horizontal loss of periodontal tissue support less than 3 mm; grade II, horizontal loss of tissue support exceeding 3 mm but not encompassing the total width of the furcation area; and grade III, horizontal through-and-through destruction of the periodontal tissue in the furcations (Hamp et al. 1975).

Furcation Classification (Heins and Canter)—A system of furcation classification based on three characteristics or the morphology of the interradicular bony deformities: (1) the locations or surface of the tooth (furca) that is involved; (II) the number of distinct bony walls in the lesion, either one, two, three, or four walls; and (III) the degree of *furcal exposure*, being either "incipient," "partial," or "complete." This system is useful in considering bone grafts or other new attachment procedures (Heins and Canter 1968).

Furcation Classification (Lindhe)—In this system, furcation involvement is measured by recording the width of interradicular bone loss by thirds. *Degree I* is horizontal loss of supporting tissues not exceeding one-third of the width of the tooth; *degree II* is horizontal loss of supporting tissues but not encompassing the total width of the furcation area; and *degree III* is horizontal through-and-through destruction of the supporting tissues in the furcation (Lindhe 1989).

Furcation Classification (Ramfjord and Ash)—This system utilizes millimeter measurements of interradicular destruction by 2 mm or more. *Class 1* is a beginning involvement not exceeding 2 mm into the furcation; *class 2* is involvement extending deeper than 2 mm but not passing entirely through the furcation; and *class 3* is a through-and-through involvement in which a probe can be passed between the roots through the entire furcation (Ramfjord and Ash 1979b).

Furcation Classification (Ricchetti)—This system is based on a linear classification that provides horizontal and vertical measurement and serves as a clinical tool for determining the approach to treatment. It is based on the relationship of the pulp chamber to the extent of horizontal furcation involvement and is divided into *class I* with a subclass Ia; *class II* with a subclass IIa; and *class III* (Ricchetti 1982).

Furcation Classification (Staffelino)—This three-class system is similar to Glickman's 1953 classification. It consists of class 1; class 2 with subclasses 2-F, 2-L, 2-M, and 2-D; and class 3. The subclasses in class 2 are referenced to those furcations with osseous destruction from the facial aspect only (2-F), lingual aspect only (2-L), mesial aspect only (2-M), or distal aspect only (2-D) (Staffileno 1969b). See also furcation classification (Glickman).

Furcation Classification (Tarnow and Fletcher)—This system records the vertical loss of interradicular alveolar bone in millimeters from the roof of the furcation to the level of radicular (alveolar) bone. It may be combined with any acceptable grade I, II, III, or other classifications. *Subclass A* is vertical bone loss of 0 to 3 mm, *subclass B* is vertical bone loss from 4 to 6 mm, and *subclass C* is vertical bone loss of 7 mm or greater (Tarnow and Fletcher 1984). These dimensions are difficult to measure when the furcation roof is subgingival; measurements would then have to be made from vertical dental radiographs (Newell 1998).

Furcation Dome—Also known as "root roof" (Matia et al. 1986). See also root roof.

Furcation Invasion—Also known as furcation involvement and referenced to the loss of periodontal attachment (bone and periodontal ligament) in furcations of multirooted teeth (See Fig. H-5) (Staffileno 1969b). See also bifurcation invasion, bifurcation involvement, furcation involvement, trifurcation involvement.

Furcation Involvement—Also known as furcation invasion, or the extension of pocket formation into the interradicular area of multirooted teeth (See Fig. F-10). It can be

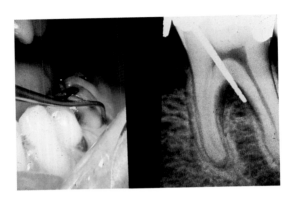

Fig. F-10

termed a "bifurcation" or "trifurcation" involvement, depending on the number of involved roots (see Figs. H-1c and V-1a) (Goldman and Cohen 1968; Larato 1970c). See also bifurcation invasion, bifurcation involvement, furcation invasion, trifurcation involvement.

G

General Adaptation Syndrome (GAS)—
This syndrome, described by Hans Selye
in 1946, comprises all the systemic reactions of the body resulting from long, continuous stress. These responses fall into
three categories: (1) the *alarm reaction*, or
the sum of all nonspecific phenomena
elicited by sudden exposure to stimuli to
which the organism is insufficiently
adapted, consisting of primary shock
(nervous stimuli) and secondary shock; (2)
the *stage of resistance*, or the sum of all nonspecific systemic reactions elicited by prolonged exposure to stimuli to which the
organism has acquired adaptations; and
(3) the *stage of exhaustion*, or the sum of all
nonspecific systemic reactions that eventually occur due to prolonged exposure to
stimuli to which adaptation was acquired
but could not be maintained (Selye 1946).

Generalized Juvenile Periodontitis (GJP)—
This classification of periodontitis in a juvenile requires the involvement of at least
four or more teeth with at least 3 mm of attachment loss, where at least two affected
teeth are second molars, cuspids, or premolars (Loe and Brown 1991). The expression GJP has been eliminated from the classification of periodontal disease and is now
considered under the all-encompassing
term *aggressive periodontitis* (Armitage
1999). See also aggressive periodontitis, juvenile periodontitis, localized juvenile
periodontitis (LJP).

Geriatric Periodontics—The rapidly growing elderly population with its many so-
cial and medical problems, often leading
to medically compromised situations, has
brought a new challenge of treating periodontitis in the aging populace. Therefore
the expression *geriatric periodontics* has
taken on a new meaning in the twenty-
first century (Pollack 1986, 1991; Greenwell and Bissada 1989). An informational
statement and position paper on geriatric
periodontics has been compiled and published (AAP 1994).

Gindex Index—This periodontal index is a
colorimetric test to measure gingival inflammation based on the hemoglobin con-
tent of saliva. The authors formed a correlation between the gindex values, the
gingival index, and crevicular fluid flow
(Abbott and Caffesse 1978). A subsequent
study found the gindex index to be unre-
liable in determining the presence or absence of gingival inflammation (Hellden
et al. 1980).

Gingiva—The part of the oral mucous membrane surrounding the teeth and adapted
to resist masticatory stresses. It consists of
the free or marginal gingiva, the attached
gingiva, and the interdental papilla
(Orban 1948a). A modern definition states
that it is the fibrous investing tissue covered by keratinized epithelium that immediately surrounds a tooth and is contiguous with its periodontal ligament and

the mucosal tissues of the mouth (AAP 2001a).

Gingival Augmentation—This is a surgical procedure designed to increase the quantity of attached gingival (See Fig. G-1a,b,c) (AAP 2001a). Specifically, it is useful to (1) create an amount of attached gingiva to reduce gum recession, (2) cover exposed root surfaces with gingiva, (3) enhance the appearance of the teeth and gum line, (4) treat root sensitivity, and (5) treat root decay. Gingival augmentation will support the dentogingival unit, increase its resistance to additional breakdown, and in many instances reconstruct the lost segment of the periodontium (Maynard 1998).

Gingival Biotype—A classification of healthy gingival contours as dictated by the distance between the marginal and interdental tissue heights. Its architecture may be considered as (1) flat, (2) average scalloped (combination flat and scalloped), and (3) pronounced scalloped, all reflected by the underlying osseous contour (Ochsenbein and Ross 1969). It had previously been stated that the osseous topography and subsequent "gingival contour" in health is dictated by the rise and fall of the adjacent cementoenamel junctions (CEJs) (Ritchey and Orban 1953a). See also gingival morphotype, periodontal biotype.

Gingival Bleeding Index (GBI)—This index is intended to record the presence or absence of gingival inflammation as determined by bleeding from interproximal gingival sulci. With the mouth divided into six segments, unwaxed dental floss is curved around both sides of the interdental papillae and moved in an incisogingival direction to determine the tendency to bleed. Bleeding is recorded as either positive or negative after waiting 30 seconds following the placement of floss. The total number of positive bleeding sites (papillae) is the GBI; no averaging is performed in this reversible index (Carter and Barnes 1974). See also reversible index.

Gingival–Bone Count Index—A subjective measurement for epidemiologic work to study periodontal disease in a population. It utilizes the reversible index of a gingi-

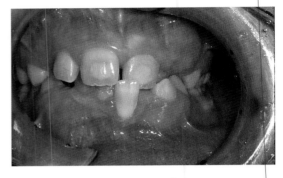

Fig. G-1a: Presurgery; central incisor

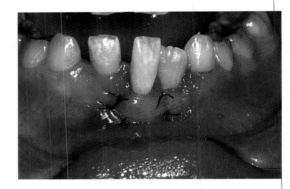

Fig. G-1b: Tissue moved from lateral incisor

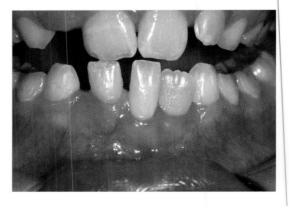

Fig. G-1c: Four weeks postoperatively

val (G) condition (0 to 3) combined with the irreversible index of bone (B) loss (0 to 5) as determined by radiographic examination. The combined G and B scores produce the composite gingival–bone count index, which may vary from 0 to 8. The use of this index is time-consuming; it is therefore rarely used in fieldwork today (Dunning and Leach 1960). See also composite index, irreversible index, reversible index.

Gingival Cleft—A narrow type of gingival deformity encountered on the marginal aspect of the gingiva and extending regularly or irregularly from the gingival margin in an apical or lateral direction, with margins that are usually thick and often rolled inward (See Fig. P-3a) (Moskow and Bressman 1965). It has also been described as a capillary slit running from the gingival margin a variable length in an apical direction across the attached gingiva and sometimes into the alveolar mucosa (Everett 1968). Simply stated, a gingival cleft is a vertical fissure in the gingiva (AAP 2001a). See also Stillman's clefts.

Gingival Contour Index—This periodontal index system records the gingival contour of both buccal and lingual margins (M) and the interproximal papillae (P). The degree of gingival contour for all three areas is recorded from 0 to 4: 0 = feather edge (M) and tightly bound down, (P) filling the interdental spaces; 1 = rolled (M) and slightly rolled/enlarged (P); 2 = rolled (M) with blunting or cratering of (P); 3a = buccal and lingual portion of (P) detached by air jet; 3b = vertical clefts in (M); and 4 = gross fibrous enlargement of (M) and/or (P) (Newman 1984). See also index of gingival architectural form.

Gingival Crevice—The shallow fissure between the marginal gingiva and the enamel or cementum (AAP 2001a). The depth of the gingival crevice varies according to location, state of eruption, and presence or absence of disease. The average depth of the normal crevice is usually less than 3 mm; however, it should not be considered abnormal if greater than 2 or 3 mm (Ramfjord and Ash 1979c; AAP 2001a). See also gingival sulcus.

Gingival Crevicular Fluid (GCF)—The tissue fluid that seeps through the crevicular and junctional epithelium, which is increased in the presence of inflammation (AAP 2001a). As early as 1817, it was believed that this tissue fluid was secreted by gingival glands, later called Serres glands (Serres 1817). The fluid was soon found to be an inflammatory exudate, which was thought to produce erosion of the tooth enamel (Bodecker 1933, 1945). The gingival crevicular fluid has been studied extensively and reported on by numerous authors, with many good overviews and reviews (Weinstein and Mandel 1964; Uitto 2003; Armitage 2004b).

Gingival Curettage—A closed procedure that includes the removal of inflamed, devitalized, contaminated tissue or foreign material from or adjacent to a lesion (See Fig. S-7a,b). In addition to debriding the soft tissue wall of a periodontal pocket, routine root instrumentation is accomplished in conjunction with the soft tissue management (AAP 1989). Its objective is pocket reduction by either (1) shrinkage, (2) new connective tissue attachment, or (3) epithelial adhesion via long epithelial attachment (Tandy 1970). See also apoxesis, closed crevicular curettage, closed curettage, curettage, root curettage, root planing, subgingival curettage.

Gingival Cyst—These cysts are located within the gingiva, most commonly in the mandibular canine-premolar area. They are believed to be derived from epithelial rests of the dental lamina (AAP 2001a). Other possible etiologies are presented in a report on gingival cysts. They may be (1) heterotopic glandular tissue (rare); (2) remnants of dental lamina, enamel organ, or epithelial islands of the periodontal ligament; (3) degenerative changes (strangulations) of proliferative epithelial rete pegs; or (4) traumatic implantations (most common) (Ritchey and Orban 1953b).

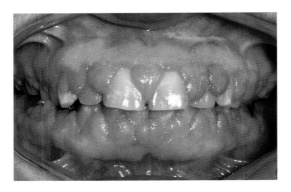

Fig. G-2: Diphenylhydantoin enlargement

Gingival Enlargement—The classic definition is an overgrowth or increase in the size of the gingiva (See Fig. G-2) (AAP 2001a, 2004). Specifically, gingival enlargement may be caused by (1) chronic or acute inflammation, (2) noninflammatory enlargement related to medications, (3) combined gingival enlargement from 1 and 2, (4) conditioned gingival enlargement as due to hormones or medical conditions, (5) neoplasms, or (6) developmental gingival enlargement (Glickman 1950b). See also gingival hyperplasia, gingival hypertrophy.

Gingival Epithelium—The integument that covers and protects the underlying periodontal structures. It consists of three components: oral epithelium, sulcular or crevicular epithelium, and junctional epithelium or the epithelial attachment (Orban 1957). See also junctional epithelium, oral epithelium, sulcular epithelium.

Gingival Extension—This is an archaic surgical procedure to manage alterations in the mucobuccal fold, such as abnormal frena attachments, deep pockets traversing the attached gingiva and ending in alveolar mucosa, extremely shallow vestibules with no room for adequate gingiva and inadequate attached gingiva to ensure good function. It was performed by incising the attached gingiva so as to allow muscle pull to draw the flap api-

cally, exposing 2 to 4 mm of marginal bone. Very often the remaining gingiva was removed with scissors. Surgical cement was applied and pushed against the wound to prevent coronal migration of the incised alveolar mucosa (Goldman et al. 1956). This periodontal surgery procedure was studied extensively both clinically and histologically by Gerald P. Ivancie (Ivancie 1957). See also displaced flap, pouch procedure, pushback procedure.

Gingival Facade—A class V restoration on single teeth that have undergone severe recession from surgery, toothbrush wear, and/or muscular/frenular pull. The restoration comprises an acrylic resin that is color adapted to the patient's normal gingiva (Larato 1970e). See also gingival prosthesis, gum veneer, party gums, prosthetic gingival veneer.

Gingival Festoons—The contour of the gingiva over the roots of the teeth, which tend to follow the cervical lines. They are especially prominent in the presence of a thin alveolar process (AAP 2001a). They have been thought to be caused by improper toothbrushing (Hirschfeld 1939) or occlusal traumatism (Stillman and McCall 1922). See also McCall's festoons.

Gingival Fiber Group—These are connective tissue fiber groups that pass from the cementum to the gingiva and traverse the gingiva itself (See Fig. D-2). They consist of the dentogingival, alveologingival, circular, transseptal, dentoperiosteal, and interpapillary fiber groups (Orban 1957). See also alveologingival fiber group, circular fiber group, dentogingival fiber group, dentoperiosteal fiber group, interpapillary fiber group, periodontal ligament, transseptal fiber group.

Gingival Hyperplasia—This refers basically to the overgrowth of the gingival tissues (See Fig. G-3). Specifically, the overgrowth of tissue results from an increase in the *number* of its elements, not the *size* of the elements, and serves no useful purpose (AAP 1947). More recently, gingival hyperplasia has been simply defined as an

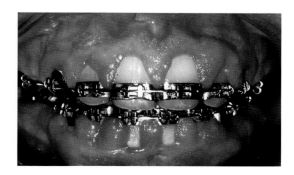

Fig. G-3: (With permission from the American Academy of Periodontology)

enlargement of the gingiva due to an increase in the number of cells (AAP 2001a, 2004). See also gingival enlargement, gingival hypertrophy.

Gingival Hyperplasia—Grade—This grading system was introduced in an attempt to categorize the degree or amount of gingival hyperplasia. *Grade I* is slight or moderate hyperplasia, where the interdental papillae have assumed a more rounded, blunt form; the gingival margin is slightly thickened, and the anatomic crowns are covered up to one-third of the vestibular surfaces. *Grade II* is marked hyperplasia; the papillae and the gingival margin are covered from one-third to one-half of the vestibular surfaces. In most cases the papillae are separated only by a V-shaped cleft. *Grade III* is severe hyperplasia; the gingiva propria covers one-half to two-thirds of the vestibular surfaces and protrudes 3 to 4 mm from the surface of the tooth. *Grade IV* is very severe hyperplasia; the hyperplastic tissue covers from two-thirds to the entire clinical crowns in one or more regions and the occlusion is rendered difficult if not prevented (Aas 1963). Another system of grading diphenylhydantoin gingival hyperplasia was presented in 1972. In this system, a grade of zero shows no hyperplasia or normal gingiva; grade I occurs when the hyperplastic gingiva covers the cervical third or less of the anatomic crowns of the anterior teeth; grade II is present when the hyperplastic gingiva extends anywhere in the middle third of the anatomic crowns of the anterior teeth; and grade III is seen when the hyperplastic gingiva covers more than two-thirds of the anatomic crowns of the anterior teeth (Angelopoulos and Goaz 1972).

Gingival Hyperplasia—Score—This system employs the following arbitrary method: a zero denotes no gingival hyperplasia; a plus sign (+) denotes gingival tissues covering one-third or less of the crown of the tooth; two plus signs (++) are recorded when gingival tissues cover between one-third and one-half of the crown of the tooth; three plus signs (+++) are noted when gingival tissues cover between one-half and three-quarters of the crown of the tooth; and four plus signs (++++) are recorded when gingival tissues cover between three-quarters and the entire crown of the tooth. This scoring system is limited to the six maxillary teeth (Davis et al. 1963). Another method of scoring gingival hyperplasia utilizes full-mouth alginate impressions for recording the thickness of the gingiva in a buccolingual direction plus the encroachment on adjacent tooth surfaces; this method measures only the maxillary and mandibular six anterior teeth. The thickness is measured as 0 = normal, 1 = thickening from the normal up to 2 mm, and 2 = thickening from the normal up to more than 2 mm. The extent of encroachment of the gingival tissues onto adjacent crowns is graded as follows: 1 = encroachment to one-third of the way to the midline, 2 = encroachment to two-thirds of the way to the midline, and 3 = encroachment up to the midline of the tooth. The maximum score using this method is 5 (Seymour et al. 1985).

Gingival Hypertrophy—In the classification and nomenclature of periodontal diseases of 1942, gingival hypertrophy, as it occurs in an inflammatory disturbance, was defined as an overgrowth of gingival tissues.

At that time, it was said that the collagenous fiber bundles and proliferating epithelium increase in number and size, along with accumulation of inflammatory products, hyperemic blood vessels, and edema (Orban 1942). More simply stated today, gingival hypertrophy is due to an increase in the size of cells (AAP 2001a, 2004). See also gingival enlargement, gingival hyperplasia.

Gingival Index (GI)— The gingival index assesses the gingival condition, clearly distinguishing between the quality of the gingiva (severity of the lesion) and its extent (quantity) as related to the buccal, mesial, distal, and lingual surfaces of six selected teeth. These teeth are the maxillary right first molar, the right lateral incisor, the left first bicuspid, and the mandibular left first molar, lateral incisor, and right first bicuspid. The grades are as follows: GI 0 = absence of inflammation (normal gingiva); GI 1 = mild inflammation with slight change in color and little change in texture; GI 2 = moderate inflammation with moderate glazing, redness, edema, hypertrophy, and bleeding on pressure; and GI 3 = severe inflammation with marked redness and hypertrophy as well as a tendency to spontaneous bleeding and ulcerations. The gingival index may be derived for each tooth (divided by 4) or for each patient (divided by 6). The gingival index does not consider periodontal pocket depth, degrees of bone loss, or other quantitative changes of the periodontium. The criteria are entirely confined to qualitative changes in the gingival soft tissues (Loe and Silness 1963). See also plaque index.

Gingival Indices—This term refers to an ordinal and arbitrary system of measurement which describes or quantitates a gingival condition (AAP 2001a; Barnes et al. 1986). See also gingival bleeding index (GBI), gingival contour index, gingival hyperplasia grade/score, gingival index (GI).

Gingival Morphotype—Also known as gingival biotype (Becker and Becker 1998).

See also gingival biotype, periodontal biotype.

Gingival Mucoperiosteal Flap—This surgical procedure involves detachment of the attached gingiva and the mucoperiosteum (alveolar mucosa and periosteum) from the underlying alveolar bone in the treatment of periodontitis (Kohler and Ramfjord 1960). See also blunt dissection, full-thickness flap, mucoperiosteal flap.

Gingival Mucosal Flap—This term refers to the removal of half the papillary gingiva, marginal and attached gingiva, and unattached vestibular gingiva, delicately dissecting these from the underlying tissues so as to leave a stump of tissue attached to the tooth and periosteum (Staffileno et al. 1962). See also mucosal flap, partial-thickness flap, split-thickness flap.

Gingival Papilla Index—The purpose of this index is to evaluate the degree of recession and/or regeneration of gingival papillae adjacent to single-tooth implants. The papillae are graded on a scale of 0 to 4. If there are no papillae or indications of a curvature of soft tissue adjacent to the implant crown, the grade is 0. A grade of 1 means that less than half the papillary height is present and that convex curvature of the soft tissue adjacent to the implant crown and adjacent tooth can be observed. Grade 2 means that at least half the papillary height is evident but not to the contact point, the papilla is not completely harmonious with the adjacent papillae between the permanent teeth, and the soft tissue is harmonious with the adjacent teeth. Grade 3 means that the papilla fills the entire proximal space and is harmonious with the adjacent papillae and also that the soft tissue contour is optimal. Grade 4 means that the papillae are hyperplastic and cover too much of the implant or the adjacent tooth and that the soft tissue contour is irregular (Jemt 1997).

Gingival-Periodontal Index (GPI)—A system for recording the periodontal status that combines both the gingival and periodontal findings of the dentition, which is divided into six segments. Only the highest score found for any one tooth in a segment is recorded for the score in that segment. The highest score for the segment, either gingival or periodontal, is used in computing the GPI. This periodontal screening examination was developed for the use of general dental practitioners in their daily practice (O'Leary et al. 1963; O'Leary 1967).

Gingival Pocket—The pathologic condition of the gingival sulcus when there are disturbances around the tooth (Orban 1957). There is no apical proliferation of the epithelial attachment. More recently, the gingival pocket has been defined as a pathologically deepened gingival crevice that does not involve loss of connective tissue attachment; this is frequently observed when there is gingival enlargement (AAP 2001a). See also periodontal pocket, sulcus depth.

Gingival Prosthesis—An appliance designed to "replace" the gingival contour in an anterior sextant, where, following periodontal surgery, the teeth have longer clinical crowns and the interproximal embrasures are open (See Fig. G-4a,b). It is made of denture acrylic material and can be used secondarily as a retainer for stabilizing mobile teeth (See Fig. P-2a,b) (Swenson and Hansen 1961). See also gingival facade, party gums, prosthetic gingival veneer.

Gingival Rebound—In osseous surgery, the regrowth of gingiva to its original preoperative level because the underlying architecture of the alveolar bone was not taken into consideration; consequently, the pockets are reformed. The gingival architecture is to some degree qualified by the architecture of the underlying bone (Ochsenbein 1958).

Gingival Recession—Commonly defined as a condition in which the location of the gingival margin is apical to the cementoenamel junction (AAP 2001a). Many authors have defined gingival recession into degrees of severity and extent in order to

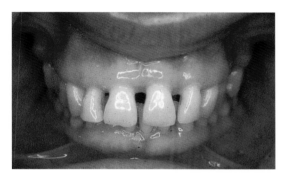

Fig. G-4a: Preprosthesis

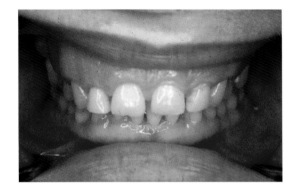

Fig. G-4b: Postprosthesis (Courtesy of Dr. Henry M. Swenson)

help the clinician to define treatment options and prognosis. In 1968, Sullivan and Atkins defined gingival recession as exposure of the root surface by an apical shift in the position of the marginal tissue. They classified it as follows: (1) deep and wide, (2) shallow and wide, (3) deep and narrow, and (4) shallow and narrow (Sullivan and Atkins 1968). Another attempt to quantify gingival recession was made in 1978 by Guinard and Caffesse, who also presented four classes: (1) narrow-shallow, (2) narrow-deep, (3) wide-shallow, and (4) wide-wide (Guinard and Caffesse 1978). In 1980, two types of gingival recession based on anatomic landmarks were described. The first is *visible recession*, which is the amount of clinically

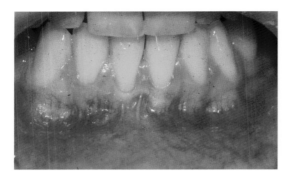

Fig. G-5a: Visible recession (With permission from the American Academy of Periodontology)

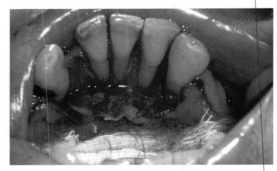

Fig. G-5c: Hidden recession surgically exposed

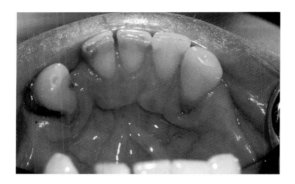

Fig. G-5b: Hidden recession

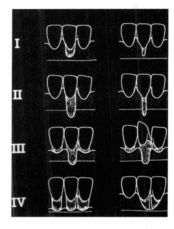

Fig. G-5d: (With permission from Blackwell Publishing)

observable root measured from the cementoenamel junction to the crest of the soft tissue margin (See Fig. G-5a). The second is *hidden recession,* or the depth of the sulcus or pocket as measured from the soft tissue margin to the epithelial attachment (junctional epithelium) (See Fig. G-5b,c) (Liu and Solt 1980). In 1985, P.D. Miller combined the four classes of Sullivan and Atkins into two (shallow and deep) and then created two additional classes, all related to the height of the interproximal bone and the relation of the gingival recession to the mucogingival junction (See Fig. G-5d). His four classifications are classes I through IV. Miller presented this classification of gingival recession to help the clinician determine the degree of root cover-

age expected during periodontal plastic surgery procedures (Miller 1985a).

Gingival Replacement—This term, as suggested by Nathan Friedman, denotes a mucogingival procedure to create a new zone of attached gingiva where none had existed. In essence, it is a procedure of replacing alveolar mucosa with gingiva. It is an archaic technique and is not currently in vogue (Friedman 1957). See also pushback procedure.

Gingival Sulcus—The gingival sulcus is the shallow groove that develops between the gingiva and the tooth surface and extends around the circumference of the tooth. It is

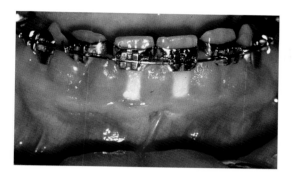

Fig. G-6a: Pregingivectomy

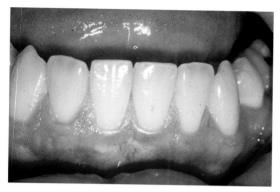

Fig. G-6c: Three-year healed gingiva

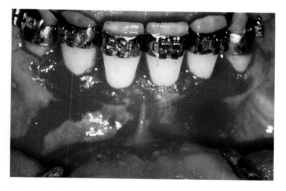

Fig. G-6b: Postgingivectomy (With permission from the American Academy of Periodontology)

bounded by the tooth on one side and the free gingiva on the other (Orban 1957; AAP 2001a). See also gingival crevice.

Gingivectomy—The periodontal surgical procedure called gingivectomy (*gingiva* meaning "gums" and *ektome* or "excision") is performed by careful resection of the unsupported gingival tissue to a point where it is firmly attached, so that a new gingival margin is established that has a shallow or minimal sulcus clinically (See Fig. G-6a,b,c). An early advocate of removing gingiva in the treatment of periodontal disease was Solomon Robicsek of Hungary. His method consisted of removing the gingiva down to the alveolar bone for altering the shape of the bone, a procedure that became known as the radical

gingivectomy (Stern et al. 1965). There is also an attempt to restore the form and function of the gingiva (Beckham et al. 1962). Briefly stated, the gingivectomy is a surgical procedure to remove excessive free gingival tissue so to enable the patient to keep the teeth clean (Ramfjord 1952a). See also external bevel gingivectomy.

Gingivitis—One form of periodontal disease in which there is inflammation of the gingiva without loss of clinical attachment (See Fig. G-7a,b) (AAP 1996b). This disease may or may not be plaque-induced. Plaque-associated gingivitis is an inflammation of the interdental and marginal gingiva that can be controlled or prevented by removing and/or inhibiting plaque accumulation. It is characterized clinically by changes in color, gingival form, position, surface appearance, and presence of bleeding and/or exudate (Mariotti 1999) Non-plaque-induced gingivitis is gingival inflammation having an etiology other than dental plaque, such as gingival diseases of specific bacterial, viral, fungal, or genetic origin, due to systemic conditions, trauma, foreign-body reactions, or other causes (Holmstrup 1999; AAP 2001a). See also periodontal diseases.

Gingivo-Muco-Myo-Skeletal Involvement—This multisyllabic term refers to those periodontal defects involving a narrow

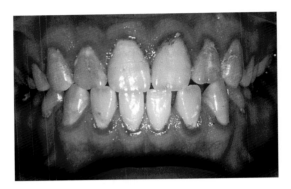

Fig. G-7a: Gingivitis (untreated)

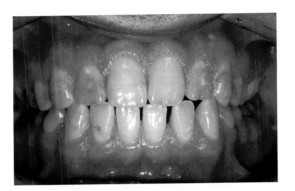

Fig. G-7b: Gingivitis (treated))

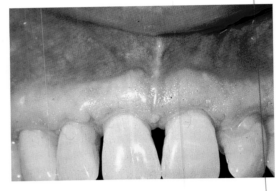

Fig. G-8a: Pregingivoplasty

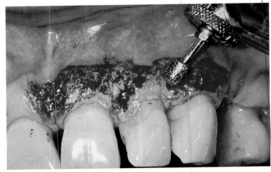

Fig. G-8b: Gingivoplasty

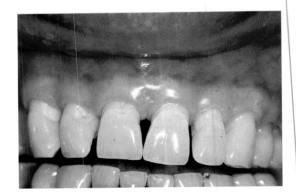

Fig. G-8c: Postgingivoplasty

zone of attached gingiva and relating to the underlying orofacial musculature and osseous structure of the maxilla and mandible. Briefly stated, it refers to those periodontal alterations associated with the mucogingival area (Hawley and Staffileno 1970). See also mucogingival defect, mucogingival problem, mucogingival surgery.

Gingivoplasty—This term, Latin "gingiva" plus Greek "plasso" to form/shape/mold, is a plastic surgical procedure to contour or reposition the gingiva to achieve a physiologic gingival contour (See Fig. G-8a,b,c). Henry Goldman is credited as having originated the philosophy and the term *gingivoplasty* as well as for the "establishment of a physiologic gingival architecture in order to maintain health, emphasizing form and function." Its objective is to reestablish gingival physiology through (1) interdental vertical grooving, (2) establishing a thin gingival margin, (3) creating festooning of the gingiva, and (4) establishing a cone-shaped interdental papilla from buccal to lingual (Goldman 1950).

Gingivosis—This is an archaic term for desquamative gingivitis (AAP 2001a). According to the 1966 World Workshop in periodontics, it was strongly recommended that the term *gingivosis*, alluding to a degenerative change and used synonymously with *desquamative gingivitis*, was inappropriate and should be discarded (AAP 1966). Historically, the term was coined in 1947 by Schour and Massler in examining postwar Italian children who were nutritionally and chronically ill. It was used then to designate a degenerative condition of the gingiva (Schour and Massler 1947). This condition was later described as a degenerative disease of the gingiva accompanied by tissue changes, meaning loss of connective tissue and ground substance, accompanied by an accumulation of edema and inflammatory exudate (Foss et al. 1953). See also chronic desquamative gingivitis (CDG), desquamative gingivitis.

Gingivostomatitis—Also known as atypical gingivostomatitis or plasma cell gingivitis, this is an allergic reaction of the gingiva characterized by a triad of symptoms: (1) erythematous gingivitis, (2) angular cheilitis, and (3) a sore, fissured tongue, or glossitis (See Fig. G-9a,b,c) (Owings 1969; Perry et al. 1973; Neville et al. 2002).

Gnatho-Thesiometer—An apparatus for recording the positions of the lower jaw in three main planes on a freely movable cast of the lower jaw. Its name is derived from the Greek *gnathos*, meaning "jaw," and *thesis*, meaning "position" (Posselt 1957).

Gomphosis—Also known as the periodontal ligament. This term was first used by Bartolomeo Eustachius, a physician and professor of anatomy in Rome (Firkin and Whiteworth 1996; Carranza and Shklar 2003) The gomphosis is a type of fibrous joint where a conical process (i.e., tooth) is inserted into a socket-like process (i.e., the alveolar bone) (Jablonski 1992). See also periodontal ligament.

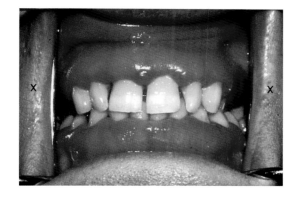

Fig. G-9b: Erythematous gingiva x, angular cheilitis

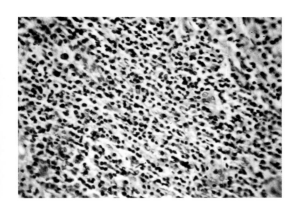

Fig. G-9a: Plasma cell (biopsy)

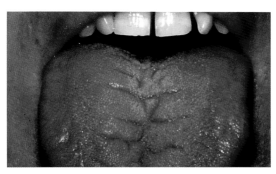

Fig. G-9c: Fissured tongue (glossitis)

Growth and Differentiation Factors—Biological mediators that regulate connective tissue maturation and proliferation as well as the synthesis of proteins and other components of the extracellular matrix. They may have great potential in stimulating periodontal regeneration in humans, yet to be described (Page 1993). Briefly stated, they are a diverse group of polypeptides that have important roles in regulating the growth and development of a variety of organs (AAP 2001a). A position paper outlining the potential of these biological mediators in periodontal regeneration has been published (AAP 1996e). See also cytokines.

Guided Bone Regeneration (GBR)—The regeneration of bone defects utilizing membranes, which may or may not include osseous implantation (Buser et al. 1993). It has also been explained as a surgical procedure that involves the placement of a cell-occlusive physical barrier between the soft tissues and the alveolar bone defect, creating a space within which a blood clot can form, with subsequent bone formation (Mellonig et al. 1998). Guided bone regeneration typically refers to ridge augmentation or bone regeneration procedures (AAP 2001a). See also periodontal regeneration, regeneration.

Guided Tissue Regeneration (GTR)—As early as 1976, a theory on the repair potential of periodontal tissues was proposed; it postulated that cells which repopulate the exposed root surface in periodontal surgery will determine the nature of the "attachment" (Melcher 1976). This theory gave rise to the term *guided tissue regeneration* (GTR), which refers to surgical procedures attempting to regenerate lost periodontal structures through differential tissue responses (see Fig. P-8a,b) (Cortellino and Tonetti 2000; Hammerle and Jung 2003). Such procedures involve the placement of various barriers in the hope of preventing epithelium and the gingival corium, in the belief that they interfere with regeneration, from populating on the root or existing bone surface (Schallhorn and McClain 1998; AAP 2001a). Guided tissue regeneration was first reported both in animals and humans in 1982 (Nyman et al. 1982a, 1982b). See also functional repair, periodontal regeneration, regeneration.

Gum Veneer—This acrylic appliance is made to cover multiple areas of root (cemental) exposure following periodontal therapy. It not only covers the root cementum and interdental spaces but also provides support to the lip and provides an acceptable "gingival" contour (See Fig. G-4a,b) (Staffileno 1964). See also gingival façade, gingival prosthesis, party gums, prosthetic gingival veneer.

H

Hawthorne Effect—This psychological term refers to a positive change in the performances of a group of people taking place in an experiment or study due to their perception of being singled out for special consideration (Random House Dictionary of the English Language 1987). In a paper on studying oral hygiene agents and procedures, Timothy J. O'Leary mentions the Hawthorne effect as one variable in analyzing results. He states that when an individual participates in an experiment, his or her behavior changes until the novelty of being a subject wears off. Thus the results of short-term studies are questionable (O'Leary 1970). This term is named after the Hawthorne Works of the Western Electric Company in Cicero, Illinois, where such an effect was observed in experiments from 1960 to 1965.

Hemisection—The removal or separation of the root with its accompanying crown portion (See Fig. H-1a,b,c) (Basaraba 1969). This procedure is most frequently performed on lower molars, but it may be performed on any multirooted tooth. The mandibular molars are sectioned in a buccolingual direction and the associated portion of the crown may be either removed or restored (See Fig R-5) (Augsburger 1976; Newell 1991; Bohnenkamp and Garcia 2004).

Hemiseptum (pl. hemisepta)—An osseous defect created by the loss of either the mesial or distal half of the interproximal bony septum (Schluger 1949a). It is also known as a one-wall interproximal defect (Goldman and Cohen 1958). See also infrabony defect, osseous defect.

Hereditary Gingival Fibromatosis—This hereditary gingival aberration is clinically presented as a diffuse, fibrous overgrowth of the gingival (See Fig. H-2). It may occur in mental retardation, epilepsy, or in abnormal conditions consisting of a group of signs or symptoms (i.e., syndromes) (Gorlin et al. 2001). It has been identified as an autosomal dominant condition (Singer et al. 1993) and is classified as one of the non-plaque-induced gingival lesions (Armitage 1999).

Hertwig Epithelial Root Sheath—This term designates the double-layered structure that occurs during root development and is formed by the union of the inner and outer epithelium. It shapes the mold into which the root dentin and subsequently the root is deposited (Orban 1957). It is named after the German zoologist Wilhelm August Oscar Hertwig (Sperber and Buckingham 2000). See also epithelial rests of Malassez.

Heterogenous Bone—This term refers to bone procured from a source other than the patient that is used in periodontal regeneration (Beube and Silvers 1934). An example of heterogenous bone is bovine bone, harvested from young calves or calf

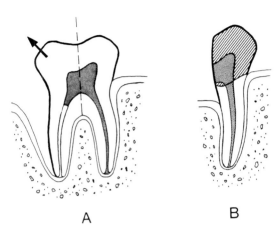

Fig. H-1a

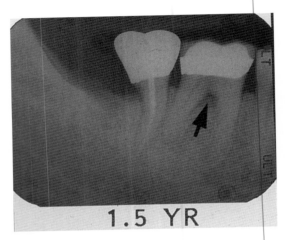

Fig. H-1c: After hemisection; arrow, furcation invasion

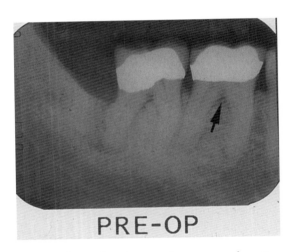

Fig. H-1b: Before hemisection; arrow, furcation invasion

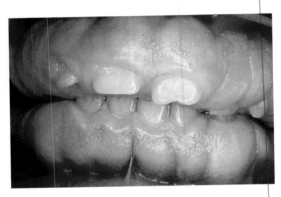

Fig. H-2

embryos and known commercially as Boplant. Synonyms for *heterogenous* include *heteroplast* and *heterograft* (Older 1967).

Heterograft—A synonym for *xenograft*, referring to a graft from a different species (Mellonig 1996). See also xenograft.

Histologic Reattachment—Restoration of the integrity of the connection between periodontal tissue and hard tooth structure. This phenomenon may be divided into (1) the attachment of the epithelium at a more coronal level than the original base of the pocket and (2) the regeneration of new periodontal ligament fibers into new cementum and accompanied by the formation of new bone. It is a synonym for *new attachment* (Rockoff et al. 1958). See also new attachment.

HIV-Associated Gingivitis (HIV-G)—This non-plaque-induced gingival lesion (Armitage 1999) is a gingivitis characterized by a fiery-red band of marginal gingiva shown by a disproportional inflammatory intensity in relation to the amount of plaque (See Fig. H-3). This gingival disease shows no pocketing or loss of attach-

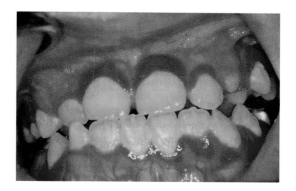

Fig. H-3: (With permission from Blackwell Publishing)

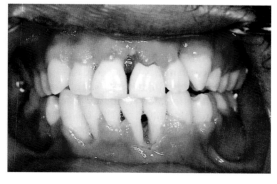

Fig. H-4: (With permission from Blackwell Publishing)

ment and elicits no response to oral hygiene measures or dental scaling (Glick et al. 1994; Murray 1994a, 1994b). See also linear gingival erythema (LGE).

HIV-Associated Periodontitis (HIV-P)—This form of periodontitis has all the gingival features of HIV- associated gingivitis plus all the signs and symptoms of a rapidly "aggressive periodontitis" (See Fig. H-4) (Armitage 1999). It is characterized clinically by severe deep pain, gingival bleeding, soft tissue necrosis, and rapid destruction of the periodontal attachment apparatus (Murray 1994a, 1994b). See also necrotizing ulcerative periodontitis (NUP).

Homograft—This type of tissue graft is taken from an operative site in one individual and grafted into an operative site in another individual of the same species. This term is synonymous with *allograft* (Hurt 1968). See also allogenic, allograft.

Horizontal Bone Loss—This phrase for loss of interdental bone in periodontitis occurs when the bone is resorbed parallel to the upper margin of the alveolar process (See Fig. H-5). According to Adolph Berger, this classification is credited to Oscar Weski, who stated that horizontal bone loss or horizontal pyorrhea is more amenable to treatment than vertical bone loss (Berger 1927). See also vertical bone loss.

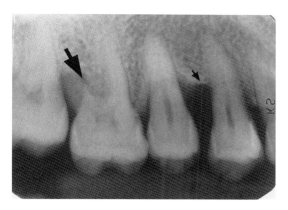

Fig. H-5: Small arrow, horizontal bone loss; large arrow, trifurcation invasion

Horizontal Continuous Suture—This suturing technique is employed when a free soft tissue autograft is to be stretched over a denuded root surface in order to establish stability and adaptation of the graft. It accomplishes three goals: (1) increases chances of revascularization, (2) eliminates dead spaces, and (3) counteracts primary contraction (Holbrook and Ochsenbein 1983). See also suture.

Horizontal Defect Dimension (HDD)—The horizontal dimension in millimeters between the surface of an "immediate implant" and the alveolar bone (socket) measured from the widest point of the socket wall (Wilson et al. 1998). See also implant-immediate, vertical defect dimension (VDD).

Horizontal Fiber Group—This group of principal fibers of the periodontal ligament course in a wavy path from the cementum to the bone (See Fig. P-4c). They are located apical to the alveolar crest fibers and transverse the periodontal ligament space at right angles to the root and bone. Their function is similar to that of the alveolar crest fibers in that they oppose lateral forces on the teeth (Orban 1957). See also periodontal ligament.

Horizontal Gingival Pedicle Graft—This is a synonym for the "lateral sliding flap" procedure of Grupe and Warren (1956) (Ratcliff 1966). See also lateral sliding flap.

Horizontal Internal Mattress Suture—This suturing technique, which preserves the esthetic results of the "curtain" techniques of Frisch, Jones, and Bhaskar (Frisch et al. 1967), is indicated when the maxillary anterior papillae are short and wide. This approach closes the flaps in the curtain technique so as to minimize gingival and interproximal recession (Newell and Brunsvold 1985). See also suture, vertical internal mattress suture.

Horizontal Lateral Sliding Papillary Flap—A surgical technique for creating attached gingiva on the buccal surfaces of a group of consecutive teeth where none previously existed. The technique is predicated on the principle of utilizing the interdental gingiva, which has morphologic and histologic characteristics of attached gingiva (Hattler 1967). A similar procedure for treating a localized problem over the buccal surface of a single tooth has been demonstrated (Cohen and Ross 1968). See also double papillae repositioned flap, interdental papillae graft, multiple interdental papilla graft.

Horizontal Sliding Flap—This is a periodontal surgical technique to correct gingival recession, which occurs as a single tooth. It is synonymous with the lateral sliding flap (Grupe 1960). See also lateral sliding flap.

Horizontal Toothbrushing Technique—In this method of toothbrushing, also known as the "crosswise" or "scrub" technique, the bristles are applied at right angles to the surface of the teeth and activated by back-and-forth horizontal strokes. The ends of the bristles are rubbed vigorously over all surfaces of the teeth and gums, in a manner similar to scrubbing a floor. It applies pressure on teeth that are prominent in the arch and may produce abrasion to the teeth and gingiva. The interdental areas are not touched by this method and bacterial plaque can remain undisturbed on proximal surfaces. This haphazard technique can be recommended only for the occlusal surfaces of the teeth (Hine 1956; Yankell and Saxer 1999; Ray 2005). See also toothbrushing technique.

Host Modulatory Therapy (HMT)—Refers to those agents (perioceutics) that can be used as adjuncts during nonsurgical or surgical procedures to improve wound healing or to stimulate regeneration of the lost attachment apparatus. The non-surgical adjuncts to HMT include systemic/topical use of nonsteroidal anti-inflammatory drugs, sub-antimicrobial-dose doxycycline, and bisphonates. The HMT adjuncts to surgical procedures include enamel matrix proteins, bone morphogenetic proteins, growth factors, and tetracyclines (Ryan 2002, 2005; AAP 2003b). See also bone morphogenetic proteins (BMP), enamel matrix proteins, growth and differentiation factors.

Iatrogenic—This term describes an abnormal mental or physical condition induced in a patient by the effects of treatment (AAP 2001a). Iatrogeny, produced by either an inadvertent or erroneous treatment, may be a result of either acts of commission or acts of omission by the therapist (Vandersall 1975). Several examples of dental iatrogenics producing periodontal defects are (1) retained black silk sutures (Manor and Kaffe 1982), (2) retained rubber dams (Abrams et al. 1978), (3) improper oral hygiene technique (Gillette and Van House 1980), and (4) retained orthodontic elastics (See Fig. I-1a,b,c; Fig. I-2a,b,c,d) (Vandersall 1971; Vandersall and Slade 1978). See also runner, wicking.

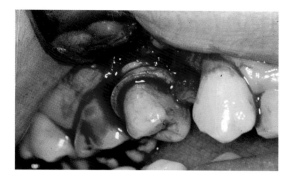

Fig. I-1b: (With permission from the American Dental Association)

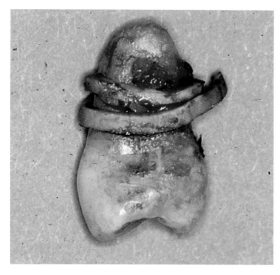

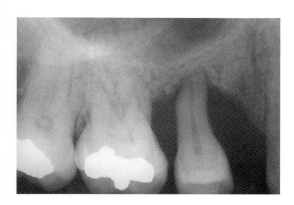

Fig. I-1a: (With permission from the American Dental Association)

Fig. I-1c

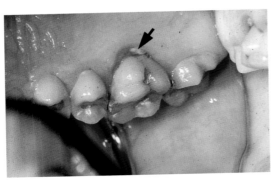

Fig. I-2a: Arrow, elastic band in situ (With permission from the American Dental Association)

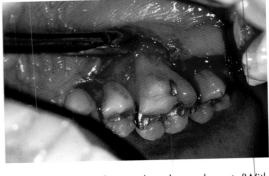

Fig. I-2c: Loss of periodontal attachment (With permission from the American Dental Association)

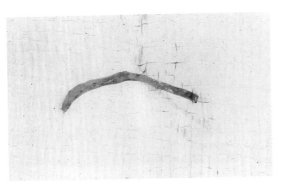

Fig. I-2b: (With permission from the American Dental Association)

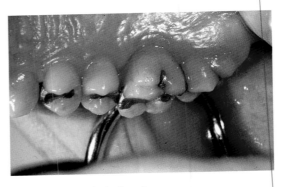

Fig. I-2d: Healed after 1 year

Iliac Crest Autograft—This type of autogenous bone graft utilizes hematopoietic bone marrow removed from the lateral or posterosuperior iliac crest (Schallhorn 1968). This approach to managing infrabony periodontal defects was fraught with complications in the 1970s and is no longer recommended for autogenous bone grafting. The reported postoperative problems were: (1) infection, (2) exfoliation and sequestration of the implanted iliac bone, (3) resorption of the root, and (4) rapid recurrence of the defect (Schallhorn 1972). See also autogenous bone graft.

Implant, Ailing—One with radiographic bone loss but no clinical inflammation when examined at 3 to 4-month mainte-

nance checks. Such an implant exhibits bone loss with pocketing; however, a lamina dura may be present at the borders of the osseous defect, indicating a state of chronicity (Meffert 1992). See also peri-implantitis.

Implant, Bladevent—These are endosseous implants that are placed directly into the bone through a small mucosal incision (See Fig. I-3). They are tapped into the bone until they are completely or almost completely in contact with bone to encourage overall retention and resist lateral forces. This is indeed an intraosseous device (Linkow 1970). These implants have been defined as having a flat, blade-shaped surface, which derives its support from its horizontal length in bone. Most

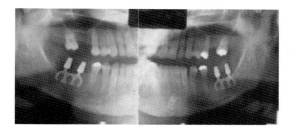

Fig. I-3: (Courtesy of Dr. Steven Blanchard)

commonly made of metal, such an implant can be perforated, smooth, fluted, textured, coated, wedge-shaped, and/or multiheaded (AAP 2001a). The parameters of their placement and management have been published (AAP 2000f).

Implant, Delayed—The placement of an endosseous implant 6 to 10 weeks following extraction, at a time when only soft tissue healing has occurred. This procedure may reduce the risk of barrier membrane exposure and minimize the effect of microorganism invasion during healing (Mayfield 1999; Minsk 2005a). See also implant, immediate; implant, late.

Implant, Dental—A biomedical device usually composed of an inert metal or metallic alloy that is placed on or within the osseous tissue (See Fig. I-4a,b). Such implants are used to replace single or multiple teeth or to serve as abutments for fixed or removable prostheses, with the goal of restoring masticatory function and/or esthetics (AAP 2001a). A position paper on the utility of employing dental implants in the treatment of full and partial edentulism has been presented (AAP 2000b). See also implant, bladevent; implant, subperiosteal; implant, vitreous carbon.

Implant, Failed—The failed implant exhibits mobility, elicits a dull sound to percussion, and radiographically reveals peri-implant radiolucency. Such an implant must be removed, since it is not functional and bone loss will continue (Meffert 1992). See also peri-implantitis.

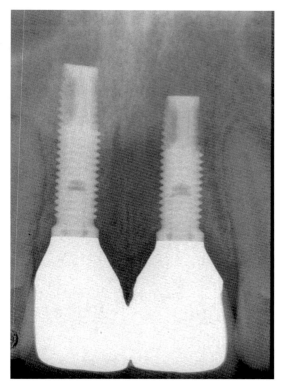

Fig. I-4a: (Courtesy of Dr. S. Jin Kim)

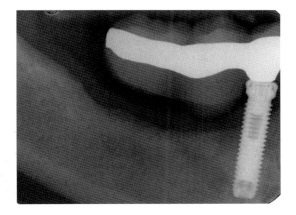

Fig. I-4b

Implant, Failing—One that exhibits radiographic bone loss, pocketing, bleeding upon probing, purulent discharge, and indications that bone loss is progressing despite therapy. However, mobility is not present (Meffert 1992). See also peri-implantitis.

Implant, Immediate—An implant during the same visit at which the tooth is extracted. It is stated that this procedure will reduce morbidity, treatment costs, and treatment time (Wilson and Weber 1993; Wilson et al. 1998). See also horizontal defect dimension (HDD); implant, delayed; implant,late; vertical defect dimension (VDD).

Implant, Late—The placement of an endosseous implant six months or more following tooth removal, a time that allows maturation of both soft and hard tissues. Substantial regeneration of the alveolar bone has occurred, allowing ideal placement and positioning of the implant and enhancing the final result (Mayfield 1999; Minsk 2005a). See also implant, immediate; implant, delayed.

Implant, Sleeper—A dental implant that cannot be used, for one reason or another, as a final restoration but that remains submerged and osseointegrated—i.e., a "sleeper" (Misch et al. 1999).

Implant, Subperiosteal—A device directly placed on the bone beneath the periosteum. It is used chiefly in an edentulous mandible and involves a two-stage surgical procedure for insertion and stability (Boyne and James 1986).

Implant, Vitreous Carbon—An implant produced by firing a phenol formaldehyde resin at a very high and carefully controlled temperature. In this process, all the noncarbon components of the resin are driven off and a pure carbon is produced in a black microcrystalline form, resulting in a pure, hard, inert material (Meffert 1977). It was first produced in 1963 and used clinically in 1969 but is now in disfavor, having been replaced by titanium and its alloys.

Incidence—A term used in statistics to represent the number of defects that may occur or accumulate in an individual or population during a given period of time. In other words, it expresses the rate at which a certain event occurs in terms of the number of new cases of a specific disease that arise within a certain period (Ramfjord 1959; Daly and Bourke 2000). See also prevalence.

Incisal Repositioning Flap—Also known as the coronally repositioned flap. It was illustrated and discussed by Charles F. Sumner in the incisal positioning of gingiva to cover the exposed root surface of a maxillary cuspid (Sumner 1969). A modification of this procedure, which first included the placement of a free soft tissue autograft to increase the width of attached gingiva, has been illustrated (Caffesse and Guinard 1978). See also coronally repositioned flap, semilunar coronally repositioned flap.

Inconsistent Bony Margin—The vertical notch-like irregularities of marginal bone with which gingiva cannot be consistent (Saari et al. 1968). In 1949, Saul Schluger stated that the pattern or flow of soft tissue is influenced by the contour of the hard tissues with which it is in contact, thus emphasizing that osseous deformities must be reshaped in order to eliminate pockets (Schluger 1949a).

Index (pl. indices)—A relative or arbitrary system of measurement that describes a quantity or condition (AAP 2001a). Such indices are appropriate for use in an individual patient or for epidemiologic studies (Barnes et al. 1986; Marks et al. 1993).

Index of Gingival Architectural Form—This index is proposed for scoring variations in gingival architectural form; its objective is to quantitate gingival topography in numerical terms. The morphology of the gingiva is recorded at three positions: the buccal margin, the papilla mesial to each tooth, and the gingival margin. Values are given of zero for ideal and 1 for a deviation, such as blunting or cratering. The mouth is divided into sextants, with scores of each sextant added and divided by the number of teeth in each sextant. The possible score for a sextant is 0 to 6, with the mouth score being the sum of the sextants (MacLeod et al. 1965). See also gingival contour index.

Index of Recession (IR)—An index that considers both the vertical and the horizontal extent of root exposure, with the former using the cementoenamel junction as a reference point. The facial and lingual sites of root exposure are assessed separately. If the vertical extent of recession encroaches into the mucogingival junction or extends beyond it into the alveolar mucosa, an asterisk is shown on the vertical score. The horizontal measurements and the criteria for scoring both dimensions are illustrated in the reference, this being an all-inclusive index of recording gingival recession on both buccal and lingual aspects (Smith 1997).

Index of Tooth Function—An index of tooth function derived by analyzing the degree of attrition on each individual tooth. Numerically it is measured as 0 = normal contour, no facets; 1 = definite enamel facets; 2 = definite enamel facets with dentin exposed; 3 = more advanced exposure of the dentin with exposure of the recessional lines of the pulp; and 4 = actual pulp exposure. The index of tooth function equals the sum of the attrition indices for each tooth divided by the number of teeth present (Davies 1956).

Inflammatory Index (II)—An assessment of the percentage of the total number of extravascular inflammatory cells in the subepithelial connective tissue within a given microscopic field. The five predetermined microscopic fields are viewed in a buccal-lingual section of tissue, with the five areas scattered throughout the specimen. They begin subjacent to the crevicular epithelium and end at the most coronal projection of the alveolar crest. Their precise location and its methodology is diagrammatically illustrated in the two articles cited here (Pihlstrom and Ramfjord 1971; Rosenberg and Ash 1974).

Infrabony Defect—This defect, defined as a pocket whose base is apical to the alveolar

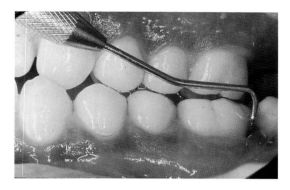

Fig. I-5a: Probing an infrabony pocket)

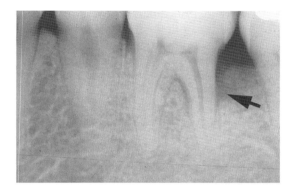

Fig. I-5b: Radiograph of infrabony pocket

crest, was described and classified by Henry M. Goldman and D. Walter Cohen in October 1959 at the American Academy of Periodontology meeting in Miami, Florida (See Fig. I-5a,b). They described such defects as having three walls, two walls, or one wall. A combination of infrabony defects may have either 3-2 walls, 3-2-1 walls, 3-1 walls, or 2-1 walls (Goldman and Cohen 1958). See also circumferential defect, crater defect, hemiseptum (pl. hemisepta), intrabony defect.

Intercuspal Position—In the science of occlusion, this term refers to the contact position of maximum intercuspation of the maxilla and mandible after closure (AAP 2001a). This is usually the most cranial position of the mandible in which the cusps and sulci of the mandibular and maxillary teeth mesh tightly. It is usually located anterior and superior to the retruded contact position (Posselt 1968). See also centric occlusion (CO), retruded contact (RC).

Interdental Bleeding Index (IBI)—An index that evaluates the health of midinterproximal gingival tissue, which is determined by placing a wooden interdental cleaner (i.e., Stim-U-Dent) horizontally between the teeth while depressing the interdental papilla 1 to 2 mm. The wooden cleaner is inserted and removed four times; then, after 15 seconds, the mouth is examined for the presence or absence of bleeding. The number of bleeding sites (index) is expressed as a percentage of the total number of sites evaluated, thus providing the IBI (Caton and Polson 1985). See also Eastman interdental bleeding index (EIBI).

Interdental Canals—Vascular channels within the interdental bone (AAP 2001a). A classic paper in 1927 by Isador Hirschfeld thoroughly describes these canals in the alveolar bone as being both linear and circular radiolucent findings, providing vascular supply to the bone; he stated that they should not be confused with radiolucency resulting from periodontal disease (Hirschfeld 1927).

Interdental Col—This is considered to be the site of least resistance (locus minoris resistentiae) to invasion by microorganisms and/or their toxins (See Fig. I-6) (Stahl 1963; Jablonski 1992). Attempts, although futile in the long term, have been made to convert the nonkeratinized stratified squamous epithelium of the interdental col to a keratinized surface (Cantor and Stahl 1965). See also col, interdental papilla.

Interdental Crater—A wide-mouthed cup or bowl-shaped defect in the interalveolar bone. The bone destruction is about equal on the roots of the contiguous teeth, with the side walls of the crater formed by marginal bone on the vestibular and lingual surfaces (Prichard 1972). The interdental crater is the most common type of osseous

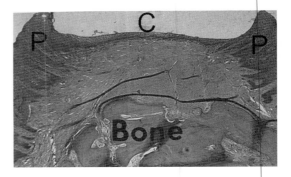

Fig. I-6: C, interdental col; P, interdental papilla

defect being twice as common posteriorly as it is anteriorly (Saari et al. 1968; Manson and Nicholson 1974). See also crater defect, interproximal crater, osseous defect.

Interdental Crest—The most coronal projection of the alveolar septum. Radiographically, the presence or absence of the crestal lamina dura has historically been suggestive of either health or disease within the deeper (bony) structures of the periodontium. However, no correlation has been found between crestal lamina dura in dental radiographs and the presence or absence of clinical inflammation, bleeding on probing, periodontal pockets, or loss of attachment (Greenstein et al. 1981). See also crestal lamina dura, lamina dura.

Interdental Denudation—A periodontal surgical technique that includes excision of all soft tissue in the interproximal region, leaving the interalveolar crestal bone exposed (Jablonski 1992). In the treatment of intrabony defects, it is believed that the retention of soft tissue might lead to epithelial downgrowth, which would line the defect before regeneration could occur. The result would lead to reformation of the osseous defect (Prichard 1977, 1983). See also interdental resection, interproximal denudation.

Interdental Grooves—The attached gingiva appears slightly depressed between adjoining teeth, which corresponds to the depression on the alveolar bone process

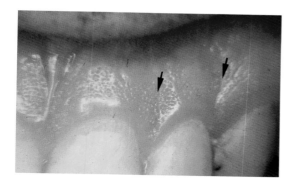

Fig. I-7a: Arrows, interdental grooves

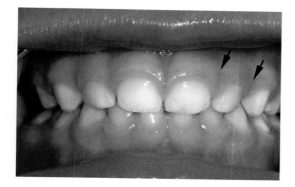

Fig. I-7b: Arrows, interdental grooves

between the eminences of the sockets (See Fig. I-7a,b). In these depressions the attached gingiva often forms slight vertical folds or grooves, whether in an adult or a child (Orban 1948a; Goldman 1949).

Interdental Papilla—The interdental papilla is that part of the gingiva (gingival papilla) that fills the space between two adjoining teeth and is limited at its base by a line drawn from the margin of the gingiva at the center of one tooth to the center of the other. It is composed of free and attached gingiva in various relations, depending largely on the topographic arrangements of the neighboring teeth. The free gingival groove separates the free from the attached gingiva (Orban 1948a; Goldman 1949). Its synonym is interprox-

imal papilla (Tarnow et al. 1992). See also col, interproximal papilla.

Interdental Papillae Graft—This surgical technique is a modification of the "double papillae repositioned flap," utilizing a new method of piecing together multiple papillae for free soft tissue autogenous grafting. While no attempt is made for root coverage in this approach, the mucogingival junction is placed more apically, thus increasing the vertical height of keratinized gingiva (i.e., gingival augmentation). This is more advantageous than the double papillae repositioned flap, which attempts to cover exposed roots and places the gingival margin more coronally with the mucogingival junction remaining in the same position (Rubelman 1977). See also double papillae repositioned flap, multiple interdental papilla graft.

Interdental Resection—This is an archaic periodontal surgical technique performed to eradicate shallow two-wall infrabony periodontal pockets to bring about tissue repair and function. It requires the complete enucleation of all the interproximal papillary tissue, dissecting loose the epithelial attachment and transseptal fibers from the proximal tooth root walls. A buccal and lingual gingival incision releases the papilla from these respective tissues and is followed by dissection of the crestal gingival fibers to free them from the underlying alveolar process. This opening of the interproximal defect improves vision of the pattern of bone resorption, facilitates root planing, and provides for complete regeneration of the interproximal tissue. The interdental socket is packed and allowed to heal (Beube 1947; Chace 1954). See also interdental denudation, interproximal denudation.

Interdental Septum (pl. Septa)—The portion of the alveolar process between adjacent teeth (See Fig. I-8a,b,c) (AAP 2001a). Radiographically, the contour and shape of the interdental septa are influenced by several factors: (1) variations in the anatomy and positions of the teeth, (2) the

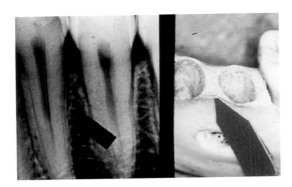

Fig. I-8a: Arrows, septa

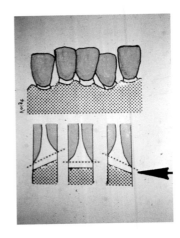

Fig. I-8c: Arrow, septa

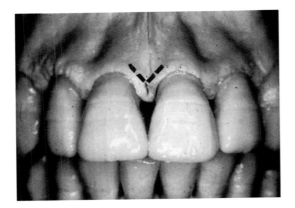

Fig. I-8b: dotted line, septum

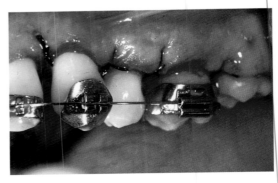

Fig. I-9a: Buccal view

state of eruption of proximating teeth, and (3) the position or inclination of the teeth in the jaws (Ritchey and Orban 1953a).

Interdental Suture—A suturing technique whereby each stitch (suture) is made with a separate piece of material (See Fig. I-9a,b). It is especially valuable when both buccal and lingual flaps are to be sutured at the same height. It produces the firmest adaptation of soft tissue to the underlying bone and tooth (Morris 1965a). See also interrupted suture, suture.

Intermediate Cementum—An area located between the root cementum and dentin which contains cellular debris trapped in a rapidly calcifying matrix. It corresponds to the time that the tooth begins to erupt.

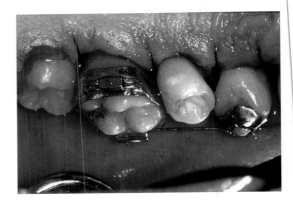

Fig. I-9b: Palatal view

It is believed that the cellular debris in fact represents portions of the Hertwig epithelial root sheath that had failed to detach from the dentin surface (El Mostehy and Stallard 1968). This layer of cementum has recently been described as being homogenous (hyaline-like) and is located from the cementoenamel junction to the apical third of the root (Ten Cate 1997). See also altered cementum, cementum, epithelial rests of Malassez, Hertwig epithelial root sheath.

Intermediate Plexus—This structure, believed to be present within the periodontal ligament, has been studied for years; controversy has existed over its presence or absence. Harry Sicher, in studying the periodontal membrane (PDM) of molars in guinea pigs and incisors in rats, believed that the dental fibers of the PDM were spliced in the middle with those fibers from the bone to those from the root cementum (See Fig. I-10a). He stated that this provided for drift, attrition, and rapid growth by unsplicing and resplicing of the fibers (Sicher 1923, 1942, 1954a, 1959). It was not until 1965 that the intermediate plexus was found not to exist and that the principal fibers of the periodontal ligament were determined to be continuous from the alveolar bone to the cementum (See Fig. I-10b) (Zwarych and Quigley 1965).

Internal Bevel Gingivectomy—Also known as the internal bevel incision. Its advantage is that it retains the greatest amount of facial tissue to cover the labial alveolar bone. In this procedure, the pocket epithelium is eliminated and, more importantly, it compensates for the fibrosis that usually accompanies a long-standing gingival inflammation (Morris 1965b). It provides exposure of additional coronal tooth structure with a reduction of excessive pocket depth in the absence of a sufficient zone of attached gingiva, with or without the need for osseous correction. Basically, it is a flap procedure (Youdelis and Smith 1976). See also internal bevel incision, in-

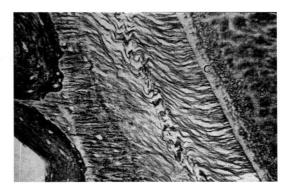

Fig. I-10a: Splicing of fibers (Courtesy of Dr. Vanchit John)

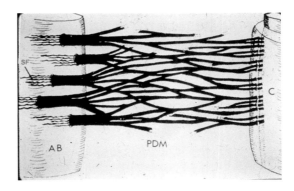

Fig. I-10b: A B—Alveolar bone, SF—Sharpey's Fibers, PDM—Periodontal membrane, C—Cementum (With permission from the Journal of Dental Research)

verse bevel incision, inverted bevel incision, reverse bevel incision.

Internal Bevel Incision—According to Bennett Klavan, Claude Nabers developed and introduced the internal bevel incision to provide a thin flap margin devoid of sulcular epithelium (Klavan 1970; Nabers 1954). Its three main objectives are to (1) remove pocket lining (epithelium), (2) conserve the relatively uninvolved outer surface of the gingiva, and (3) produce a sharp, thin flap margin for adaptation to the bone-tooth junction (Takei and Carranza 1996). It is also known as the reverse bevel incision because its bevel is in reverse position as that of a gingivectomy incision. See also inverse bevel incision, inverted bevel incision, reverse bevel incision.

Internal Mattress Suture—This technique of closing wound margins is used whenever esthetics is a concern. It is achieved by assuring that the suture material does not overlie the edges of the flap but lays below (i.e., internal mattress) the flap margins. Depending upon the vertical or horizontal penetration points of the suture needle, you are able to place either a "vertical internal mattress suture" or a "horizontal internal mattress suture" (Newell and Brunsvold 1985). See also horizontal internal mattress suture, vertical internal mattress suture.

Interpapillary Fiber Group—This group of gingival fibers interdigitates with the dentogingival and dentoperiosteal fibers. They are easily viewed in labiolingual microscopic sections of the interdental gingival septa when cut at right angles to the surface of the col. These fibers provide integrity to the papillae and are thought to provide an integral pathway for the spread of the inflammatory process in chronic gingivitis (Melcher 1962). See also gingival fiber group.

Interproximal Crater—The interproximal crater is essentially a shallow "two-wall infrabony pocket" (Goldman and Cohen 1958). It has been said to develop by the loss of bone between the facial and lingual cortical plates (Schluger 1949a) and is reported to be the most commonly found bony defect in periodontitis (Saari et al. 1968). Two-thirds of all mandibular osseous defects are represented by interproximal craters and are twice as common posteriorly as they are anteriorly. (Manson and Nicholson 1974). See also crater defect, infrabony defect, interdental crater, osseous defect.

Interproximal Denudation—This approach to the management of interproximal osseous defects was presented in 1964 by Perry A. Ratcliff and George T. Raust. The procedure was accomplished by exposing the interproximal bony defect without ex-posing the thin buccal and lingual surfaces of the alveolar process, with the objective of creating a "new attachment" (Ratcliff and Raust 1964). It is similar to the original interdental resection of Frank E. Beube (Beube 1947). See also interdental denudation, interdental resection, papillectomy.

Interproximal Papilla—Also known as an interdental papilla. It is referenced in a publication concerned with the presence or absence of the interproximal papilla (interdental papilla) when there is loss of the interdental bony crest. Measurements were made from the base of the contact area to the crest of bone to determine the presence or absence of the interproximal papillae in humans (Tarnow et al. 1992). See also interdental papilla.

Interradicular—The area between the roots of a multirooted tooth, having the following boundaries: (1) *coronal*, the apical surface of the root trunk or roof; (2) *apical*, the root apices; and (3) *lateral*, established by a plane across the lateral heights of contour of two adjacent roots of the same tooth (Heins and Canter 1968). Another definition is the area of root separation or furcation chamber bordered coronally by the base of the root trunk or roof, laterally by the roots, and apically by the remaining periodontium (Saadoun 1985).

Interradicular Fiber Group—This group of principal fibers of the periodontal ligament, located within the furcation of multirooted teeth, traverse from the crestal bone of the interradicular septum to the cementum (See Fig. I-11). Their function is to resist the forces of luxation (pulling out) or tipping of the tooth (Orban 1957). See also periodontal ligament.

Interrupted Periosteal Suture—The apical positioning of partial-thickness flaps is best achieved by utilizing the periosteal suturing technique. This approach to flap stabilization may be by either a continuous sling suture or an interrupted periosteal suture. However, if the latter method is utilized, the sutures may be dif-

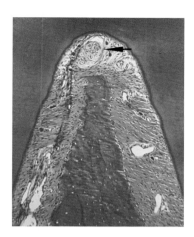

Fig. I-11: Arrow, interradicular fiber group

ficult to find and remove at the postoperative visit unless gut sutures are used (Douglas 1976). See also periosteal suture, suture.

Interrupted Suture—This suturing technique is utilized when tissue positioning is not a problem and both surgical sides need the same tension, as in a buccal and lingual papillary coaptation. Separate pieces of suture material are utilized in closing each papilla (wound margins) (Dahlberg 1969). See also interdental suture, suture.

Intrabony Defect—An osseous defect surrounded by bony walls on three sides, with the tooth root forming the fourth wall. The walls may be at different levels coronally, forming combinations with other defects, but only the "inside" of the defect, or the part that is apical to all three bony walls, is "within" bone, or intrabony. The intrabony defect is not a circumferential defect; there is an osseous wall or step on each side of the root (Prichard 1972; Larato 1970b). An editorial on proper terminology for osseous defects has been written (Weinberg and Eskow 2000b). See also circumferential defect, infrabony defect, osseous defect.

Intracrevicular—This term refers to restorative margins placed into and confined within the gingival crevice. It is more limiting and descriptive than *subgingival margin* (Maynard and Wilson 1979; Wilson and Maynard 1981). More specifically, *intracrevicular* was said to refer to the placement of a dental restoration in that space bounded by the tooth and the sulcular epithelium without infringing on the junctional epithelium (Nevins and Skurow 1984; Nevins and Cappetta 1998).

Inverse Bevel Incision—This surgical incision is performed during the process of flap evaluation. The incision is placed in an attempt to produce a thinned gingival margin to the flap, leaving behind inflamed cervicular epithelium and connective tissue attached to the tooth (Friedman and Levine 1964). It was illustrated in 1957 by Claude L. Nabers and has been described as a scalloped incision, about 20 degrees to the long axis of the tooth, starting 1 to 2 mm from the gingival margin and ending at the crest of the alveolar bone (Zamet 1967). See also internal bevel incision, inverted bevel incision, reverse bevel incision.

Inverted Bevel Incision—According to Melvin L. Morris, this incision removes the epithelial lining and 1 or 2 mm of gingival height in preparation for flap elevation. It is performed as an internal gingivectomy, which results in a flap with a smooth, thin gingival margin. It is also known as the inverse and internal bevel incision (Morris 1965b). See also internal bevel incision, inverse bevel incision, reverse bevel incision.

Iontophoresis—A method of facilitating the transfer of ions by means of an electrical potential into soft and hard tissues of the body for therapeutic purposes (Walton et al. 1979). A more current definition is the act or process of introducing therapeutic agents into tissues using an electrical current or electrochemical gradient (AAP 2001a). A review of its periodontal application in managing cervical dentinal sensitivity has been published (Gillam and Newman 1990).

Irregularity Index—This dental index measures the horizontal linear displacement of the anatomic contact points of the six mandibular anterior teeth. Using a dental cast of the lower anterior teeth and a dial caliper accurate to 0.1 mm, the horizontal linear distance between adjacent contact points is determined for the six teeth. Five measurements are made between teeth 22 and 23, 23 and 24, 24 and 25, 25 and 26, and 26 and 27. The scale for degree of severity is 0 = perfect alignment, 1 to 3 = minimal irregularity, 4 to 6 = moderate irregularity, 7 to 9 = severe irregularity, and 10 = very severe irregularity (Little 1975).

Irreversible Index—This classification assesses the damage caused by the disease rather than the disease itself. Once an irreversible index score is established, it cannot decrease in value at future examinations. Examples of irreversible indices are the Periodontal Disease Index (PDI), Periodontal Index (PI), and Decayed-Missing-Filled Index (DMF). With the exception of measuring bone loss, the measurement of periodontal variables is mainly reversible (Barnes et al. 1986). See also reversible index.

J

Junctional Epithelium—This phrase replaced the term *epithelial attachment* when Hubert Schroeder and Max Listgarten stated that it was derived from the reduced enamel epithelium (See Fig. J-1) (Schroeder and Listgarten 1971). Irving Stern later described the relationship of the primary attachment (ameloblasts) to the tooth as formed by the basal lamina and hemidesmosomes (Stern 1981). This tissue, capable of forming and replacing itself continuously throughout life, consists of single or multilayered nonkeratinizing cells that adhere to the tooth surface at the base of the gingival crevice (AAP 2001a). See also epithelial attachment.

Juvenile Periodontitis—A disease of the periodontium that occurs in an otherwise healthy adolescent and is characterized by a rapid loss of alveolar bone around more than one tooth of the permanent dentition. Two forms of the disease have been described: (1) localized, where the affected teeth are the first molars and cuspids, or (2) generalized, where most of the dentition is affected. The amount of destruction is not commensurate with the quantity of local irritants present (Baer 1971). This condition was formerly called periodontosis, but in 1969 the term *juvenile periodontitis* was suggested, since there was no proof of any degenerative process, as implied by the suffix *-osis* (Butler 1969). More recently, it was decided to discard classification ter-

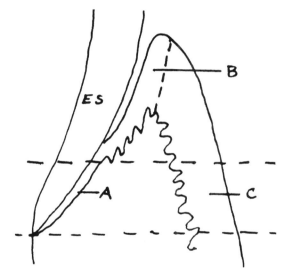

Fig. J-1: A, junctional epithelium or epithelial attachment; B, sulcular or crevicular epithelium; C, attached gingiva; ES, enamel space

minologies that were age-dependent or that required knowledge of rates of progression (i.e., localized or generalized juvenile periodontitis). Accordingly, highly destructive forms of periodontitis that were classed under "early-onset periodontitis" are now all classified as "aggressive periodontitis" (Armitage 1999). See also aggressive periodontitis, early-onset periodontitis, generalized juvenile periodontitis (GJP), localized juvenile periodontitis (LJP), parodontosis, periodontosis.

K

Karolyi Effect—An effect named after Moritz Karolyi, a Viennese dentist of Hungarian descent, who first described the possible role of hyperfunction of the masticatory muscles in eliciting traumatic occlusion as a cause of pyorrhea (periodontitis). He recommended its correction by grinding the occlusal surfaces and the use of bite planes at night. Karolyi introduced the current concept of bruxism but never used the term (Karolyi 1901; Carranza and Shklar 2003). See also bruxism, bruxomania.

Keyes Technique—The Keyes approach to treating periodontal disease nonsurgically was made popular in 1978 with Paul Keyes' introduction of the microbiologically modulated periodontal therapeutic (MMPT) procedure. It consisted of the following steps: (1) traditional methods of scaling, root planing, and oral hygiene instructions; (2) application to the gingiva of a paste consisting of baking soda and sodium bicarbonate with water and hydrogen peroxide; (3) irrigation of pockets with a water-and-salt solution (Epsom salt and magnesium sulfate could be used as a salt substitute); (4) application of fluoride to roots; (5) tetracycline 250 mg q.i.d. in severe cases for two weeks; and (6) monitoring of subgingival microbial flora by phase-contrast or dark-field microscopy to measure disease activity and determine the effectiveness of treatment (Keyes et al. 1978a, 1978b; Keyes and Rams 1983). This treatment regimen was challenged by many. In 1983, it was shown that results obtained by the Keyes technique of oral hygiene were not significantly different from conventional oral hygiene procedures and that patients treated surgically had significantly better periodontal health than those treated nonsurgically, as indicated by both clinical and bacteriologic criteria (Greenwell et al. 1983). A committee appointed by the American Academy of Periodontology in 1984 expressed serious doubt that any scientifically valid conclusions could be derived from the Keyes technique. The committee's membership consisted of E.P. Barrington, W. Becker, L. Berg (consultant), C.W. Finley (AAP president), M.G. Newman, S.S. Socransky, and S.S. Stahl (AAP 1984). The current understanding of the role of the Keyes technique in periodontal therapy has been published (AAP 1998d). See also microbiologically modulated periodontal therapy (MMPT).

Kobayaski–Ash Plaque Index—This plaque index is a modification of the Shick-Ash plaque index. Using Bismark Brown as a disclosing solution, the degree of plaque present is expressed numerically by P0, P1, P2, P3, or P4. P0 is an absence of dental plaque. P1 is dental plaque on one of the interproximal surfaces or on the middle of the facial or lingual gingival marginal aspect of the tooth and not covering more than one-third of the gingival half of the facial or lingual surface. P2 is dental plaque on two interproximal surfaces or any two gingival marginal surfaces but not covering more than one-third of the gingival half of the facial or lingual surface of the crown of a tooth. P3 is dental plaque extending from mesial to distal and not covering more than one-third of the gingival half of the facial or lingual surfaces of the crown of a tooth. P4 is plaque covering one-third to two-thirds of the gingival half of the facial or lingual surface of the crown of a tooth (Kobayaski and Ash 1964). See also Shick-Ash plaque index.

L

Labiogingival Notch—This is an anatomic variant of the permanent maxillary central incisor, which appears as a "notch" in the facial enamel, affecting the gingival contour. It appears as a depression in the enamel, close to the cementoenamel junction, and can occur as a shallow depression to a deep groove. This defect should be considered a *locus minoris resistentiae*, or a possible source of plaque accumulation and potential periodontal problems (Ben-Bassat and Brin 2001). See also facial radicular groove.

Lamellar Bone—Lamellated or lamellar bone is mature bone whose fibrils are arranged in different directions in adjacent lamellae. This change in fibril direction, which produces the lamellar pattern, increases the resistance of bone to mechanical forces, especially shearing forces (Weinmann and Sicher 1955). This type of bone is well structured to withstand force and is the bone of choice for implant longevity, being a structured load-bearing bone (Misch 1988). See also bundle bone, woven bone.

Lamina Dura—This term refers to the radiographic image of the alveolar bone proper, the cortical bone that surrounds the root of a tooth and into which are embedded Sharpey's fibers of the periodontal ligament (Elfenbaum 1958). Its considerable variations may occur due to the shape and position of the root and/or changes in angulation of the x-ray beam (Manson 1963). See also alveolar bone proper, crestal lamina dura, cribriform plate.

Laminin—This term refers to a high-molecular-weight glycoprotein composed of three polypeptide chains organized in a cross-like manner. It is a principal component of the basal lamina, and the functional domains of this molecule have an affinity for cell surface receptors and extracellular matrix components (AAP 2001a). Laminin is a chemoattractant to epithelial cells and promotes their growth (Terranova et al. 1986). A review of laminin and its place in periodontal regeneration has been published (Abdallah et al. 1988). See also fibronectin.

Laser—This term is an acronym for light amplification by stimulated emission of radiation. The laser is capable of mobilizing immense heat and power when it is focused at close range; it is used as a tool in surgical procedures, diagnosis, and physiologic studies (AAP 2001a). The lasers most commonly used in dentistry are CO_2, with a wavelength of 10,600 nm, and Nd:YAG, with a wavelength of 1,064 nm. The former has a wavelength in the "far infrared" and the latter in "near infrared" (Pick and Powell 1993). A position paper (AAP 1996d) and an informational paper (AAP 2002b) on the use of lasers in periodontics have been published.

Lateral Repositioned Flap—This surgical procedure is a modification of Grupe and Warren's basic lateral sliding flap. The difference is that an adjacent edentulous area serves as the donor tissue. Its indications are to manage the loss of gingival tissue width on teeth adjacent to edentulous areas, especially on mandibular cuspids, and to correct the distobuccal recession of gingiva on maxillary molars (Rosenberg 1963; Robinson 1964; McFall 1967; Pfeifer and Heller 1971). See also contiguous pedicle graft, edentulous area pedicle graft, sliding flap.

Lateral Sliding Flap—The lateral sliding flap is a synonym for "sliding flap," which was coined and presented by Harold E. Grupe and Richard F. Warren, Jr. (See Fig. L-1a,b,c). Its purpose was to cover areas of localized gingival recession and to increase the quantity and quality of attached gingiva. The gingiva is moved from an adjacent donor site to the recipient site while maintaining its blood supply. It was also discovered that these flaps would attach to denuded root surfaces (Grupe and Warren 1956). Many variations of this procedure have appeared in the literature by authors who have modified incision placement, flap design, and movement. See also modified sliding flap, sliding flap.

Leonard Toothbrushing Technique—Harold J. Leonard advocated an up-and-down motion of brushing over the facial surfaces of clenched posterior teeth for tooth cleaning and gingival stimulation. The bristles are placed at right angles to the teeth and rest partly on the gingiva without forcing. A slight mesiodistal movement is made to produce a slight blanching of the gingiva. The bristle ends remain virtually on the spot where they are placed but do not pass over the tooth and gingival, as in the scrubbing technique. When so used, this method penetrates the interdental embrasures deeply, producing a deep vibratory massage. One must be cautious about carrying the brush too high into the alveolar mucosa (Leonard 1939; Ray 2005).

Ligamentum Circulare Dentis—This group of circular fibers in the gingiva was first

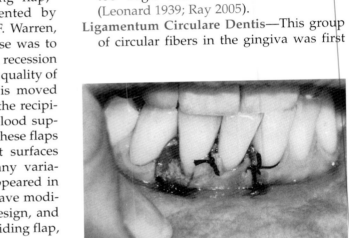

Fig. L-1b: Sutured flap

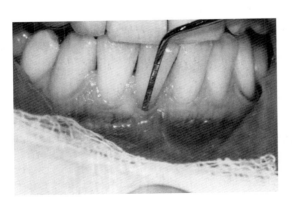

Fig. L-1a: Preoperative view

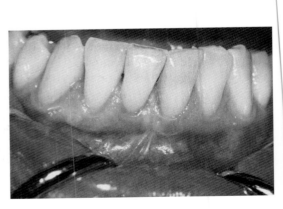

Fig. L-1c: Postoperative view

identified and named by Rudolph Albert Kolliker of Wurtsburg, Germany. He made extensive studies in histology and embryology, identified the osteoclast, and elucidated dental and oral tissues, including the fibrous systems of the gingiva (Kolliker 1867; Carranza and Shklar 2003). In 1953, these fibers were studied more thoroughly and named the "circular fiber group" of the gingival fiber network (Arnim and Hagerman 1953). See also circular fiber group.

Linear Gingival Erythema (LGE)—This type of gingival erythema is present as a distinct red band on the gingival margin in patients infected with the human immunodeficiency virus (HIV) (See Fig. L-2) (Holmstrup and Westergaard 1998). It does not resolve with dental scaling/prophylaxis and is disproportionate to the amount of plaque (Winkler et al. 1989). This nonplaque gingivitis is often associated with a lack of bleeding upon probing (See Fig. H-3) (Robinson et al. 1994). See also HIV-associated gingivitis (HIV-G).

Lingual Approach—In 1976 an approach to managing mandibular osseous defects (i.e., craters) from the lingual was described for the following reasons: (1) facial aspect is limited by a thick shelf, shallow vestibule, and an external oblique ridge; (2) root trunks are shorter on the facial than the lingual; (3) mandibular teeth are lingually inclined, placing the lingual furcations more apical than facial; (4) interdental craters are usually located more lingual, directly below contact area; (5) lingual embrasures are wider than facial; (6) lingual bone is thicker; (7) there is more attached gingiva on lingual; and (8) there is greater vestibular depth on lingual (Tibbetts et al. 1976). See also palatal approach.

Local Extension of the Vestibular Trough—This term is synonymous with the pouch and pushback procedures; both are considered archaic and no longer performed (Goldman et al. 1956). See also pouch procedure, pushback procedure.

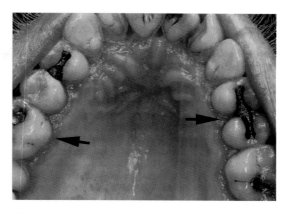

Fig. L-2: Arrows, LGE (With permission from Blackwell Publishing)

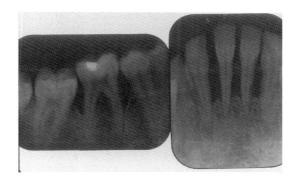

Fig. L-3)

Localized Juvenile Periodontitis (LJP)—This classification of periodontitis has been defined as periodontal involvement of at least one first molar and at least one incisor or second molar and two or fewer cuspids or premolars with 3 mm or more of attachment loss (See Fig. L-3) (Loe and Brown 1991). Balint Orban and Joseph Weinmann introduced the name *periodontosis* for this disease, limited to teenagers and young adults, and described it as occurring in three stages, degeneration of the cervical fibers of the periodontal ligament, epithelial migration, and pocket formation (Orban and Weinmann 1942). Localized juvenile periodontitis is now considered to be an "aggressive" periodontitis, being either localized or generalized depending on the percentage of sites involved or the degree of loss of clinical attachment (Armitage 1999). See also aggressive periodontitis, generalized juvenile periodontitis (GJP), juvenile periodontitis, periodontosis.

Long Centric—This term, as used in the study of occlusion, refers to the area between centric relation and centric occlusion moving along a horizontal flat level. The Pankey-Mann-Schuyler group stated this horizontal distance should be between 0.5 and 1.0 mm (Mann and Pankey 1959). Simply stated, two years later, long centric was defined as a range of noninterfering contact from centric relation distally to a convenient relation slightly anterior (Ramfjord 1961). See also freedom in centric.

Long Junctional Epithelium—Refers to the adaptation and adherence of the junctional epithelium to the root surface following various therapeutic procedures, which apparently can be maintained for many years without any regrowth of bone (Hirschfeld 1962). It has been said that this type of wound healing is a *locus minoris resistentiae* and is prone to the ravages of the oral flora and future periodontal breakdown and pocket formation (Barrington 1981; Magnusson et al. 1983). On the other hand, long junctional epithelial adhesion has the ability to retain its position on the tooth surface over long periods. Long junctional epithelium has responded well to the challenges of plaque and its toxic products when compared to the naturally occurring connective tissue attachment (Beaumont et al. 1984). This clinical phenomenon is considered to be repair and *not* new attachment (Yukna and Lawrence 1980). See also repair.

Loss of Attachment (LOA)—The apical shift of the junctional epithelium and apical migration of the connective tissue attachment with concomitant loss of alveolar bone utilizing the CEJ as a fixed reference point. It is a more relevant and precise way to examine alterations in "attachment" levels than simply probing for pocket depth. The procedure of determining the LOA requires two measurements: (1) from the gingival margin to the bottom of the clinical pocket and (2) from the gingival margin to the cementoenamel junction (Lindhe 1989).

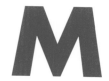

Macroperiodontometer—This is an instrument for measuring horizontal tooth mobility of incisors, cuspids, and first bicuspids that is especially adapted for use in the maxillary arch. It consists of a dial indicator mounted on an impression and adapted with the indicator's pointer to the labial or buccal surfaces of the teeth to be measured. Measurements are made in hundredths of a millimeter (0.01 mm) (Muhlemann 1954, 1960). See also microperiodontometer, periodontometry.

Magnetostrictive—The conversion of 60-HZ, 120-V current in an ultrasonic dental unit, which continually alters the shape of a (magnetostrictive) bimetallic stack of nickel-cobalt alloys. The resulting 25,000 contractions and expansions per second produce an ultrasonic wave, moving the tip in an elliptical motion of approximately 0.0015 cm. The magnetostrictive effect was discovered by James Prescott when he observed that certain ferromagnetic metals change their length under the influence of a magnetic field (Brown et al. 1987). The current status of ultrasonics in periodontics has been published (AAP 2000c). See also ultrasonics, vibratory.

Malalignment Index—This index is used to measure both the rotation and displacement alignment of all sextants in the mouth and is scored with either 0, 1, or 2 as follows: 0 = ideal alignment with no apparent deviation from the ideal arch line as projected through the contact points; 1 = minor malalignment, minor rotation, angle formed by a line projected through contact points is less than 45 degrees, minor displacement, contact points are moved in the same direction, from ideal, less than 1.5 mm; 2 = major malalignment, major rotation, angle formed by line projected through contact points is 45 degrees or greater; major displacement, contact points are moved in same direction from ideal, by 1.5 mm or more. The malalignment index is the sum of all scores for all sextants (Van Kirk and Pennell 1959).

Margin Index (MI)—This index records the location of crown margins of bridge retainers. It is built on the principles similar to those underlying the plaque index and the gingival index. Each of the four areas of the crowned tooth is given a score from 0 to 3, which is the MI for the area. The margin index system is as follows: 0 = restoration margin more than 2 mm above the gingival margin; 1 = restoration margin less than 2 mm above the gingival margin; 2 = restoration margin level with the gingival margin, and 3 = restoration margin below the gingival margin (Silness 1970).

Margin of the Gingiva—Balint Orban gave this nomenclature to the coronal border of the free or marginal gingiva (Orban 1948a). See also free gingiva, marginal gingiva.

Marginal Gingiva—This term refers to that part of the free gingiva that is localized at the labial, buccal, and lingual aspects of the teeth (See Fig. F-4) (Orban 1948a). See also free gingiva.

Marginal Line Calculus Index (MLC-I)—The marginal line calculus index scores only supragingival calculus formed in the cervical area along the marginal gingiva on the lingual side of the four lower incisors. The cervical band of calculus is further divided into two parts by an axial line bisecting the incisal edge of the incisors, resulting in a mesial and distal half of the calculus deposit. In order to simplify the procedure, only 0, 12.5, 25, 50, 75, or 100 percentages are used. The mesial and distal percentage of calculus deposition is averaged and the means of the four teeth are averaged to give the patient's score. The strength of this index is to reduce experimental times in testing calculus inhibitors, and it permits a more precise evaluation of the effects of supragingival calculus on the marginal gingiva (Muhlemann and Villa 1967).

Materia Alba—This phrase refers to a soft white (from the Latin *albus*, for "white") mass of material consisting of food debris, desquamated epithelial cells, and bacterial aggregates. The materia alba serves as a medium for bacterial growth; however, it is not organized or strongly adherent to the tooth. (Friedman 1962b). See also tooth accumulated material (TAM).

Mattress Suture—A suturing technique where the suture enters the flap at or near the mucogingival junction and exits the flap through the interdental papilla. In this approach, more of the suture lies on top of the flap and is thus able to hold the full extent of the flap in close proximity to the underlying bone or periosteum. This aids in healing and flap reattachment and reduces the chance of postoperative bleeding (Dello Russo 1998). This suture is also beneficial in closing a flap over a bone graft, since the suture is directly over the papilla or flap and never contacts the graft (Takei 1991). See also horizontal internal mattress suture, suture, vertical internal mattress suture.

Maximum Intercuspation—This term refers to the complete intercuspation or interdigitation of the opposing teeth independent of the condylar position (AP 1994). It is also referred to as the *acquired centric occlusion* or *habitual centric occlusion*. See also centric occlusion (CO).

McCall's Festoons—This refers to "lifesaver"-shaped enlargements of the marginal gingiva that occur primarily on the facial surfaces of the anteriors and bicuspids. These semilunar enlargements were named after John Oppie McCall, who, along with Paul R. Stillman, believed occlusal traumatism to be an etiologic factor (Stillman and McCall 1922). Later studies could not substantiate or show evidence that festoons were initiated by occlusal disharmonies (Posselt 1959). See also gingival festoons.

Meta-Analysis—*Meta* is a Greek term meaning "after, behind, beyond, or among." In periodontics, meta-analysis refers to an assessment technique that quantifies data from several studies and allows scoring based on the quality of the reporting in the individual studies. In other words, it is a statistical procedure for combining data from a number of studies and investigations in order to analyze the therapeutic effectiveness of specific treatments and plan future studies. Data obtained from combined studies must be compatible to be evaluated by this method (Antczak-Bouckoms 1993).

Microbial Mass Index—This index measures the microbial masses collected from the buccal, mesial, and lingual surfaces of all six year molars; if these are absent, the twelve year molars are used. Using a glass slide with a cover slip under 600x magnification, the number of microbes and their motility are recorded. The numbers are recorded as 0 = no microbes/cells, 1 = 1 to 15 microbes/cells, 2 = 5 to 15 microbes/cells, 3 = 15 or more microbes/cells. The motility is recorded as 0 = no motility, 1 = mild motility, 2 = medium motility, and 3 = much motility (Dunkin 1966).

Microbiologically Modulated Periodontal Therapy (MMPT)—This phrase refers to the 1978 *Keyes technique* of treating periodontal disease nonsurgically. It specifically directs attention to the microscopic evaluation/reevaluation phase of treatment, *microbiologically*, and makes reference to additional treatment if response had not been successful by including antibodies or a repeat of the regimen, *modulated* (Keyes 1982; Rams et al. 1985). See also Keyes technique, monitored and modulated therapy (MMT).

Microcosm—This term refers to the oral microbial flora that colonizes on the crowns of teeth. This was the term Sumter S. Arnim at the University of Houston used while studying dental plaque through a phase-contrast microscope. Dr. Armin stated one is able to observe a tiny microscopic world or "microcosm" in plaque, which aptly conveys the ecologic import of this pathobiologic unit, or "little world" (Arnim 1959, 1964). See also animalcules, plaque (dental).

Microperiodontometer—This is an instrument for measuring the mobility of all teeth, in contrast to the limited application of the macroperiodontometer. The dial is very small, it is tedious to use, the technique is difficult to learn, and the results are not very reproducible (Muhlemann 1960). A similar instrument was designed to allow measurement of tooth mobility in all areas of the dental arch to ten-thousandths of an inch (0.0001 in.). This prototype was found to produce results as reproducible or at least equal to those obtained with the macroperiodontometer of Muhlemann (O'Leary and Rudd 1963). See also macroperiodontometer, periodontometry.

Modified Bass Toothbrushing Technique—The "vibratory motion" technique of toothbrushing introduced by Charles C. Bass has been modified by clinicians and patients (Bass 1948). This modification is the addition of a rolling stroke of the brush away from the gingiva following the vibratory movement. This additional or modified stroke is supposed to lift debris away from the gingiva (Perry and Beemsterboer 2001). See also Bass toothbrushing technique.

Modified Distal Wedge—This surgical procedure is a modification of the traditional proximal wedge (Kramer and Schwarz 1964) or distal wedge (Robinson 1966) procedure. It was designed to obtain primary intention healing of the soft tissue in furcation areas of molars adjacent to edentulous regions. It provides easy flap manipulation for the visualization of osseous architecture, enabling definitive pocket elimination, and establishes soft tissue adaptation with total coverage of the furcation (Pollack 1980). See also distal wedge, proximal wedge.

Modified Sliding Flap—Harold E. Grupe introduced the modified sliding flap in 1966 due to the potential sequelae of donor site complications while performing the lateral sliding flap (Grupe 1966a). A submarginal incision was placed on the donor site to prevent gingival recession and possible exposure of a root dehiscence. According to Walter B. Hall, these surgical sequelae were a concern of Balint Orban, who tried the procedure and found a dehiscence on the root of the donor site. Orban's experience became the basis for this modification (Hall 1984). See also lateral sliding flap, sliding flap.

Modified Stillman's Toothbrushing Technique—In this technique of toothbrushing, the bristles are placed onto the attached gingiva with light pressure to effect blanching at a 45 degree angle apically to the long axis of the tooth. The brush is then rotated occlusally with a slight twisting of the brush handle. It involves *no* rotary, sulcular, scrubbing, or vibratory motions, as in Stillman's toothbrushing technique. The vibratory action of the bristles is supplemented by a movement of the brush toward the line of occlusion (Hirschfeld 1939; Allen 1993b; Ray 2005). See also Stillman's toothbrushing technique.

Modified Widman Flap (MWF)—This surgical procedure, named for Leonard Widman, a Swedish dentist, is performed by a scalloped, repositioned, mucoperiosteal flap, accomplished with an internal bevel incision (reverse bevel incision) that provides access for root preparation. It is designed to maintain as much of the interdental papilla as possible in order to effect primary closure whenever possible (Everett et al. 1971; Ramfjord 1977). Because the crevicular epithelium is removed at the time of the initial incision, maximal healing and "reattachment" with new attachment is facilitated and anticipated (Ramfjord and Nissle 1974). It has been compared to open subgingival curettage to facilitate new attachment; it is a type of repositioned mucoperiosteal flap (Caffesse 1980). See also open flap curettage.

Molar Uprighting—This term refers to orthodontically changing the long axis of a molar tooth that has inclined/drifted out of occlusion, both inter and intra-archwise. It also helps maintain dental, skeletal, and facial vertical support and enhances oral hygiene procedures; it may also prevent overpreparation of teeth and obviate the need for endodontic therapy (Brown 1973; Ingber 1974). Brown and Ingber have substantiated positive changes from molar uprighting, which may occur to the bone and soft tissue as a result of forced eruption/molar uprighting. Attention has been brought to the adverse changes which may occur to the furcation of molars with moderate periodontal involvement (Burch et al. 1992). See also forced eruption.

Monitored and Modulated Therapy (MMT)—This expression is a synonym for the Keyes technique or microbiologically modulated periodontal therapy (MMPT). It is has two main goals: (1) to evaluate whether the disease is active or not (monitored) and (2) to eliminate bacterial plaque with oral hygiene and perhaps systemic drugs (modulated) (Chace and Keyes 1981). See also Keyes technique, microbiologically modulated periodontal therapy (MMPT).

Mucoalveolar Gingival Surgery—This term is a synonym for the following procedures designed to deepen the vestibular trough, reposition or increase the zone of attached gingiva, or a combination involving both the alveolar and gingival mucosa: pushback, pouch, mucobuccal fold extension, vestibuloplasty, and mucogingival surgery. *Mucoalveolar gingival surgery* is said to be the only term histologically and topographically accurate to represent this list of terms (Beckham et al. 1962). See also mucobuccal fold extension, mucogingival surgery, pouch procedure, pushback procedure, vestibuloplasty.

Mucobuccal Fold Extension—This is an archaic term for the procedure to increase the vestibular depth and extend the mucobuccal fold. Varaztad Hoveness Kazanjian, an oral surgeon and physician, is credited with the first approach to extend the mucobuccal fold in edentulous patients (Kazanjian 1924, 1935). In the 1930s, Dr. Kazanjian was considered by many to be "the father of modern plastic surgery" (Herschfeld 1984). Nathan Friedman described the procedure as making incisions at the mucogingival line while dissecting the mucosa away from the periosteum and pushing it apically. This mucosal flap is apically positioned to (1) remove muscle pull, (2) establish good form and function, (3) increase the zone of attached gingiva, and (4) deepen the vestibule. It is a modification of the original frenectomy (Friedman 1957). See also frenectomy, frenulumectomy, gingival extension, gingival replacement, mucobuccal fold resection.

Mucobuccal Fold Resection—This is a synonym for the archaic procedure known as the mucobuccal fold extension (Whinston 1956). See also mucobuccal fold extension.

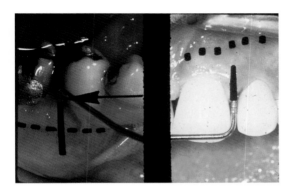

Fig. M-1: left: tip of probe beyond MGJ; right: tip of probe within the AG

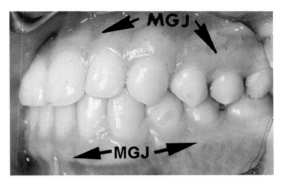

Fig. M-2a

Mucogingival Defect—This term, as defined by Henry M. Goldman, exists when (1) pocket depths extend below the level of attached gingiva, (2) high frenums are attached into the marginal gingival, and (3) there are problems of lateral food impaction and difficulty with oral hygiene in the presence of shallow vestibules (See Fig. M-1) (Goldman 1953). A modern definition of mucogingival defects is when there are developmental and acquired aberrations in the morphology, the position and/or the amount of gingiva surrounding teeth (Maynard 1998). This statement has been elucidated by Maynard, in his four classifications of periodontiums, by describing the most resistant periodontium in evolving mucogingival defects. They are: type I, normal or ideal dimension of keratinized tissue (3 to 5 mm) with relatively thick periodontium; type II, thinner keratinized gingiva (less than 2 mm) with reasonably thick bone (periodontium); type III, normal or ideal dimension of keratinized gingiva (3 to 5 mm) but with thin bone roots palpated; and type IV, thin keratinized tissue (less than 2 mm) with thin labiogingival dimensions of underlying bone (Maynard 1998). The American Academy of Periodontology has described mucogingival defect as "any deviation from the normal anatomic relationship between the gingi-

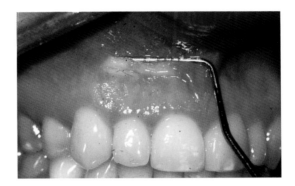

Fig. M-2b: (MGJ) demonstrated with probe

val margin and the mucogingival junction (MGJ)" (AAP 2000d). See also gingivo-muco-myo-skeletal involvement, mucogingival problem.

Mucogingival Junction—A scalloped line that separates the attached gingiva from the alveolar mucosa (See Fig. M-2a,b) (Orban 1948a). It has been shown that the mucogingival junction remains stationary or in a constant relationship throughout life (See Fig. A-6) (Ainamo 1978). See also alveolar mucosa, attached gingiva, mucogingival line.

Mucogingival Line—This is a scalloped line separating gingiva and alveolar mucosa (See Fig. M-3a,b). It is caused by the difference in their structure. The attached gin-

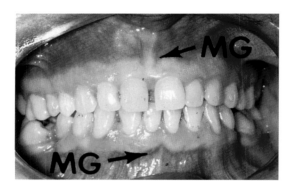

Fig. M-3a: MG, mucogingival line (Courtesy of Dr. Vanchit John)

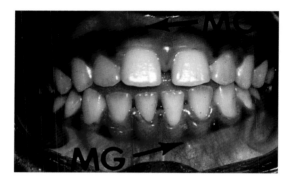

Fig. M-3b: MG, mucogingival line (Courtesy of Dr. Vanchit John)

giva is stippled, firm, and thick, lacking a separate submucous layer; it is immovably attached to the bone and has no glands. The alveolar mucosa is thin and loosely attached to the periosteum by a well-defined submucous layer of loose connective tissue; it may contain small mucous glands. The structural differences also cause the color difference between the pale pink gingiva and dark red lining mucosa (Orban 1948a; Goldman 1949). See also alveolar mucosa, attached gingiva, mucogingival junction.

Mucogingival Problem—Also known as a mucogingival defect. J. Gary Maynard has described it as a "developmental and acquired aberration in the morphology, the position and/or the amount of gingiva surrounding teeth" (Maynard 1998). Another term or synonym is *mucogingival deformity,* which is defined as a "departure or deviation from the normal dimension and morphology of, and/or interrelationship between gingiva and alveolar mucosa; the abnormality may be associated with a deformity of the underlying bone" (AAP 2000f, 2001a). See also gingivo-muco-myo-skeletal involvement, mucogingival defect.

Mucogingival Surgery—This is a dated/archaic expression and has been replaced by *periodontal plastic surgery* (Miller 1988; Miller and Allen 1996) and more recently by *oral plastic surgery* (Miller 2003). However, when Nathan Friedman coined the expression *mucogingival surgery,* it was defined as surgery to (1) preserve gingiva, (2) remove aberrant frenulum or muscle attachments, and (3) increase the depth of the vestibule (Friedman 1957). These were surgical procedures utilized to resolve problems involving the interrelationships between gingiva and alveolar mucosa, such as pockets extending apical to the mucogingival junction, malpositioned frena, and inadequate vestibular depth. Henry M. Goldman was the first to describe the "purpose" of mucogingival surgery before it became popularized with Friedman's publication. He stated, "mucogingival surgery was performed to facilitate the elimination of facial pockets with their base apical to the mucogingival line, to release tension on the gingival margin and to create space for the toothbrush" (Goldman 1953). These procedures were performed only to reestablish functionality and were not concerned with esthetics. A paper entitled "Historical Development of Mucogingival Surgery" has been published (Nery and Davies 1976). See also mucoalveolar gingival surgery, oral plastic surgery, periodontal plastic surgery.

Mucoperiosteal Flap—This surgical term refers to the detachment of the gingiva and mucoperiosteum from the teeth and the underlying bone, exposing the necks of the teeth and the alveolar process. Its purpose is to have an open view and access for the removal of granulomatous tissue and root debridement; it has been called a "flap procedure for debridement" (See Fig. F-8) (AAP 1989). Based on the variations of incisions for this flap, it may be curved, triangular, trapezoidal, or rectangular in shape (Luebke and Ingle 1964). See also blunt dissection, full-thickness flap, gingival mucoperiosteal flap.

Mucosal Flap—This is a surgical expression for the split-thickness and/or partial-thickness flap. This procedure, considered to be protective to the underlying bone, was studied extensively in the 1960s (Staffileno 1960, 1969a; Staffileno et al. 1962, 1966). See also apically displaced split flap, gingival mucosal flap, partial-thickness flap, split-thickness flap.

MUDL Rule—This expression is commonly used in the selective grinding of a malocclusion. It is used when the mandible must be repositioned in a retruded position from habitual centric. The MUDL letters refer to grinding the mesial (M) incline of the upper (U) cusp (usually lingual cusp) and the distal (D) incline of the lower (L) cusp (usually buccal cusp). This procedure will move the cusp tips mesially (Bjorndahl 1958). See also BULL rule.

Multiple Interdental Papilla Graft—This mucogingival surgery procedure is directed at increasing the attached gingiva where there is either an absence of gingiva or an inadequate amount of it. The donor site in this technique is the adjacent papilla(e). This approach to gingival augmentation has been demonstrated by Arthur B. Hattler and Herman Corn (Hattler 1967; Corn 1980). Gingival augmentation of an entire sextant using this technique has been demonstrated by Gordon L Douglas (Douglas 1976) and David Hoexter (Hoexter 1999). See also interdental papilla graft.

Myofascial Face Pain (MFP)—MFP is among the most common types of temporomandibular disorders (TMD). It is characterized by aches in the jaw, face, or surrounding area as well as pain on palpation at three or more of 20 specific facial muscle sites. It is often associated with and must be differentiated from fibromyalgia (Raphael et al. 2000; Raphael and Marbach 2001). See also temporomandibular disorders (TMD).

Myofascial Pain Dysfunction Syndrome (MPD)—This syndrome has been defined as a collection of medical/dental conditions affecting the temporomandibular joint (TMJ) and/or the muscles of mastication and contiguous components (AAP 2001a). The cardinal signs and symptoms of MPD are (1) pain in the preauricular area or masticatory muscles, (2) limitation of mandibular movement, (3) tenderness in the masticatory muscles, and (4) clicking or popping of the TMJ (Butler et al. 1975; Mercuri et al. 1979). See also Costen Syndrome, temporomandibular disorders (TMD).

N

Nasmyth's Membrane—This term refers to the primary enamel cuticle, which is approximately 1 μ thick; it is a product of the ameloblasts following enamel formation (Wertheimer and Fullmer 1962). It is also referred to as the enamel cuticle, ameloblastic cuticle, or epithelial cuticle. (Skillen and Mueller 1927). It is named after Alexander Nasmyth, a Scottish surgeon who lived in London (Sperber and Buckingham 2000). See also primary cuticle.

Navy Periodontal Disease Index (NPDI)—This index is part of the Navy periodontal screening examination (NPSE) and measures the spread of inflammation around the circumference of a tooth. It consists of two parts: (1) the *gingival score* assesses inflammation, color, consistency, density, enlargement, and bleeding and (2) the *pocket score* measures tissue destruction as determined by pocket depth (Hancock, and Wirthlin 1977). The highest combined gingival/pocket score for any one tooth is the patient's NPDI (Grossman and Fedi 1974). See also Navy periodontal screening examination (NPSE).

Navy Periodontal Screening Examination (NPSE)—This screening examination consists of two parts: (1) the Navy periodontal disease index (NPDI) and (2) the Navy plaque index (NPI). Both parts of this examination include measuring only six teeth: the maxillary right first molar, left central incisor, left first bicuspid, the mandibular left first molar, right central incisor, and the right first bicuspid. These are the same six teeth used in the periodontal disease index (PDI) (Ramfjord 1959; Grossman and Fedi 1974). See also Navy periodontal disease index (NPDI), Navy plaque index (NPI).

Navy Plaque Index (NPI)—This index is one part of the Navy periodontal screening examination (NPSE). The NPI, following the use of disclosing wafers or a solution to expose plaque, measures plaque in the cervical areas of the tooth in contact with the gingival margin. The areas measured and the scores given are the mesial proximal surface (M-3), the distal proximal surface (D-3), the facial or gingival surface (G-2), and the facial or lingual surface (R-1) if plaque is not in contact with the gingival tissue. The highest total for any of the six teeth scored is the patient's NPI (Hancock and Wirthlin 1977; Grossman and Fedi 1974). See also Navy periodontal disease index (NPDI), Navy periodontal screening examination (NPSE).

Necrotizing Periodontal Diseases—This category of periodontal diseases includes necrotizing ulcerative gingivitis (NUG) and necrotizing ulcerative periodontitis (NUP) (See Figs. N-1 and N-2) (Armitage 1999). It was decided by committees that these two diseases might be different stages of the same infection and currently

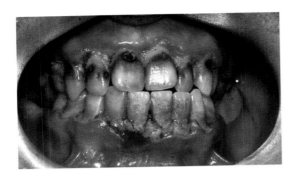

Fig. N-1

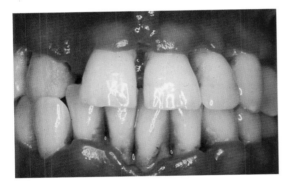

Fig. N-2: (Courtesy of Dr. Vanchit John)

there is not enough data to place them in separate disease categories; therefore the term *necrotizing periodontal diseases* is the preferred designation for NUG and NUP (AAP 1999a). See also necrotizing ulcerative gingivitis (NUG), necrotizing ulcerative periodontitis (NUP).

Necrotizing Ulcerative Gingivitis (NUG)— This form of necrotizing periodontal disease is an infection characterized by gingival necrosis presenting as "punched-out" papillae, with gingival bleeding and pain (See Figs. N-1 and A-3). A fetid breath and a pseudomembrane covering the gingiva may be a secondary diagnostic feature of NUG (Rowland 1999). See also acute necrotizing ulcerative gingivitis (ANUG); acute ulcerative gingivitis, necrotizing periodontal diseases, trench mouth, ul-

ceromembranous gingivitis, Vincent's angina infection.

Necrotizing Ulcerative Periodontitis (NUP)— This form of necrotizing periodontal disease is an infection causing necrosis of gingival tissue, periodontal ligament, and alveolar bone (See Fig. N-2). The lesion is most commonly observed in individuals with systemic conditions including but not limited to HIV infection, severe malnutrition, and/or immunosuppression. (Novak 1999; AAP 1999a). The signs and symptoms include localized ulcerations/necrosis of gingival tissue, exposure and rapid destruction of alveolar bone, spontaneous gingival bleeding, and severe radiating pain from the jaw. (Glick et al. 1994). See also HIV-associated periodontitis (HIV-P), necrotizing periodontal diseases.

New Attachment—The reunion of connective tissue with a root surface that had been deprived of its periodontal ligament. This reunion occurs by the formation of new cementum with inserting collagen fibers. The formation of new bone is not necessarily a condition of new attachment. In addition, new attachment to a root surface may be mediated through epithelial adhesion (junctional epithelium) or connective tissue adhesion (Mellonig 1992, 1998; AAP 1989). The early periodontal literature used the terms *new attachment* and *reattachment* interchangeably (Stones 1934; Barnes and Schaffer 1960). A thorough historical review on new attachment was published in 1987 (Card et al. 1987). See also histologic reattachment.

Nonspecific Plaque Hypothesis—This hypothesis proposes that the etiologic mechanism in periodontitis is related to the total plaque mass and that therefore reducing the amount of plaque (by therapeutic means) will diminish disease activity. The severity of inflammation is directly related to the overall quantity of plaque bacteria in the mouth. When plaque accumulation exceeds the host's defense capabilities, inflammation is thought to occur (Theilade 1986). Willoughby D. Miller, the first oral microbiologist with formal training, was likely the first to discuss the nonspecific plaque hypothesis in his classic book *The Microorganisms of the Human Mouth* (Miller 1890). He believed that the disease was not caused by a specific bacterium but by a complex array of bacteria normally present in the oral cavity (Carranza and Shklar 2003). See also specific plaque hypothesis.

Nonworking Side—In the study of occlusion, this term refers to the disoccluding side of the occlusion during the shift of the mandible toward the working/ chewing or bolus side. It is synonymous with *balancing side* (Posselt 1968). See also balancing side.

Nonworking Side Interference—In the study of occlusion, this term is synonymous with *balancing side interference*. According to a 1965 publication, molar teeth with nonworking or balancing interferences exhibit a greater amount of bone loss, mobility, and pocket depth (Yuodelis and Mann 1965). The nonworking side is also known as the nonfunctional side, or the side away from which the mandible moves during lateral excursions (AAP 2001a). See also balancing side interference.

Oblique Fiber Group—This group of principal fibers of the periodontal ligament, being the largest group, pass from the cementum outwardly and coronally to insert into the alveolar bone. They lie between the horizontal and apical group of fibers and function to absorb occlusal forces (Orban 1957). See also periodontal ligament.

Oblique Rotated Flap—This is a mucogingival surgery technique directed to the management of gingival clefts or denuded root surfaces involving two adjacent teeth, as often observed in the mandibular anterior region (See Fig. O-1). This defect is often characterized by gingival recession, little to no attached gingiva, a shallow vestibule, and chronic marginal inflammation (Pennel et al. 1965). This procedure is a modification of the sliding-flap operation (Grupe and Warren 1956), the lateral repositioned flap (Robinson 1964), and the edentulous area pedicle graft (Corn 1964). (See Fig. P-3). Peter Rubelman classified this flap as an interdental (single-papilla) pedicle graft (Rubelman 1977). See also edentulous area pedicle graft, interdental papilla graft, lateral repositioned flap, sliding flap.

Occlusal Trauma—The microscopic lesion within the periodontium resulting from traumatic occlusion. According to most authors, it comprises thrombosis, hyalinization or necrosis of the periodontal liga-

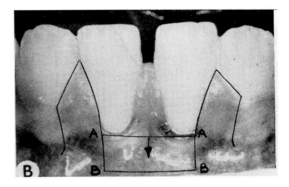

Fig. O-1: (With permission from the American Academy of Periodontology)

ment, and resorption of the alveolar bone and cementum (Muhlemann et al. 1956). Pathologic changes are not observed in the gingival tissues or the junctional epithelium (Wentz et al. 1958). The term *occlusal trauma* should not be used to signify the forces placed on the teeth (AAP 1966). See also trauma from occlusion, traumatic occlusion.

Occlusion Feature Index (OFI)—This index was originally developed at the National Institute of Dental Research in 1957 to score only the morphologic form of the teeth with no information on occlusal disharmonies. It reportedly considers the *crowding* of the lower anterior arch from canine to canine (0-3), the *interdigitation* of

101

the right premolar-to-molar area from the buccal aspect with teeth in occlusion (0-2), the *vertical overbite* as measured by that portion of the lower incisors covered by the upper central incisors in occlusion (0-2), and the *horizontal overjet* from the labial surface of the upper incisors to the labial surface of the lower incisors as measured in occlusion with a small ruler (0-2). The numbers for each group are recorded and added, with a possible range from 0 to 9 (Poulton and Aaronson 1961). A correlation was shown to exist between the OFI and the periodontal index (PI) of Russell (Russell 1956). See also periodontal index (PI).

Odontexesis—This is an archaic expression (*odont*, meaning "tooth," and, from the Greek, *xesis*, meaning "scraping") for scaling, root curettage, and/or root planing (Ingle 1952; Halik 1969). See also apoxesis, root curettage, root planing, scaling.

Odontoplasty—A procedure devised to reshape a tooth in order to correct the errors in tooth form that have occurred naturally or which, because of changes in the gingival margins, have become a factor in the further progress of periodontal disease (Cohen and Chacker 1964). This term was mentioned in 1958 by Henry M Goldman for the removal of tooth substances in managing furcation involvement so as to give a desired occlusal-cervical concavity to the horizontal defect in an incipient furcation. (Goldman 1958). See also furcaplasty.

Onlay Graft—This is a soft tissue graft designed to augment ridge defects in the apicocoronal plane of space to gain ridge height and width. They are thick "gingival grafts" derived from the partial or total thickness of the palate, containing lamina propria and submucosal tissues (Seibert 1983a, 1983b; Seibert and Louis 1996). See also ridge augmentation.

Onplant—This is a new device designed to provide anchorage for orthodontic tooth movement. It is a disk, textured and hydroxylapatite-coated on one side, with an internal thread on the other. It is placed on palatal bone and, after integration, can be connected to the teeth for anchorage. It can provide absolute anchorage to move a tooth toward it and provide sufficient anchorage to molars to prevent anterior migration without moving the implant (Block and Hoffman 1995).

Open Contacts—This term refers to a space between adjacent teeth that allows the impaction of food and endangers the periodontal health (level of attachment) of adjacent teeth. It is suggested that intrabony lesions are associated with factors causing food impaction (Larato 1971), and the relationship between open contact food impaction and periodontal breakdown is known (Hancock et al. 1980).

Open Flap Curettage—This surgical procedure is also recognized as the modified Widman flap technique. The main advantages are the possibility of obtaining a close adaptation of the soft tissues to the root surface while causing minimum trauma to the exposed alveolar bone and soft connective tissues. It also results in less exposure of the root surfaces, which is an advantage in treating the anterior segments (Lindhe 1989). See also modified Widman flap (MWF).

Open Probing Attachment Level (OPAL)—This is a procedure performed during the guided tissue regeneration (GTR) technique. Using the cementoenamel junction as a fixed reference point, measurements of the vertical depths of periodontal defects undergoing GTR procedures are taken at the time of surgical instrumentation and upon removal of the barrier membrane (Murphy 1995b). See also open probing clinical attachment, open probing new attachment.

Open Probing Clinical Attachment—This is a procedure performed during healing of guided tissue regeneration. This term describes the tissues that are measured at *reentry* of furcations, following six months of healing in guided tissue regeneration in class II and class III furcation involvement. The measured new attachment in the molar furcations reflects tissue that is firm, resistant to probing forces, and possesses the consistency of a rubber dam. It is not bone (Becker et al. 1988). See also open probing attachment level (OPAL), open probing new attachment.

Open Probing New Attachment—This phrase refers to tissue sounding/exploring during the reentry of guided tissue regeneration (GTR) procedures in molar furcation involvements. The term *open probing new attachment* describes the type of tissue evident at reentry. If the new tissue is not bone, it is termed *open probing new attachment*, reflecting the fact that there was a coronal gain of new attachment (Becker et al. 1987). See also open probing attachment level (OPAL), open probing clinical attachment.

Open View Operation—This surgical flap operation presented by James L. Zemsky in 1926 was very similar in design and purpose to the modified Widman flap, mucoperiosteal flap, and open flap curettage of modern periodontics. It represented an unobstructed field of operation by an elevated full-thickness flap to remove all diseased and affected periodontal structures and completely eliminate the pyorrhea pockets. It accomplished the removal of "infected and sharp edges of bone" and eradicated "foci of infection" (Zemsky 1926). See also modified Widman flap (MWF), mucoperiosteal flap, open flap curettage.

Oral Epithelium—The lining of the oral cavity protecting the gingiva and hard palate with keratinized epithelium and nonkeratinized epithelium covering the alveolar mucosa and floor of the mouth, soft palate, lips, cheek, and tonsils (Orban 1948a, 1957; Jablonski 1992). See also gingival epithelium.

Oral Hygiene Index (OHI)—This reversible index is a quantitative assessment of the oral hygiene of individuals or groups; it consists of a debris index (DI) and a calculus index (CI). Twelve numerical determi-

nations (six from buccal and six from lingual) are made for both the DI and CI from six sextants of the mouth. The DI and CI scores range from 0 (no debris, no calculus), 1 (soft debris covering not more than one-third of the tooth and calculus covering not more than one-third of the tooth), 2 (soft debris covering more than one-third, but not more than two-thirds of the tooth, and calculus covering more than one-third but not more than two-thirds of the tooth) and 3 (debris covering more than two-thirds of the tooth and calculus covering more than two-thirds of the tooth (Greene and Vermilion 1960). See also oral hygiene index simplified (OHI-S), reversible index.

Oral Hygiene Index Simplified (OHI-S)—This index is similar to the oral hygiene index (OHI); however, only six tooth surfaces are scored for the (DI-S) and (CI-S) rather than twelve, as in the OHI. The teeth examined are four posteriors and two anteriors: the first fully erupted tooth distal to the second bicuspid (usually the first molar) in each arch and the maxillary right central incisor and the mandibular left central incisor. The buccal surfaces of the selected upper molars and only the labial surfaces of the incisors are scored. The combined DI and CI from these six surfaces give rise to the OHI-S (Greene and Vermilion 1964). See also oral hygiene index (OHI), reversible index.

Oral Mucosa—The oral mucosa can be divided into three distinct zones: the *specialized mucosa*, the *masticatory mucosa*, and the *lining mucosa*. The base of the tongue contains the specialized mucosa; the gingiva and hard palate makeup the masticatory mucosa; and the lining mucosa covers the floor of the mouth, cheek, soft palate, and alveolar mucosa, which is separated from the gingiva by the mucogingival junction (Orban and Sicher 1946; Orban 1948a).

Oral Plastic Surgery—This phrase is replacing the term *periodontal plastic surgery* (Miller 1988) to encompass reconstructive, esthetic, and functional surgery other than that involving the periodontium. Some examples would be sinus lift grafting, intraoral autogenous block grafting, ridge augmentation and preservation, edentulous ridge expansion, distraction osteogenesis, and vestibular deepening in dentulous and edentulous subjects (Miller 2003). See also mucogingival surgery, periodontal plastic surgery.

Orogranulocytic Migratory Rate Index (OMRI)—This periodontal index is determined by counting the number of orogranulocytes (polymorphonuclear leukocytes, or PMNs) present in a series of sequential collections of oral mucus. Orogranulocytes are functionally competent PMNs in the layer of isotonic mucus covering all free surfaces of the oral cavity. It is based on the fact the OMR reflects a correlation between inflammation and vascularization of gingival and periodontal tissues (Klinkhamer 1968a, 1968b). This index did not gain wide popularity owing to difficulties in reproducibility and low correlations with other accepted clinical indices (Hase and Reade 1979).

Orthodontic Extrusion—See also vertical extrusion.

Orthodontic Intrusion—This orthodontic procedure is an attempt to intrude periodontally diseased teeth into the alveolus to generate new connective tissue attachment on a previously diseased root surface. Gingival inflammation must be eliminated and the root surfaces scaled (planed) to make it possible for new cementum to form on previously infected root surfaces. The biomechanical forces and oral hygiene must be kept under control to achieve the desired result of new attachment (Melsen et al. 1988).

Osseointegration—A direct structural and functional connection at the light microscopic level between ordered living bone and the surface of a load-carrying implant (Branemark 1995). Dr. Per-Ingvar Branemark is credited with having coined this term in 1982 (Darle 2003). According to

the American Academy of Implant Dentistry, it is described as a "contact established without interposition of non-bone tissue between normal remodeling bone and an implant entailing a sustained transfer and distribution of load from the implant to and within and bone tissue" (AAID 1986). See also biointegration, fibroosseous integration, functional ankylosis.

Osseous Coagulum—An osseous graft procedure introduced by R. Earl Robinson in 1969. The coagulum is derived by using a #6 or #8 round bur running at 25,000 to 35,000 rpm and collecting bone dust (cortical or cancellous) blood, and saliva. The source of the bone dust may be an exostosis, tori, heavy marginal ridges, or adjacent sites undergoing osseous correction (Robinson 1969). The theory behind this technique is as follows: (1) the smaller the particle size, the more certain its resorption and replacement, (2) mineralized fragments can induce osteogenesis, (3) an intraoral approach is more desirable than an extraoral approach, and (4) slight overpacking is preferred. Before this term was introduced in 1968, at the AAP meeting in Miami, Florida, this procedure was called *bone dust grafting*. R. Earl Robinson initially presented this procedure to the Northwestern University Post Graduate Section on December 7, 1967; it was therefore the first coagulum procedure to be reported. This technique is similar to the earlier bone chip augmentation (Nabers and O'Leary 1965, 1967). See also bone blending, osseous filtration.

Osseous Defect—This term is a synonym for *bony defect*, being an alteration in the contour of normal/healthy alveolar supporting bone resulting from inflammation, trauma, or other injury (See Fig. O-2). Such defects include the following: infrabony/ intrabony, hemiseptums, inconsistent bony margins, interdental craters, fenestrations, dehiscences, furcation involvements, and/or circumferential defects (Stahl et al. 1963; O'Connor and Biggs

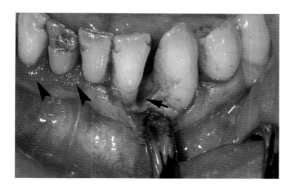

Fig. O-2: Arrow, osseous defect; delta point, gingivoplasty incision (With permission from Elsevier Publishing)

1964; Saari et al. 1968; Larato 1970a,b,c,d; Rees et al. 1971). See also bony defect.

Osseous Filtration—This is a technique devised in 1974 for obtaining and conserving autogenous osseous material for reimplantation into bony defects. The particles of surgically removed osseous tissue are trapped in a filtration mechanism placed into the suction line. These particles are subsequently retrieved and used as autogenous graft material (Bierly and Sottosanti 1974). See also bone blending, osseous coagulum.

Osseous Graft—Osseous grafting is the surgical placement of various biological or inert substances into periodontal intrabony/infrabony defects with the goal of reconstructing a lost attachment apparatus (Adams 1966; Gara and Adams 1981; Rosen et al. 2000). These substances have been referred to as "implants" in the older literature but should not be confused with the titanium endosseous implants of the twenty-first century (AAP 2000a). See also allograft, alloplast, autogenous bone graft, heterograft, xenograft.

Osseous Resection—The removal of osseous deformities and the creation of a physiologic parabolic bony contour that will mimic the final anticipated gingival architecture (Schluger 1949a; Carnevale and Kaldahl 2000). Saul Schluger stated

that the pattern of behavior of the soft tissue is conditioned by the hard tissue with which it comes into contact. Osseous resection has further been stated to include osteoplasty and osteoectomy (or ostectomy) (Friedman 1955). The principle of osseous resection was defined in the Spanish literature in 1935 by Fermin A. Carranza Sr., when he explained the exact manner in which the removal of alveolar bone might expedite the treatment of periodontal pockets (Carranza 1956; Carranza and Shklar 2003). See also ostectomy, osteoplasty.

Osseous Surgery—This term refers to those periodontal surgical procedures that include *resective* (subtractive) procedures, *regenerative* (additive) procedure or a combination of both, any of which may be employed to modify the bony support of the tooth (Mills and McDonnell 1998). A comprehensive review on resective and regenerative osseous surgery has been published (Wirthlin 1987).

Ostectomy—A periodontal surgical procedure that removes supporting alveolar bone, a part of the attachment apparatus, in order to eliminate a periodontal pocket and establish good physiologic gingival contour (Friedman 1955). The American Academy of Periodontology has described it as the removal of some alveolar (supporting) bone, which changes the position of crestal bone on the tooth root. It is performed to reshape deformities caused by periodontitis in the marginal and interalveolar bone (AAP 1989). The literature also shows this word to be spelled as *osteoectomy* (Friedman 1955). See also attachment apparatus.

Osteocementum—This term refers to cellular cementum, which resembles bone in that formative cells are incorporated in lacunar spaces from which canaliculi radiate. It is porous, and derives its name from its morphologic resemblance to bone (Kerr 1961). See also cellular cementum.

Osteoconduction—A graft material that acts as a passive matrix, like a trellis or scaffolding, upon which new bone forms to cover a defect. It facilitates "fill" from adjacent bony margins of the defect (Wirthlin 1987).

Osteoinduction—This term refers to the ability of a material to induce chemotaxis, mitosis, and differentiation of mesenchymal cells into chondroblasts and osteoblasts (Urist et al. 1967). This has also been described as a process by which new bone is induced to form through the action of factors contained within the grafted bone, such as proteins or growth factors (Mellonig 1998). See also bone morphogenetic protein (BMP).

Osteoplasty—The periodontal surgical procedure of removing nonsupporting alveolar bone. Nathan Friedman has described it as "a plastic procedure in which the periodontal pocket is eliminated and the bone reshaped in order to achieve physiologic contour of the bone and the gingiva overlying it . . . in this operation the bone that is reshaped is not part of the attachment apparatus, thus no bony support of the tooth or teeth is lost" (Friedman 1955). It may also include vertical grooving or festooning (Ochsenbein 1958) and radicular blending (Carranza 1990). See also festooning, radicular blending, vertical grooving.

Overlapped Flap—This surgical flap is utilized to cover implant fixture installation while avoiding several complications arising from the standard Le Fort I ostectomy approach for exposure of the edentulous ridge. The buccal and palatal or lingual

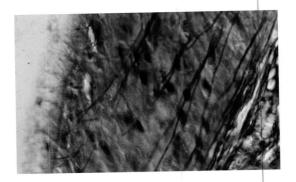

Fig. O-3

flap overlaps itself, providing proper tissue coverage, avoiding bacterial contamination, reducing postoperative edema and ecchymosis, and facilitating easy suture removal (Langer and Langer 1990).

Oxytalan Fiber—This type of connective tissue fiber is a normal constituent of the human periodontal ligament and gingiva (See Fig. O-3). It may be related to elastic fibers and is so named because of its resistance to acid hydrolysis. It was discovered in 1958 (Fullmer and Lillie 1958). Such fibers have been found to be larger and more numerous in functional than nonfunctional periodontal ligaments (PDLs) (Fullmer 1961). They have also been found to provide structural integrity and distribution of forces over a wider area of the PDL and may also help stabilize blood and lymph vessels (Edmunds et al. 1979). See also elaunin fibers.

P

Palatal Approach—This surgical approach is a method of approaching osseous craters from the palatal aspect of the maxillary molars; it presents several advantages over the buccal approach. These benefits are (1) a greater quantity of keratinized tissue on the palate, (2) greater surgical access to wider palatal embrazures than buccal, (3) utilizes the cleansing effect of the tongue on the palate, and (4) involves less postsurgical bone resorption on the palate owing to the presence of more cancellous bone than on buccal (Ochsenbein and Bohannon 1963, 1964). See also lingual approach.

Palatal Flap—Tissue elevation to gain access to palatal osseous defects is accomplished through several types of palatal flaps. These may be mucoperiosteal or full thickness flaps (AAP 1989), mucosal/partial thickness or split thickness flaps (Staffileno 1969a), or the modified partial-thickness flap, also called "ledge and wedge" (Ochsenbein 1958; Ochsenbein and Bohannon 1963, 1964).

Palatal Groove—Also known as the palatogingival groove, a defect originating in the region of the cingulum of upper incisors and extending toward the cemento-enamel junction (CEJ), often terminating there. However, it occasionally extends past the CEJ and onto the root, serving as a nidus for bacterial plaque deposition and likely periodontal involvement (Bacic

et al. 1990). See also cinguloradicular groove, distolingual groove, palatogingival groove, palatoradicular groove, radiculolingual groove.

Palatogingival Groove—A developmental anomaly of the maxillary incisors that begins in the central fossa, crosses the cingulum, and extends varying distances apically onto the root surface. This groove is often a factor predisposing to the development of a localized periodontitis. It was first reported in 1968 to draw attention to the association between this groove and a localized periodontal breakdown (Lee et al. 1968). See also cinguloradicular groove, distolingual groove, palatal groove, palatoradicular groove, radicular lingual groove.

Palatoradicular Groove—Also known as the palatogingival groove. It usually begins in the central fossa of the maxillary central and lateral incisors, crosses the cingulum, and extends varying distances down the root. Because of the enamel extension along with the groove, it may be a factor in the progression of localized periodontal disease (Kogan 1986; Hou and Tsai 1993). See also cinguloradicular groove, distogingival groove, palatogingival groove, palatal groove, radiculolingual groove.

Papilla Bleeding Index (PBI)—In this index, the sulcus is swept with a blunt periodontal probe and the amount of papillary bleeding recorded 20 to 30 seconds after each quadrant has been probed. The amount of bleeding is scored from 1 (minimal) to 4 (profuse); the PBI is the average bleeding score across all papillae examined, as follows: 0 = no bleeding, 1 = only one bleeding point present, 2 = several isolated bleeding points present, 3 = interdental triangle filled with blood, and 4 = profuse bleeding spreading toward the marginal gingiva. The PBI is the average bleeding score across all papillae examined (Saxer and Muhlemann 1975; Marks et al. 1993).

Papilla Preservation Technique—A periodontal surgery designed to conserve the interdental papilla when placing implant material interdentally, either in the anterior or posterior dentition, in order to treat periodontal defects. Healing occurs by primary intention. Because the papilla is retained by this technique, soft tissue craters do not develop. In order to improve the postoperative soft tissue contour, this flap design may be used in surgeries that do not require graft placement (Takei et al. 1985, 1989; Takei 1991; Cortellini et al. 1995; Cortellini 1999).

Papillary Bleeding Score (PBS)—The PBS is determined on all papillae anterior to the second molars, disregarding readings on the buccal and lingual gingival margins. Following placement of a Stim-U-Dent interproximally, a PBS score of 0 to 5 is determined as follows: 0 = no bleeding, 1 = edematous and reddened gingiva but no bleeding, 2 = bleeding without flow, 3 = bleeding with flow along the gingival margin, 4 = copius bleeding, and 5 = spontaneous bleeding. A distinguishing feature of the PBS is that two examiners must agree on their findings of bleeding (Loesche 1979; Marks et al. 1993).

Papillary Height Classification—This system allows for easy means to assess progressive degrees of interdental papillary loss using readily observed anatomic landmarks for reference and assisting future communications among clinicians and researchers. It consists of four divisions: normal, interdental papilla fills embrasure space to the apical extent of the interdental contact point/area; class I, the tip of the interdental papilla lies between the interdental contact point and the most coronal extent of the interproximal CEJ (space is present but the interproximal CEJ is not visible); class II, the tip of the interdental papilla lies at or apical to the interproximal CEJ but coronal to the apical extent of the facial CEJ (the interproximal CEJ is visible); class III, the tip of the interdental papilla lies level with or apical to the facial CEJ (Nordland and Tarnow 1998).

Papillary Marginal Attached Index (PMA)—A numerical system for recording gingival health primarily in children, satisfying the criteria of simplicity, speed, accuracy, quantitativeness, and reproducibility. The "P" represents that part of the gingiva that fills the interproximal space between two teeth (papillae); the "M" represents the free gingival collar on the labial, buccal, and lingual aspects of the teeth (marginal gingiva); and the "A" is that part of the gingiva which is firmly attached to the underlying tooth and bone and stippled on the surface (attached gingiva). The severity of inflammation in this reversible index is indicated on a scale of 0 to 4; in its original form, only the labial gingiva of the six lower anterior teeth was examined (Schour and Massler 1947; Massler and Schour 1949; Massler 1967).

Papillary Marginal Gingivitis Index (PMGI)—A combination of the P-M-A index of Massler and Schour and the G.I. by Loe and Silness. Only the papillae and margins on the facial and lingual gingiva of natural teeth are scored on a scale of 0 to 3, as follows: 0 = no inflammation or normal gingiva; 1 = mild inflammation or slight change in color (erythema) and little change in texture; 2 = moderate inflammation with moderate glazing, redness, edema, and enlargement as well as bleeding on pressure with a blunt instrument; and 3 = severe inflammation with marked redness and enlargement as well as a tendency for spontaneous bleeding and ulceration. The individual score is the number of all inflammatory scores divided by the number of papillary and marginal units examined per subject (De La Rosa and Sturzenberger 1976; Massler and Schour 1949; Loe and Silness 1963).

Papillary Marginal Index (PM)—This index utilizes bleeding upon gentle probing as the initial sign of periodontal disease. Using a modified PMA index, a gingivitis survey is determined by examining the labial sides of the interdental papillae (P) and the free marginal gingiva (M) from cuspid to cuspid of both arches. A hooked explorer is placed not more than 1 mm under the free marginal gingiva and between the sides of the papillae to arrive at a score of 0 to 3, as follows: 0 = no bleeding, 1 = bleeding upon probing but no color change or swelling, 2 = bleeding on probing with color change but no swelling, and 3 = bleeding on probing with color change and swelling. In order to avoid confusion with the PMA index of Massler and Schour, the PM index was renamed the sulcus bleeding index (SBI) in 1971 (Muhlemann and Mazor 1958). See also sulcus bleeding index (SBI).

Papillary Marginal Recession Index (PMR)—This system is a modification of the PMA index of Massler and Schour, where the value for "A" (attached gingiva) was omitted and an "R" for gingival recession was inserted, producing the PMR index. The "R" for recession is recorded whenever the cementoenamel junction is exposed, with the results given as percentages of teeth affected by both gingival inflammation and recession (Stahl and Morris 1955). See also papillary marginal attached index (PMA).

Papillectomy—The surgical removal of the entire papilla (Ratcliff 1966; AAP 2001a). In the older periodontal literature, it is equated with "interdental resection" on non-apically positioned flaps when the objective of treatment was new attach-

ment. See also interdental denudation, interdental resection, interproximal denudation.

Papillon-LeFevre Syndrome—This syndrome consists of an advanced periodontal disease in children with concurrent skin lesions consisting of hyperkeratosis palmoplantaris (See Fig. P-1a,b,c,d). It is also known as PPKPD syndrome or palmarplantar hyperkeratosis with periodontal destruction (Giansanti et al. 1973; Gorlin et al. 2001; Ahuja et al. 2005). It is inherited in an autosomal recessive gene and named after its discoverers M.M. Papillon and Paul LeFevre (Papillon and LeFevre 1924). It is classified among the genetic disorders under "Periodontitis as

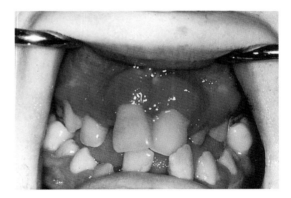

Fig. P-1a: Gingival inflammation and tooth migration/extrusion

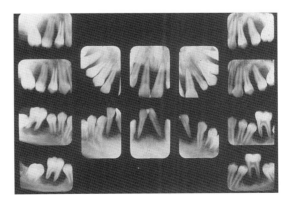

Fig. P-1b: Radiographic image

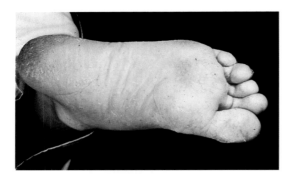

Fig. P-1c: Plantar hyperkeratosis

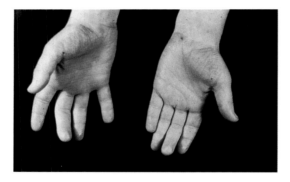

Fig. P-1d: Palmar hyperkeratosis (Illustrations P-1a,b,c,d courtesy of Dr. John R. Billen; with permission from Elsevier Publishing)

a Manifestation of Systemic Diseases" in the new classification system of periodontal diseases (Armitage 1999).

Paradentium—This term was suggested by Oskar Weski, a German physician and dentist, for the complex tissue structures that hold the teeth in position; namely, the gingiva, alveolar bone, periodontal ligament, and cementum (Weski 1921). It is now known as the periodontium. See also periodontium.

Paradontosis—This term was used by Kurt H. Thoma and Henry M. Goldman for Bernhard Gottleib's diffuse alveolar atrophy or juvenile periodontitis. They also believed that the disease was degenerative, not inflammatory, and of systemic origin in which the bone was affected first. They described parodontosis as a generalized involvement of the permanent dentition of young people between the ages of 14 and 25 years (Thoma and Goldman 1937, 1940). See also juvenile periodontitis.

Parafunction—This term is synonymous with all contact movements of the maxillary and mandibular teeth other than the functional movements. This includes bruxism, clenching, and any other disordered or perverted functions/movements of the maxillomandibular occlusion. It was a term suggested and introduced in the German literature by W. Drum (Drum 1950). See also bruxism, clenching.

Partial-Thickness Flap—This periodontal surgical procedure involves the elevation of a flap while leaving some connective tissue and periosteum on the bone. An inverse bevel incision is utilized without contacting the alveolar crest margin, but the blade passes externally to the periosteum. The flap is reflected, leaving the bone surface covered by periosteum and a layer of connective tissue (Barrington 1973). Harry Staffileno and coworkers have published extensively on the healing, histology, and cellular mobilization of the partial- or split-thickness flap (Staffileno 1960, 1969a; Staffileno et al. 1962, 1966). See also gingival mucosal flap, mucosal flap, split-thickness flap.

Party Gums—This is a prosthetic device to correct definite esthetic problems of major concern to the patient in the anterior segment of the dentition (See Fig. P-2a,b). It reestablishes gingival contour to correct gingival recession from vigorous toothbrushing and/or major periodontal surgery (See Fig. G-4a,b) (Risch et al. 1977). See also gingival facade, gingival prosthesis, gum veneer, prosthetic gingival veneer.

Passive Eruption—This term refers to tooth exposure secondary to apical migration of the gingiva. It occurs in four stages: stage

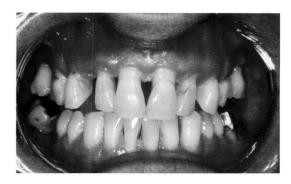

Fig. P-2a: Preparty gums

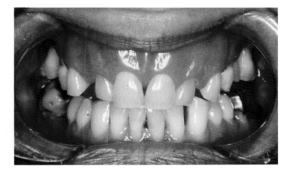

Fig. P-2b: Post-party gums (Courtesy of Dr. W. Peter Nordland)

I, gingival margin and junctional epithelium are on enamel; stage II, gingival margin is on enamel and the junctional epithelium is partially on enamel and cementum; stage III, gingival margin is at the cementoenamel junction and the junctional epithelium is totally on cementum; and stage IV, gingival margin and junctional epithelium are totally on cementum (Gargiulo et al. 1961). See also active eruption, altered passive eruption, delayed passive eruption.

Patient Hygiene Performance Index (PHP-I)—This index was developed to assess an individual's ability to eliminate plaque and debris. Following the application of a disclosing solution, five surfaces (mesial, distal, and three divisions in the middle third

of the tooth: cervical, central, coronal) on six teeth (maxillary right first molar, right central incisor, left first molar, and the mandibular left first molar, left central incisor, and the right first molar) are evaluated for cleanliness. The scale is either 0 for no debris or 1 for the presence of debris. The range is 0 to 5 per tooth. The scores for all individual teeth are added and divided by the number of teeth examined. No score will be higher than 5 (Podshadley and Haley 1968).

Pedicle Flap—This is a surgical procedure intended to repair a gingival defect or cleft with either a full- or partial-thickness flap attached to the donor site by a "pedicle" with a nutrient supply (See Fig. P-3a,b,c). It is a synonym for the sliding flap of Grupe and Warren (1956) and has been studied both clinically and histologically by numerous authors (Patur and Glickman 1958; Wilderman and Wentz 1965; Sugarman 1969). See also pedicle graft, sliding flap.

Pedicle Graft—This surgical procedure refers to all flaps, full or partial thickness, that are raised from an area with a base attached to the donor site and in which the free margin is moved (Wilderman 1967). It is also known as *pedicle flap, sliding flap, lateral sliding flap, horizontal sliding flap,* etc. See also pedicle flap, horizontal sliding flap, lateral sliding flap, sliding flap.

Pergingival GTR—This expression refers to placing a barrier membrane, which has been perforated with a 3 mm hole, around a dental (titanium) implant for the purpose of guided tissue regeneration (GTR). The prefix *per,* meaning "through," explains the technique of pergingival GTR (Jovanovic 1996).

Pericementum—This is an archaic expression for the periodontal ligament. John Oppie McCall called it a cushioning medium that softens the shock transmitted to the alveolar bone when pressure is applied to a tooth (McCall 1939). See also periodontal ligament.

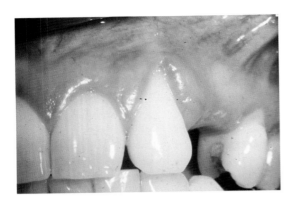

Fig. P-3a: Before surgery

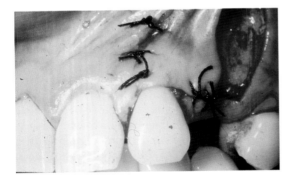

Fig. P-3b: Surgery

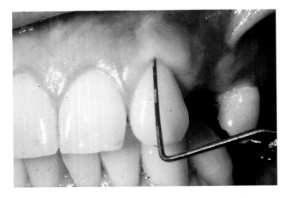

Fig. P-3c: After surgery (Courtesy of Dr. Clifton E. Nakatani)

Peri-Implantitis—An infection of the peri-implant epithelium and connective tissue potentially resulting in marginal bone loss and implant failure (Berman 1989; Meffert 1996; Mombelli and Lang 1998; Klinge et al. 2005). The breakdown of the peri-implant soft tissue cuff progresses to the loss of bone, as in periodontitis, both clinically and radiographically. The associated bacteria and inflammatory processes are remarkably similar in peri-implantitis and periodontitis (Listgarten 1999). See also implant, ailing; implant, failed; implant, failing.

Period Prevalence—This statistical term refers to the number of illnesses existing at any time within a "specified period" and is related to the average number of persons exposed to the risk during that period. In short, the object is to show the total number of cases of a sickness that existed during a given interval (Daly and Bourke 2000). See also prevalence.

Periodontal Biotype—This expression attempts to relate the morphology of the periodontium to tooth form as either being "thin" or "thick." Based on the assessment of a ratio between crown length and crown width in the upper central incisors, the periodontal biotype is considered *thin* if the teeth are long and narrow and *thick* if the teeth are short and wide (Olsson and Lindhe 1991). See also gingival biotype, gingival morphology.

Periodontal Destructive Syndrome—This term is suggested as an inclusive phrase or syndrome for all periodontal diseases. It is based on the fact that the term *periodontal diseases* labels a pattern of morbid signs and symptoms whose etiologies are not fully understood. Descriptive modifiers, such as *adult, juvenile, rapidly progressive*, and so on could still be used to specifically label the periodontal destructive syndrome (Rethman 1993).

Periodontal Diseases—This is a general term describing specific diseases that affect the gingiva and supporting connective tissue and alveolar bone that anchor the teeth in the jaws (Williams 1990). They are usually referenced to gingivitis and periodontitis, two inflammatory diseases affecting the surrounding and supporting tissues of the teeth (Armitage 1996, 1999, 2002, 2004a). See also gingivitis, periodontitis.

Periodontal Disease Index (PDI)—A composite index designed to meet the needs of both the epidemiologist and the clinician. The six teeth examined are the maxillary right first molar, left central incisor, left first bicuspid, mandibular left first molar, right central incisor, and right first bicuspid. The clinical exam includes gingival, calculus, and pocket findings as well as occlusal/incisal wear, tooth mobility, contact, and presence of plaque. An index for each parameter can be determined or values for all six teeth can be totalled and divided by six for the individual's PDI (Ramfjord 1959). The score from only the mesial surface of the six selected teeth can be taken as representative of all surfaces of the tooth, a considerable simplification (Ash et al. 1964).

Periodontal Disease Rate (PDR)—This index is based on the presence of one or more of the following criteria for periodontal disease: (1) gingival necrosis/hypertrophy or inflammation encircling the tooth or a purulent exudate from the gingival crevice, (2) a gingival crevice depth of 3 mm or more, (3) tooth mobility greater than 1 mm in any direction, and (4) roentgenographic evidence of resorption of alveolar bone extending more than 3 mm apically from the cementoenamel junction. The PDR is derived by dividing the total number of teeth affected by periodontal disease by the total tooth population of the individual patient (Sandler and Stahl 1959).

Periodontal Dressing—A material applied over a surgical wound primarily for the following reasons: (1) protection of the wound area, (2) enhancement of patient comfort, (3) maintenance of a debris-free area, and (4) control of bleeding (Levin

1980). Its synonym and archaic term is periodontal *pack* (AAP 2001a). See also Baer-Sumner fat pack, cyanoacrylates, Ward's Wonderpak, zinc-oxide eugenol dressing, zinc-oxide noneugenol dressing.

Periodontal-Endodontic Lesion—The progression of a marginal periodontitis to the apex of a root or to the emergence of an accessory canal inducing a secondary pulpal involvement (Carranza 1990). Essentially, it is periodontal disease involving the dental pulp by progressive destruction of the periodontal tissues in an apical direction. The progression of periodontitis apically involving the lateral canals is most imminent (Rubach and Mitchell 1965; Simon et al. 1972; John et al. 2004; Rotstein and Simon 2004). A classification of periodontal endodontic lesions has been described in five categories of involvement: (1) primary endodontic lesion, (2) primary endodontic lesion with secondary periodontal involvement, (3) primary periodontal lesion, (4) primary periodontal lesion with secondary endodontic involvement, and (5) a true combined lesion (Simon et al. 1972). See also endodontic-periodontal lesion.

Periodontal Flap—A surgical term for that part of the gingiva and oral mucosa that is separated from the teeth and alveolar bone by horizontal and/or vertical incisors yet remains attached to the rest of the alveolar mucosa in at least one area (Bahat and Handelsman 1991). Flap descriptions have been numerous and reflect multiple varieties and name changes from the literature over the years. See also mucoperiosteal flap, mucosal flap.

Periodontal Index (PI)—This index is for use only in epidemiologic field operation studies to determine the population characteristics of periodontal disease. The clinical criteria for scoring the gingival/periodontal status range from 0 (normal) to 1 (mild gingivitis), 2 (generalized gingivitis), 6 (gingivitis with bone loss up to half the length of the root) and 8 (advanced destruction with loss of masticatory function and bone loss over half of the length of the root). All teeth except the third molars are examined. The PI for a patient is derived by adding the scores of all the teeth and dividing by the number of teeth present (Russell 1956). See also composite index.

Periodontal Index (pl. Indices)—Periodontal indices are descriptive values, usually numerical with maximum and minimum limits, to evaluate both the need for periodontal therapy and the effectiveness of different therapeutic regimens. The scores may be *reversible* (able to increase or decrease during specified time periods) or *irreversible* (unable to decrease in value on subsequent examinations). Likewise, periodontal indices may measure the entire mouth (full mouth) or be localized to a pre-determined number or surfaces of teeth (partial or simplified) (Barnes et al. 1986; Marks et al. 1993).

Periodontal Ligament—This ligament, one portion of the attachment apparatus, is a connective tissue investing layer containing collagenous fibers that connect the tooth to the alveolar bone and is continuous with the gingival connective tissue (See Fig. P-4a,b,c,d). It is called the periosteum of cementum. The groups of fibers making up the investing layer are (1) gin-

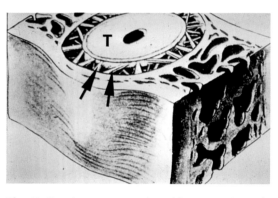

Fig. P-4a: Arrows, periodontal ligament; T, tooth

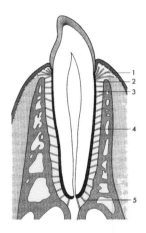

Fig. P-4c: 1, gingival fibers; 2, alveolar crest fibers; 3, horizontal fibers; 4, oblique fibers; 5, apical fibers

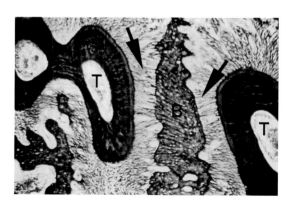

Fig. P-4b: Arrows, periodontal ligament; B, alveolar bone; T, tooth

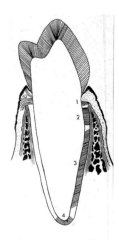

Fig. P-4d: 1, alveolar crest fibers; 2, horizontal fibers; 3, oblique fibers; 4, apical fibers

gival, (2) transseptal, (3) alveolar crest, (4) horizontal, (5) oblique, (6) apical, and (7) interradicular (Orban 1957). The functions of the periodontal ligament include bone forming, nourishing, and tooth supporting (Cupit 1904), sensory (Waugh 1904) transmission of occlusal forces, attachment of tooth to bone, maintaining good relationship of gingival tissues, resisting occlusal forces, and providing a soft tissue casing to protect vessels and nerves (Glickman 1972). The periodontal ligament has also been known as the alveolar periosteum, alveolodental ligament, cemental ligament, desmodent, dental periosteum, gomphosis, paradonto, pericementum, peridentium, periodontium, peridental membrane, and periodonto (Cordero 1966). See also alveolodental ligament, attachment apparatus, periodontal membrane.

Periodontal Maintenance (PM)—This is the preferred term for those procedures formerly referred to as supportive periodontal therapy (Schallhorn and Snider 1981) or periodontal recall (Ogilvie 1967) and includes maintenance of dental implants (AAP 1989, 2000f). A position paper on periodontal maintenance (PM) has been published which states that PM is usually instituted following periodontal and implant therapy and continues at varying intervals for the life of the dentition or its implants replacements. PM may temporarily be discontinued and surgical or nonsurgical therapy reinstituted if recurrent disease or pathosis is detected (AAP 2003a). See also periodontal maintenance therapy (PMT), periodontal recall, prophylaxis (dental), supportive periodontal therapy (SPT).

Periodontal Maintenance Therapy (PMT)— This term implies that once a state of periodontal (oral) health has been established, periodic treatment is necessary for continued health in the supporting structures of the teeth. The PMT assumes that adequate therapy has been provided for whatever periodontal disease existed (Shick 1981).

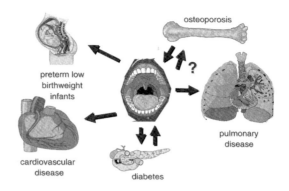

Fig. P-5: (With permission from Elsevier Publishing)

PMT has been classified in four parts: (1) preventive PMT, designed to prevent the inception of disease in individuals without periodontal pathosis; (2) trial PMT, designed to maintain borderline conditions; (3) Compromise PMT, designed to slow the progression of disease in patients who cannot undergo or afford therapy; and (4) Posttreatment PMT, designed to prevent recurrence of a disease which was arrested and originally managed through proper and adequate therapy (Schallhorn and Snider 1981). See also periodontal recall, prophylaxis (dental), supportive periodontal therapy (SPT).

Periodontal Medicine—This term is used to describe the interaction between periodontitis and certain systemic diseases and conditions, such as cardiovascular disease, delivery of low-birth-weight babies prematurely, and reduced control of diabetes (See Fig. P-5) (Newman 1998; AAP 1998b; Williams and Offenbacher 2000; Cohen 2000; Kennedy and Cohen 2000; Paquette 2004; Scannapieco 2005). Periodontal medicine is also known as *oral-systemic* (Glick 2005). See also systemic periodontitis.

Periodontal Membrane—Also known as the periodontal ligament. However, because anatomically the majority of the fibers take part in the process of connecting the two surfaces (bone and root surface) rather than separating them as is the function of a membrane, it is more accurate to describe this as a *ligament* and not a *membrane* (Noble 1969). Rudolph Kronfeld was the first to measure the thickness of the periodontal membrane (PDM) in functioning (thick PDM) and nonfunctioning teeth (thin PDM). Kronfeld found that the PDM was thicker near the alveolar margin and apex and thinnest below the middle of the root (Kronfeld 1931). Edgar David Coolidge later measured the average width of the periodontal membrane to be 0.23 mm at the alveolar crest, 0.17 mm at midroot, and 0.24 mm near the apex of the root (Coolidge 1937). Again, the functions of the periodontal membrane (also known as the periodontal ligament) are (1) formative, (2) supportive, (3) nutritive, and (4) sensory (Noble 1969). See also periodontal ligament.

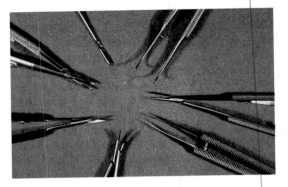

Fig. P-6: (With permission from Elsevier Publishing)

Periodontal Microsurgery—Periodontal surgery performed under optical magnification, providing increased visual activity for delicate, atraumatic handling of soft and hard tissues with microsurgery instruments to achieve primary wound closure (See Fig. P-6) (Tibbetts and Shanelec 1994). Dennis A. Shanelec of Santa Barbara, California, is regarded as the founder, pioneer, and developer of periodontal microsurgery. He and Leonard S. Tibbetts, Jr., of Arlington, Texas, have contributed greatly to the literature on periodontal microsurgery (Tibbetts and Shanelec 1994, 1998; Shanelec and Tibbetts 1996; Belcher 2001).

Periodontal Plastic Surgery—Those procedures performed to correct or eliminate anatomic, developmental, or traumatic deformities of the gingiva or alveolar mucosa so as to provide functional and esthetic results (Miller 1988; Miller and Allen 1996). The term encompasses treatment of the following: (1) shallow vestibule (vestibular deepening), (2) aberrant frenum (frenectomy), (3) marginal tissue recession (soft tissue grafting), (4) excessive gingival display (crown lengthening),

(5) deficient ridges (ridge augmentation), (6) prevention of ridge collapse following extraction of periodontally involved teeth (atraumatic extraction and/or GBR), (7) lost interdental papilla (papillary reconstruction) and (8) unerupted teeth requiring orthodontic movement (surgical exposure) (Miller 1993). This surgical term has been used in the earlier literature on reconstructive periodontal surgery (Seibert 1970); however, P.D. Miller, Jr. is credited with popularizing the procedure; his name is therefore associated with the term (Miller 2003). See also mucogingival surgery, oral plastic surgery.

Periodontal Pocket—The dictionary definition of periodontal pocket is simply a gingival sulcus deepened into the periodontal ligament apically to the original level of the resorbed alveolar crest (Jablonsky 1992). Balint Orban has classified periodontal pockets into three types: I, a gingival pocket, pseudopocket, or false pocket, as found in gingivitis; II, a periodontal pocket or a pathologically deepened pocket, characterized by displacement of the epithelial attachment along with root resorption, bottom of pocket coronal to alveolar crest; and III, intraalveolar, intraosseous, or intrabony pocket where the bottom of the pocket extends apically to the margin of the alveolar crest (Orban 1948b). A modern definition, as stated by the American Academy of Periodontology, refers to a periodontal pocket as a deepened fissure between a tooth and the crevicular epithelium, limited at its apex by the junctional epithelium. It is an abnormal apical extension of the gingival crevice caused by migration of the junctional epithelium along the root as the periodontal ligament is detached by the disease process (AAP 2001a). See also gingival pocket, sulcus depth.

Periodontal Pocket Bleeding Index (PPBI)—The PPBI is based upon probing utilizing a probe with a fixed pressure whose tip is 0.63 mm in diameter. The index is determined by a *grade of 0* where no bleeding occurs from the pocket after probing with a force of 0.75 N or a *grade of 1* where bleeding occurs within 30 seconds after probing with a force of 0.75 N (van der Velden and De Vries 1978; van der Velden 1979, 1980).

Periodontal Probe—Its use was first described by F.V. Simonton of the University of California, San Francisco (See Fig. P-7a,b) (Simonton 1925), when he and others referred to it as a periodontometer (Carranza and Shklar 2003). The periodontal probe is a calibrated instrument with millimeter markings used to measure the depth and determine the configuration of a periodontal pocket (Easley 1967; Tibbetts 1969). It has been shown that in general, a gentle force of about 0.25 N (25 g) will elicit little discomfort (Bulyhuis et al. 1998). This probing force can be clinically determined by applying the probe tip to your fingernail bed, where it will initiate blanching (Greenstein 1990, 2005). In addition to estimating the depth of sulci and periodontal pockets, the periodontal probe may be used to quantify bacterial plaque (Silness and Loe 1964); quantify gingival inflammation (Loe and Silness 1963); measure the relationship of pocket depth to the mucogingival junction and the gingival width (Bowers 1963) (See Fig. M-1); measure gingival recession (Guinard and Caffesse 1978; Caffesse and

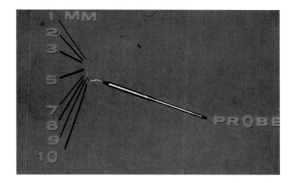

Fig. P-7a

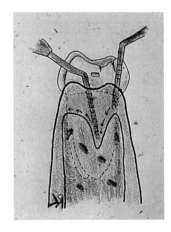

Fig. P-7b

Guinard 1978); measure the thickness of soft tissue over edentulous ridges, tuberosities, or retromolar areas (Tibbetts 1969); and measure attachment levels (Silverton and Burgett 1976). A literature review on periodontal probing has been published (De Waal et al. 1986). See also bone sounding, transgingival probing.

Periodontal Recall—This term is frequently associated with periodontal maintenance therapy (PMT), where emphasis is placed upon managing the oral health of a patient who had already been treated for periodontitis and would thus be vulnerable to periodontal breakdown. It affords the clinician the opportunity to reinforce the patient's role in plaque control in addition to performing the necessary instrumentation and examination of the hard and soft tissues. It should not be confused with the procedure known as dental prophylaxis (Chace 1951; Ogilvie 1967). See also periodontal maintenance (PM), periodontal maintenance therapy (PMT), prophlaxis (dental), supportive periodontal treatment (SPT).

Periodontal Regeneration—The restoration of new alveolar bone, new cementum, and a new periodontal ligament on a region of the root that had been deprived of its attachment apparatus (See Fig. P-8a,b). This new unit restores the architecture and function of the periodontal attachment apparatus (AAP 1989, 2005b; Wang and Cooke 2005). In addition, the gingival structures have also been said to be included in periodontal regeneration (Garrett and Bogle 1993). See also functional repair, guided bone regeneration (GBR), guided tissue regeneration (GTR), regeneration.

Periodontal Risk Calculator (PRC)—This is a computer-based tool for assessing a patient's risk of experiencing periodontal disease and for predicting disease onset and progression. It is based on mathematically derived algorithms assigning relative weights to the various known risks that enhance a person's susceptibility to periodontitis (Page et al. 2002; Persson et al. 2003; Page et al. 2004). See also risk factor.

Periodontal Screening and Recording (PSR)—In June 1992, the American Dental Association and the American Academy of Periodontology jointly developed and launched the PSR program in the United States (ADA/AAP 1992). The PSR is a modification of the Community Periodontal Index of Treatment Needs (CPITN), used to assess the state of periodontal health in a rapid and effective manner and to motivate patients to seek necessary and complete periodontal assessment and treatment (Lo Frisco and Bramson 1993;

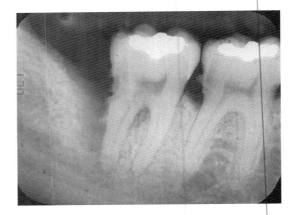

Fig. P-8a: Preperiodontal regeneration

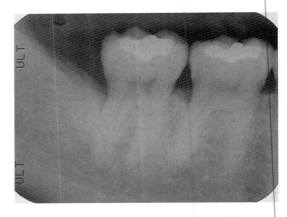

Fig. P-8b: Four years after periodontal regeneration

Salkin et al. 1993; Knocht et al. 1995, 1996). See also community periodontal index of treatment needs (CPITN), periodontal screening and recording (PSR) probe.

Periodontal Screening And Recording (PSR) Probe—The PSR probe was designed by George S. Beagrie of Vancouver, Canada, and Jukka Ainamo of Helsinki, Finland, in 1980 for use in periodontal screening and recording (See Fig. P-9) (Emslie 1980). The PSR probe was described by the World Health Organization (WHO) in the Technical Report Series #621 and originally referred to as the

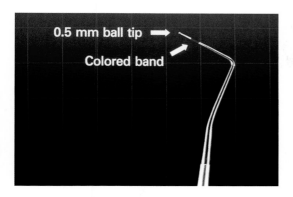

Fig. P-9: (With permission from Blackwell Publishing)

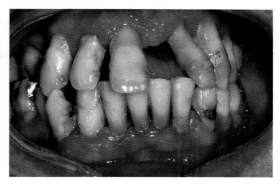

Fig. P-10a

WHO #621 probe (WHO 1978). It consists of a knurled handle 3.5 mm in diameter, weighs 4.5 g, and has a spherical working tip 0.5 mm in diameter with a 0.25 mm neck that gradually tapers from the handle. It has black bands between 3.5 and 5.5 mm from the end of the probe to assist in determining the PSR. The original WHO #621 had two additional gradation marks at 8.5 and 11.5 mm. These last two gradations were subsequently removed (WHO 1978; Emslie 1980). See also community periodontal index of treatment needs (CPITN), periodontal screening and recording (PSR).

Periodontics—The branch of dentistry which deals with the diagnosis, treatment, and prevention of pathologic conditions affecting the roots and the supporting and surrounding tissues of the teeth and dental implants. The goal of periodontal therapy is to preserve the natural dentition and maintain periodontal health, comfort, esthetics, and function. The currently accepted clinical signs of a healthy periodontium include the absence of redness, swelling, bleeding on gentle probing, and exudates; maintenance of the functional periodontal attachment over a period of time; and immobile dental implants (AAP 1988, 2001a).

Periodontitis—An inflammatory disease of the periodontium characterized by in-

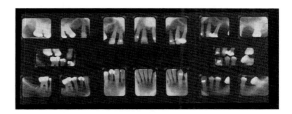

Fig. P-10b

flammation of the gingiva and adjacent attachment apparatus, illustrated by loss of clinical attachment due to destruction of the periodontal ligament and loss of the adjacent supporting bone (See Fig. P-10a,b) (AAP 1996b). It may also be expressed as being localized (having less than 30 percent of sites involved) or generalized (having more than 30 percent of sites involved). The severity of clinical attachment loss (CAL) can be described as slight (1 to 2 mm CAL), moderate (3 to 4 mm CAL), or severe (5 mm or more CAL) (Armitage 1999). See also gingivitis, periodontal diseases.

Periodontium—This term is used to describe the supporting tissues of the teeth, divided into two tissue systems: (1) *The attachment apparatus*, consisting of the cementum, alveolar bone, and periodontal ligament, and (2) *the gingiva* (See Fig. P-11a,b) (AAP 2001a). Harold Keith Box, of Canada, is credited with originating the

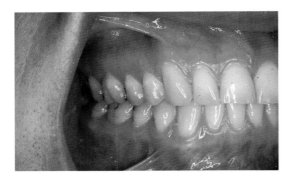

Fig. P-11a: Right, healthy clinical periodontium

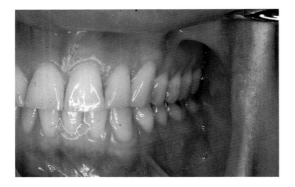

Fig. P-11b: Left, healthy clinical periodontium

term *periodontium* to designate all the supporting structures of the teeth as a group (Box 1940). This term was then adopted by the 1949 nomenclature committee of the American Academy of Periodontology (Lyons et al. 1950). A thorough review of the structure and function of the four tissue compartments of the periodontium (i.e., gingiva, periodontal ligament, alveolar bone, and cementum) has been described. A healthy periodontium is shown in Fig. P-11a,b (Hassell 1993; Cho and Garant 2000). See also paradentium.

Periodontoclasia—This archaic term from the Greek (*-klosis*, meaning "breaking") refers to a breaking down of the investing tissues of a tooth (Leonard 1936). It was accepted by the American Dental Associa-tion's nomenclature committee as a preferred term, replacing its synonyms *pyorrhea alveolaris* and *Riggs' disease* (ADA 1943). This disease was defined as indicating nonspecifically and collectively all destructive and degenerative diseases of the periodontium. Again, in 1949, it was known as a disease in which mobility, migration, elongation, and tooth loss occurred as a result of destruction of the supporting tissues (Glickman 1949). See also pyorrhea alveolaris.

Periodontometry—This is the measuring of tooth mobility, subjectively, achieved through an intricate instrument designed by Hans R. Muhlemann of Switzerland. It is called a *periodontometer* and was originally developed in an attempt to find a method for quantitative evaluation of the so-called bone factor of Glickman (Muhlemann 1951). The periodontometer was also used to determine the magnitude of oral muscular forces transmitted to the crowns of teeth (Muhlemann 1960). *Caution:* The term *periodontometer* as used by F.V. Simonton (1925) referred to the periodontal probe. See also macroperiodontometer, microperiodontometer.

Periodontoplasty—An archaic term referring to all plastic modifications of the periodontium, where the junctional epithelium either approximates or lies apical to the mucogingival junction. The pockets may be deep or shallow and may be infrabony or suprabony (Ariaudo and Tyrrell 1960).

Periodontosis—In 1971, periodontosis was defined as a disease of the periodontium occurring in an otherwise healthy adolescent and characterized by a rapid loss of alveolar bone about more than one tooth of a permanent dentition. There are two basic forms in which this occurs: (1) the only teeth affected are the first molars and incisors (See Fig. L-3) and (2) the more generalized form, which may affect most of the dentition. The amount of destruction manifest is not commensurate with the amount of local irritants present

(Benjamin and Baer 1967; Baer 1971). Periodontosis was described as early as 1920 by Bernhard Gottleib, who called it "diffuse atrophy of the alveolar bone" (Gottleib 1920). E. Wannenmacher was the first to describe this disease as inflammatory in nature; he called it "paradontitis marginales progressiva" (Wannenmacher 1936, 1938; Carranza and Shklar 2003). The term *periodontosis* was introduced in 1942 by Balint Orban and Joseph P. Weinmann (Orban and Weinmann 1942). Today, periodontosis is referred to as an aggressive periodontitis (Armitage 1999). See also aggressive periodontitis, diffuse alveolar atrophy, juvenile periodontitis.

Perioscopy—The process of localizing and removing subgingival biofilm and root deposits with the vision and magnification provided by the dental endoscope. It can be thought of as an extension of traditional scaling and root planing with vision and magnification in those sites that do not respond fully to scaling alone (Stambaugh et al. 2002; Stambaugh 2002). Many lesions on single-rooted teeth can be treated successfully with perioscopy, resulting in a significant reduction of probable pocket depth and a gain in the calibrated attachment level (Stambaugh 2002). The term *perioscopy-clean* refers to a root surface free of all visible calculus, including calculus embedded in the root surface when viewed by direct vision with the endoscope.

Periosteal Fenestration—This surgical technique, as used in mucogingival surgery, was introduced in 1957 by R. Earl Robinson of San Mateo, California. It is a procedure to modify the vestibular extension operation which involves a second incision denuding bone at the apex of the wound, exposing a band or strip of bone. The objective is to create scar formation in the alveolar mucosa which helps maintain the marginal and mucogingival correction. Periosteal fenestration is suggested as a descriptive term for the second incision procedure. (Robinson 1957, 1961).

See also periosteal incision, periosteal separation.

Periosteal Incision—This surgical term is also known as periosteal fenestration, as used during mucogingival procedures. An incision is made below the inferior border of a free soft tissue autograft for the goal of extending the depth of the vestibular fornix (Zingale 1974). See also periosteal fenestration, periosteal separation.

Periosteal Retention—This term refers to maintaining the periosteum over alveolar bone in conjunction with a split thickness or mucosal flap procedure (i.e., periosteal retention procedure) (Bohannon 1962b; Wilderman 1963; Staffileno et al. 1966). See also mucosal flap, split-thickness flap.

Periosteal Separation—The objective of this surgical procedure is to eliminate pockets by (1) stabilizing an adequate zone of attached gingiva, and (2) eliminate high frenum attachments (See Fig. P-12a,b,c). The procedure creates an island of bare bone 4 to 5 mm wide to a level which determines the desired amount of vestibular deepening. The process separates the mentalis muscle from its insertion, thus preventing the rejoining of these fibers to their previous level (Corn 1962). According to P.D. Miller Jr., this is a dated procedure with the advent of the free soft tissue grafting procedures (Miller 1993). See also periosteal fenestration, periosteal incision.

Periosteal Suture—A suturing technique that involves immobilizing a partial-thickness flap or a free soft tissue autograft in a new position by utilizing the subjacent and/or adjacent periosteum to anchor the flap or graft (See Fig. D-1b) (Kramer et al. 1970). See also interrupted periosteal suture, suture.

Physiologic Architecture—The osseous contour of the interradicular bone when it is placed coronal (incisal) to the radicular bone, even though the architecture becomes flatter posteriorly (Selipsky 1976; AAP 2001a). It is known that the contour of the marginal bone in normal periodon-

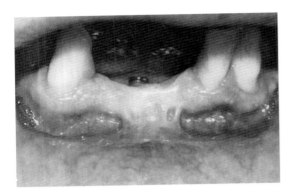

Fig. P-12a: Before surgery

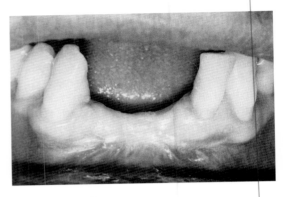

Fig. P-12c: After surgery

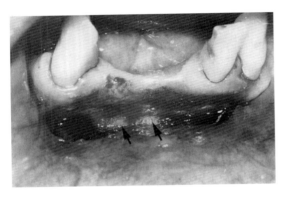

Fig. P-12b: Arrow, exposed periosteum

tium very closely follows the shape of the cementoenamel junction (See Fig. I-8c) (Johnson, RL 1976). See also positive architecture, scalloped architecture.

Physiologic Regeneration—This term characterizes the same phenomenon as occurs in "creeping attachment," in which there is postsurgical movement of the gingiva coronally. It is entirely unpredictable in its occurrence and amount of root coverage expected (Goldman et al. 1960). See also coronal migration, creeping attachment, secondary root coverage.

Physiologic Toothbrushing Technique—A technique of toothbrushing introduced in 1940 by T. Sidney Smith that involves brushing from the occlusal/incisal area toward the gingiva in a "physiologic" fashion similar to the normal excursions of food during eating. It was an attempt to duplicate what was believed to be nature's self-cleansing mechanism, when the downward flow of food over the smooth surfaces of the buccal and lingual surface would remove plaque. Very soft bristles were swept over the crown and gingiva to give a "physiologic" stimulation to the free gingiva and interproximal tissue. Smith also suggested a few gentle horizontal strokes to clean the portion of the sulci directly over the bifurcations of the roots. This technique was highly advocated by Dickson Gabriel Bell in 1948 and is often called the Smith-Bell technique or simply the Bell toothbrushing technique (Smith 1940; Bell 1948; Yankell and Saxer 1999; Ray 2005). See also Bell toothbrushing technique.

Piezoelectric—A term describing ultrasonic energy from a crystal system that expands and contracts when an electric current is applied. The low electromagnetic interference is not hazardous to cardiac pacemakers. The principle of the piezoelectric effect was first shown by Pierre Curie in 1880, when he was able to produce positive and negative electrical charges on the surface of quartz crystals under pressure. If electrical energy is applied across a piezoelectric substance, measurable changes in length occur (Brown et al. 1987; Ewen and Sorrin 1964; Firkin and Whitworth 1996). A position paper on ultrasonics in periodontal therapy, including piezoelectric energy, has been published (AAP 2000c).

Plaque Assessment Scoring System (PASS)—A simplified technique for determining the presence of bacterial plaque without the use of a disclosing solution. The technique is as follows: (1) Five teeth are selected, four first molars and one maxillary incisor; (2) substitute may be made of teeth missing; (3) teeth are divided into four areas—mesial, distal, buccal, and lingual; (4) a periodontal probe is swept 1 mm into the sulcus around each quarter of the tooth; (5) the score is positive only if plaque is visible; and (6) twenty possible plaque surfaces are inspected. The PASS is equal to the percentage of surfaces positive for plaque, which is derived by dividing the plaque-covered surfaces by the total number of surfaces examined. This method has the advantages of evaluating subgingival plaque, taking less time, and requiring no predisclosing solution (Butler et al. 1996).

Plaque Control Record—This is a method of assessing the patient's plaque-control skills. Once the dental plaque is stained, all plaque at the dentogingival junction on the mesial, distal, facial, and lingual surfaces of all teeth is scored as present or absent. The plaque control record (index) is derived by dividing the number of plaque-containing surfaces by the number of available surfaces and multiplying by 100. Soft accumulations *not* at the dentogingival junction are not recorded. The objective is to reach 10 percent or less of the available tooth surfaces stained (O'Leary et al. 1972).

Plaque (Dental)—Dental plaque is a highly variable entity resulting from the colonization and growth of microorganisms on the surfaces of teeth and oral soft tissues and consisting of a number of microbial species and strains embedded in an extracellular matrix (See Fig. G-7a).

Clinically, plaque is found supragingivally and subgingivally as well as on oral surfaces including restorations and oral appliances (Fischman 1986). It is defined by the AAP as an organized mass, consisting mainly of microorganisms, that adheres to teeth, prosthesis, and oral surfaces and is found in the gingival crevice and periodontal pockets. Other components include an organic polysaccharide-protein matrix consisting of bacterial by-products such as enzymes, food debris, desquamated cells, and inorganic components such as calcium and phosphate (AAP 2001a). See also animalcules, tooth accumulated material (TAM).

Plaque-Free Zone—This is an area coronal to the junctional epithelium in a periodontal pocket that is devoid of bacterial plaque. Jans Waerhaug stated there is a certain space between the deepest point of the calculus and the bottom of the clinical pocket (Waerhaug 1952, 1954). Again in 1979, Waerhaug said the distance from plaque to bone was never found to be less than 0.5 mm and never more than 2.7 mm (Waerhaug 1979). This zone was also described as an area between the apical border of the plaque and the most coronal part of the periodontal fibers in a periodontal pocket (Saglie et al. 1975). This zone has also been studied utilizing scanning and transmission electron microscopy (Brady 1973).

Plaque Index—This index measures the amount of plaque on six predetermined teeth: the maxillary right first molar, right lateral incisor, left first bicuspid, mandibular left first molar, left lateral incisor, and right first bicuspid. The scores are graded as 0 = no plaque; 1 = a film of plaque adhering to the free gingival margin and adjacent area of the tooth, where the plaque may be seen in situ only after application of disclosing solution or by using the probe on the tooth surface; 2 = moderate accumulation of soft deposits within the gingival pocket or on the tooth and gingival margin which can be seen with the naked eye; and 3 = abundance of soft matter within the gingival pocket and/or on the tooth and gingival margin. Each of the four surfaces of the tooth (buccal, lingual, mesial, and distal) is given a score from 0 to 3. The scores from the four areas of the tooth are added and divided by four in order to give a plaque index for the tooth. By adding the indices for the teeth and dividing by six one obtains the plaque index for the patient (Silness and Loe 1964). See also gingival index (GI).

Platelet-Rich Plasma (PRP)—This is an autologous gel of packed platelets secured from whole blood via high centrifugation. PRP has been shown to accelerate and enhance by two to three times the body's natural speed of wound healing compared with that of normal surgical sites (Marx et al. 1998). The separation of platelet-poor plasma from other blood constituents produces a cell pack of concentrated platelets. This platelet-rich gel contains two important growth factors: platelet-derived growth factor (PDGF) and TGF-B (Carlson and Roach 2002). The growth factors in the PRP have been shown to accelerate wound healing and have been called an analogous alternative to "fibrin glue" (Whitman et al. 1997). The use of PRP in periodontics has been shown to facilitate guided tissue regeneration (Cho et al. 1995), placement of osseointegrated implants (Whitman et al. 1997), and alveolar ridge and sinus augmentation (Kassolis et al. 2000). See also growth and differentiation factors.

POH—This abbreviation was introduced to periodontics by Charles Cassedy Bass in 1954 for encouragement and instructions in toothbrushing; it refers to personal oral hygiene (Bass 1954). In 1966, Sumter S. Arnim stated that the purpose of an oral hygiene program is the preservation of oral health; another way of defining POH (Arnim 1966). See also Bass toothbrushing technique.

Point Prevalence—A statistical term referring to the number of illnesses that exist at a specified "point" in time and relating to the number of persons exposed to the risk at that time. An example might be: "How many cases of the flu were in existence last Monday?" (Daly and Bourke 2000). See also epidemiology, incidence, prevalence.

Positive Architecture—The position of the interproximal bone in relation to the radicular bone. It occurs where the interproximal bone is coronal to the buccal and lingual radicular bone, leading to the concept of *physiologic bone form*. The osseous architecture becomes flatter posteriorly, but the interradicular bone is never more apical than the radicular bone. In establishing positive architecture in a molar, a molar is treated as having either one or two roots, depending on the height of the furca (Selipsky 1976; Schluger 1949a; Ochsenbein 1958, 1986). See also physiologic architecture, reverse architecture.

Postural Position—In the study of occlusion, this expression refers to the "physiologic" rest position of opening between the maxillary and mandibular teeth when the muscles of mastication are in equilibrium. It is present when the person is either sitting or standing in an upright position. This is a muscle-guided position as compared with the tooth-guided position of centric occlusion or the ligament-guided position of retruded contact. The postural or physiologic rest position is usually 2 to 4 mm below the intercuspal position. This distance is known as the free-way space (Ramfjord and Ash 1966). See also centric occlusion (CO), free-way space, rest position, retruded contact (RC).

Pouch Procedure—This term refers to two distinctly different surgical procedures, each with its own objective. The first pouch procedure (pouch I), which is now obsolete, was mentioned in 1953 by Saul Schluger for increasing the width of attached gingiva and deepening the vestibule. It consisted of elevating a full thickness flap, placing a surgical pack between the flap and bone (instead of on top of the cut edges, as is done in the pushback procedure), and allowing the tissue to granulate under the pack, thus deepening the vestibule. The goal was to reposition and extend the vestibular fornix (Friedman 1957). The second reference to a pouch procedure (pouch II) is for augmentation of an edentulous ridge by incorporating autogenous connective tissue (Seibert 1993). See also pouch II displaced flap, gingival extension, local extension of the vestibular trough, pushback procedure, ridge augmentation.

Precocious Periodontitis—This expression was suggested to replace the term periodontosis, since the disease occurs primarily early in child/adolescent development (Sugarman 1977). However, in the twenty-first century, this term, together with *periodontosis*, has been replaced by *aggressive periodontitis* in order to discard classification terminologies that were age-dependent or required knowledge of rates of progression (Armitage 1999). See also aggressive periodontitis.

Pregnancy Gingivitis—A gingival inflammation that occurs during pregnancy, being self-limiting and transient (See Fig. P-13). The gingival tissues return to their healthy state postpartum, when estrogen and progesterone levels reach baseline values (Loe and Silness 1963, 1964; Loe 1965; Cohen et al. 1969). Today it is classified as a gingival disease modified by and associated with the endocrine system (Armitage 1999).

Prepubertal Periodontitis—A form of juvenile periodontitis affecting the primary or mixed dentition of young individuals prior to the onset of puberty, from ages 1 through 12 years. It is a genetically based periodontitis, involving defective leukocyte adherence. It occurs in two forms: (1) localized, showing a limited pattern of less rapid periodontal involvement with little to no gingival inflammation, and (2) generalized, showing an acute fiery-red proliferative gingival inflammation (marginal and attached) with rapid destruction of the alveolar bone (Page et al. 1983b).

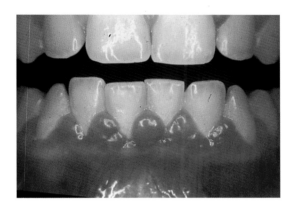

Fig. P-13: Pregnancy gingivitis

This condition is now classified under aggressive periodontitis (Armitage 1999). See also aggressive periodontitis, early-onset periodontitis.

Presuturing—The manipulation of palatal/donor tissue in the free soft tissue autograft technique. It involves placing suture material onto the donor-site tissue prior to separation for immediate placement (suturing) into the recipient site. This enables rapid management of the grafted tissue to the recipient site, thus minimizing trauma and facilitating healing (Becker 1967). See also suture.

Prevalence—The number of events or defects in an individual or population at a specified time. It may be said prevalence describes the static situation actually existing at a specified *point* in time or over a specified *period*. In contrast, *incidence* measures a changing situation over a defined period, or the number of cases of sickness arising over a given interval (Ramfjord 1959; Daly and Bourke 2000). See also incidence, period prevalence, point prevalence.

Preventive Occlusal Adjustment—The correction of an occlusion of a dentition that seems to present abnormal occlusal relationships but no signs of trauma in order to prevent future damage to the periodontal attachment apparatus (Glickman 1971). Clinicians and researchers cannot agree on the advisability of this practice and it is *not* considered acceptable in the treatment of periodontal disease today. This procedure has also been called prophylactic occlusal adjustment (Zander 1971).

Preventive Treatment Visit (PTV)—This term was coined to denote both preventive (P) and active treatment (T), which may be necessary during the periodontal recall or maintenance appointment (Wagenberg 2005). See also periodontal maintenance (PM), periodontal recall, periodontal maintenance therapy (PMT), prophylaxis (dental), supportive periodontal therapy (SPT).

Primary Cuticle—A film on the enamel of unerupted teeth, being the last product secreted by ameloblasts following enamel formation. It is calcified and slightly more resistant to acid and alkali than the enamel and tends to be worn away after eruption, particularly in areas exposed to abrasive foods. It is also called cuticle A and is about 1 μ thick (Wertheimer and Fullmer 1962; Jablonski 1992). See also Nasmyth's membrane, secondary cuticle.

Primary Occlusal Trauma—Trauma resulting from excessive occlusal forces applied to a tooth with normal bone height (See Fig. P-14). The changes produced by primary occlusal trauma do not alter the connective tissue attachment or initiate pocket formation (AAP 1989, 2001a; Carranza and Newman 1996). See also secondary occlusal trauma.

Prognosis—This may be defined as a forecast or prediction of the probable course of a disease and the chances of recovery from a planned treatment (Carranza and Newman 1996; AAP 2001a). The specific types of prognosis, as determined by the overall dentition, individual teeth, patient's health, and so on, have been divided into good, fair, poor, questionable, and hopeless (McGuire 1991, 2000).

Prognostic Factor—An environmental behavioral or biologic factor which, when

Primary Occlusal Trauma

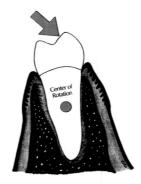

Center of Rotation

Fig. P-14: (With permission from Blackwell Publishing)

present, directly affects the probability of a positive outcome of therapy rendered for the disease. An example of a prognostic factor is the extent of presenting disease. On the other hand, smoking may be considered to be both a risk factor and a prognostic factor (Armitage 1996). See also risk factor.

Prophylaxis (Dental)—The cleaning of teeth in the dental office, including removal of plaque, material alba, calculus, and stains from the exposed and unexposed surfaces of the teeth by scaling and polishing as a preventive measure for the control of local irritative factors (Jablonski 1992; AAP 2001a). Prophylaxis is not to be confused with periodontal recall, periodontal maintenance therapy (PMT), or supportive periodontal therapy (SPT). See also periodontal maintenance (PM), periodontal maintenance therapy (PMT), periodontal recall, supportive periodontal therapy (SPT).

Prosthetic Gingival Veneer—This prosthetic device is constructed to compensate for the loss of gingiva following periodontal surgery in the anterior sextant of the maxillary arch. Early radical surgeries involved the removal of excessive amounts of gingiva, resulting in exposure of root surfaces and leading to esthetic and very often phonetic defects. Later on, crylic veneers were fabricated to cover the root surfaces and large interdental spaces, thus affording a more normal appearance (See Figs. G-4a,b and P-2a,b) (Orban 1945; Staffileno 1964). See also gingival facade, gingival prosthesis, party gums.

Proximal Wedge—A surgical flap procedure specifically designed for the periodontal lesion often found on the proximal aspect of a tooth adjacent to an edentulous area; the aim is to encourage healing by primary intention (Kramer and Schwarz 1964). See also modified distal wedge, distal wedge.

Pull Syndrome—The detaching movement of the marginal gingiva and interdental papillae transferred from the lip by the frenum when a slight "pull" is placed on the lip (Mirko et al. 1974). See also tension test.

Pushback Procedure—This is an archaic surgical procedure designed to deepen the vestibule, increase the attached gingiva, eliminate pockets, eliminate frena attachments, prevent food impaction, and create room (space) for oral hygiene. It was devised by Lewis J. Fox for the management of pockets that extended into the alveolar mucosa; it was also called the gingival replacement procedure (Friedman 1957). The details were outlined in 1956 by Henry M. Goldman and colleagues, which included removing the attached gingiva, apically displacing (pushback) the alveolar mucosa, placing a periodontal pack directly over the exposed bone, and changing the dressing weekly for 10 to 12 weeks until the vestibule was deepened (Goldman et al. 1956). This procedure is also known as a (1) displaced flap, (2) apically displaced flap, (3) gingival extension operation, (4) local extension of the vestibular trough, and (5) complete denudation. An illustration of the procedure appears in a 1966 publication (Kramer and Kohn 1966). See also complete denudation, gingival replacement, pouch procedure.

Pyorrhea Alveolaris—The word *pyorrhea* is derived from the Greek *pyon*, meaning "pus," and –*rhoia*, meaning "flow"; in other words, a discharge of pus from the alveolus (Jablonski 1992). The term was introduced into the United States by Frederick Henry Rehwinkle, a German physician, during a meeting of the American Dental Association in Chicago in 1877 (Rehwinkle 1877; Merritt 1921; Carranza and Shklar 2003) Oskar Weski suggested changing the term *pyorrhea alveolaris* to *paradentose* (Weski 1932). Then in 1937 the American Academy of Periodontology abandoned the term *pyorrhea alveolaris* in favor of *periodontal disease* (AAP 1937). See also periodontoclasia.

Quigley-Hein Plaque Index—This periodontal index records the presence of plaque on the labial/buccal and lingual surfaces of all teeth except the third molars and is performed following a 30-second rinsing with a disclosing solution of basic fuchsin. Dental plaque is registered on a scale of 0 to 5, with 0 revealing no plaque, 1 showing flecks of stain at the gingival margin, 2 showing a definite line of plaque at the gingival margin, 3 revealing stained plaque at the gingival third of the crown, 4 revealing two-thirds of the surface stained, and 5 having greater than two-thirds of the surface stained. An index for the entire mouth is determined by dividing the total score by the number of surfaces examined (Quigley and Hein 1962; Turesky et al. 1970).

R

Radectomy—This term for the resection or removal of one or more roots of a multi-rooted tooth was first reported in 1886 by Greene Vardiman Black (Black 1886; Bergenholtz 1972). This rather archaic term is more commonly replaced by *root amputation* or *root resection* (AAP 2001a). See also root amputation, root resection.

Radical Subgingival Curettage—This procedure was advocated by A.B. Riffle for the gross removal of tooth substance near the cementoenamel junction during root planing or root curettage. He felt that the cervical area of a tooth degenerated and that the necrotic material had to be removed until the tooth was so hard that a sharp instrument could remove no more (Riffle 1956). Scientific and clinical evidence now seems to negate this theory (Halik 1969). See also rifflizing.

Radicular Blending—In the removal of alveolar bone during osteoplasty, radicular blending is an extension of vertical grooving (See Fig. R-1). It is an attempt to gradually contour the bone over the entire radicular surface providing a smooth, blended surface for good flap adaptation. It is purely an osteoplastic technique (Carranza and Newman 1996). See also festooning, osteoplasty, vertical grooving.

Radicular Enamel—This term was used by Bernard S. Moskow to refer to all enamel formations that may occur on root surfaces. These enamel deposits were always

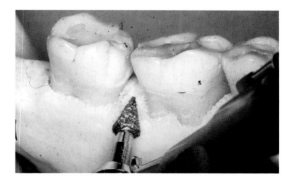

Fig. R-1

found on molar teeth, the majority occurring in the maxillary molars, and they are invariably found in the furcation area or directly adjacent to it (Moskow 1971). See also cervical enamel projection (CEP), enamel pearl.

Radiculolingual Groove—This dental anomaly is also known as the palatogingival groove. It usually starts in the region of the cingulum of maxillary anterior teeth and proceeds apically along the surface of the root for varying distances, frequently toward the distal portion of the tooth. It is especially of interest not only to the periodontist (serving as a nidus for plaque accumulation and potential periodontal detachment) but also to the endodontist in determining a differential diagnosis when symptoms occur (August 1978). See also cinguloradicular groove, distolingual groove, palatal groove, palatogingival groove, palatoradicular groove.

Radisectomy—The vital root resection of a multirooted tooth, due to periodontal involvement, in an attempt to preserve the vitality of the remaining pulpal tissue (Grossman 1981). Some degree of success without the intervention of endodontic therapy has been reported (Haskell and Stanley 1972; Smukler and Tagger 1976; Tagger and Smukler 1977). See also root amputation.

Raetzke's Pouch—This is a periodontal surgical procedure for covering localized areas of root exposure with a free connective tissue graft placed into a previously made "envelope." By undermining the adjacent tissue with a partial- (split-) thickness incision, the tissue graft is placed inside the envelope covering the area of root (cementum) exposure. This approach maximizes collateral circulation of the graft from the underlying and overlying vascular tissue. There are no vertical incisions (Raetzke 1985). This approach for covering isolated areas of root exposure has also been called the *supraperiosteal envelope* (Allen 1994). See also envelope technique, supraperiosteal envelope.

Random Burst Hypothesis—This theory attempts to explain that periodontally diseased sites may undergo cycles of exacerbation and spontaneous remission. This suggests that at least some forms of periodontal disease may be characterized by cycles of bacterial attack followed by a reparative host response (Goodson et al. 1982).

Rapidly Progressive Periodontitis (RPP)—This is a destructive form of periodontitis affecting young individuals ranging in age from puberty to 35 years; it is characterized by acute and quiescent phases and an inconsistently generalized pattern of destruction (Page et al. 1983a). It was established by R.C. Page and H.E. Schroeder

as a distinct clinical entity dominated by *Bacteroides gingivitis* (BG), *Actinobacillus actinomycetecomitans* (AA) and *Fusobacterium nucleatum* (FN) (Page and Schroeder 1982). This form of periodontitis is now catalogued as an *aggressive periodontitis* (Armitage 1999). See also aggressive periodontitis, early-onset periodontitis.

Rear Resorption—This is a pathologic process by which an area of necrosis occurs in the periodontal ligament from excessive pressure, resulting in bone resorption on the marrow or endosteal side. The result is reconstruction of the periodontal ligament but also thinning and fragmentation of the bone (Gottlieb 1942). See also frontal resorption, undermining resorption.

Reattachment—This term has been defined in two ways, depending on the date of the periodontal literature studied. Over fifty years ago, it was described as ". . . a new attachment of the soft tissue wall of a periodontal pocket to the corresponding root surface from which it had been detached previously by periodontal disease" (Ramfjord 1952b). This phenomenon is, in the true sense, new attachment. The modern definition for reattachment is "to attach again, the reunion of connective tissue with a root surface on which viable periodontal tissue is present; the area of reattachment is not affected by bacterial contamination" (Mellonig 1992; AAP 2001a). For example, a surgical flap may expose portions of the root that were not affected by disease. The flap will "reattach" to the surgically exposed root surface (Mellonig 1990). See also new attachment.

Refractory Periodontitis—This form of periodontitis has been said to recur in multiple sites after apparently appropriate therapy. These sites presumably continue to be infected by periodontal pathogens (Caton 1989). As a result of a consensus from the 1999 International Workshop for a Classification of Periodontal Diseases and Conditions, the "refractory" designation can be applied to all forms of periodontitis (e.g., refractory chronic periodontitis, refractory aggressive periodontitis, etc.) and not simply one disease entity. This separate disease category has been eliminated (Armitage 1999).

Regeneration—This term refers to the growth and differentiation of new cells and intercellular substance to form new tissue or parts (Jablonski 1992). More simply stated, it may be explained as the reproduction or reconstitution of a lost or injured part (AAP 2001a). See also guided bone regeneration (GBR), guided tissue regeneration (GTR), periodontal regeneration.

Relaxed Flap—This surgical procedure is an elevation of a periodontal flap when vertical incisions are used. It is then possible to move the flap either obliquely or laterally into a different position (Dello Russo 1998). See also envelope flap.

Repair—The healing of a wound by tissue that does not fully restore the architecture or function of a part (Mellonig 1992, 1998; AAP 2001a). The production of a long junctional epithelium, which does not fulfill the goal of (periodontal) regeneration at best, could be considered an example of repair (Yukna and Lawrence 1980). See also functional repair, long junctional epithelium.

Replaced Flap—This surgical procedure is achieved by an internal bevel incision to produce a partial-thickness flap in order to gain access to the underlying defect, with the use of releasing incision if necessary. Following degranulation of the defect, the flap is "replaced" in its original position on the root surface (Klavan 1970). See also surgical curettage, unrepositioned mucoperiosteal flap.

Repositioned Alveolar Ridge Mucosal Flap—A surgical procedure for managing bone loss on the proximal side of a tooth, utilizing the soft tissue covering an edentulous alveolar ridge. This ridge flap is composed of masticatory mucosa and contains sufficient elasticity from both buccal and lingual surfaces that circula-

tion is maintained. The soft tissue covering the edentulous ridge is an ideal source of tissue for flap procedures when it is repositioned to approximate a tooth (Hiatt 1967).

Repositioning of the Attached Gingiva—A surgical technique of apically positioning a mucoperiosteal flap utilizing one vertical incision placed mesially to the area of the deepest pocket. There is no sulcular incision and the gingiva is trimmed to a depth of at least 2 mm (Nabers 1954). In 1962, Nathan Friedman, in an attempt to retain the entire zone of attached gingiva, placed two vertical incisions in the apically repositioned flap (Friedman 1962a). This term is an archaic name for the apically positioned flap, because "reposition" implies that the flap is returned to its normal (original) site or position (Jablonski 1992; Corn 1968). See also apically positioned flap, apically repositioned flap.

Rest Position—This term, as used in the study of occlusion, refers to that position of the mandible when the mandibular musculature relaxes to tonic contraction, with the body in an upright or standing position. There is usually a space of 2 to 5 mm between the incisor teeth in the rest position (Sicher 1954b). An electromyographic definition, stated by the Academy of Denture Prosthetics in 1956, appears in a 1962 article by J. Garnick and S.P. Ramfjord. It reads, "The (physiologic) rest position is the mandibular position assumed when the head is in an upright position and the involved muscles, particularly the elevator and depressor groups, are in equilibrium in tonic contraction, and the condyles are in neutral, unstrained position" (Garnick and Ramfjord 1962). See also electromyography, postural position.

Retention Index (RI)—This index was introduced to assess the retentive factors in a mouth that facilitate the accumulation of bacterial plaque in the gingival area. These influencing factors may be supra- and subgingival calculus, ill-fitting mar-

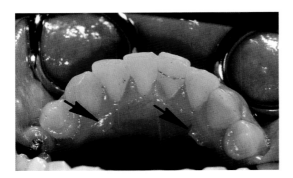

Fig. R-2: Arrows, retrocuspid papillae

gins of dental restorations, and carious lesions. This index is built on principles similar to those of the gingival and plaque indexes. The criteria for the retention index are as follows: 0 = no caries, no calculus, no imperfect margins near the gingival; 1 = supragingival cavity, calculus, or imperfect margins; 2 = subgingival cavity, calculus, or imperfect margins; and 3 = large cavity, abundant calculus, or grossly insufficient marginal fit of dental restorations in a supra- and/or subgingival location (Bjorby and Loe 1967; Loe 1967). See also gingival index (GI), plaque index.

Retrocuspid Papillae—These papillae are circumscribed soft prominences in the area of the gingiva or at the mucogingival junction on the lingual aspect of the mandibular canine region (*retro*, from the Latin, means "located behind") (See Fig. R-2). They are made up primarily of thin-walled vessels and appear hamartomatous in development, seeming to be lymphatic in nature (Everett et al. 1965). Isadore Hirschfeld was the first to describe them as a small, round mound of gingiva located on the lingual aspect of the mandibular cuspids (Hirschfeld 1947).

Retrograde Periodontitis—A tissue-destructive process that proceeds from the apical region toward the gingival margin, with the source of toxic materials originating from a diseased pulp. It may be char-

acterized by tooth mobility, pocket formation, gingival suppuration, gingival inflammation, and alveolar bone loss. It is a lesion that progresses in the opposite direction of a marginal periodontitis (Simring and Goldberg 1964). See also endodontic-periodontal lesion.

Retruded Contact (RC)—In the study of occlusion, this term refers to the position of the mandible in relation to the maxilla when both condyles are in the most retruded posterior position from which the mandible can make lateral posterior border movements. This position is *ligament*-guided, as compared to centric occlusion which is *tooth*-guided (Posselt 1968). Centric occlusion (CO) equals retruded contact (RC) in only about 10% of persons with natural, healthy, harmoniously functioning occlusions. The remaining 90% of people have an intercuspal position or centric occlusion (CO) about 0.25 to 2.25 mm anterior to the retruded contact (RC) position (Sicher 1954b). See also centric occlusion (CO), centric relation (CR), intercuspal position, terminal hinge axis.

Reverse Architecture—A morphologic relationship when the interdental gingiva or bone is located apical to its midfacial and midlingual margins (AAP 2001a). This condition induces the coronal growth of gingiva and subsequent recurrence of pocket depth (Heins 1969). Clifford Ochsenbein in 1986 altered the spelling of "reverse" to "reversed" and reiterated that "reversed architecture" may occur in the gingiva as well as the bone (Ochsenbein 1986). See also physiologic architecture, positive architecture, scalloped architecture.

Reverse Bevel Incision—This surgical incision, in preparation for a periodontal flap, is made parallel to the long axis of the tooth and is placed at least 0.5 mm away from the gingival margin so as to assure complete removal of all crevicular epithelium. It was initially described by Leonard Widman in 1918 but was alluded to previously by A. Cieszinski (Ramfjord 1977; Widman 1917, 1918; Cieszinski 1914; AAP 1989). See also internal bevel incision, inverse bevel incision, inverted bevel incision.

Reversible Index—The reversible index is a measurement of conditions that can be changed. Their scores or indices can either decrease or increase upon subsequent examinations. The reversible index accesses active disease rather than permanent damage, as measured by irreversible indices. Examples of reversible indices are the oral hygiene index (OHI), oral hygiene index simplified (OHI-S), plaque control record, Eastman interdental bleeding index (EIBI), and gingival bleeding index (GBI) (Barnes et al. 1986). See also irreversible index.

Ridge Augmentation—A surgical procedure on an edentulous ridge that had collapsed from either an extraction, endodontic infection, or accident in order to restore normal form, color, and contour. The newly augmented ridge will allow either the placement of a tooth implant (Buser et al. 1993; Nevins and Mellonig 1994) or a fixed bridge of a normal size to be placed and abutted against the restored ridge (Seibert 1993). The former two references illustrate ridge augmentation without and with osseous implantation, respectively. The latter reference demonstrates correction of deformed ridges by soft tissue augmentation only prior to prosthetic procedures using two approaches. They are either the "pouch" procedure or the "onlay" graft. The pouch procedure is a surgery involving the soft tissues under the defect (buccolingual ridge especially) to expand the contour of the ridge laterally, and a suitable augmentation material is placed into the pouch to maintain the expanded contour in the area (Seibert 1993). The onlay grafts are free soft tissue autografts of various sizes/dimensions placed over a specially prepared recipient bed (Seibert 1983a, 1983b; Seibert and Louis 1996). Jay S. Seibert was the first to demonstrate use of the onlay graft to correct ridge deformities (Seibert 1980). See also guided bone regeneration, onlay graft.

Ridge Defects (Classification)—Alveolar ridge defects have been classified two ways. The classical approach, introduced by Jay S. Seibert, is by classes: class I occurs with buccolingual loss of tissue associated with normal ridge height in an apicocoronal dimension, class II exhibits apicocoronal loss of tissue with normal ridge width in a buccolingual dimension, and class III occurs when there is a combination of buccolingual and apicocoronal loss of tissue, resulting in loss of both normal height and width (Seibert 1983a). A modification of this classification using types was described by E.P. Allen and colleagues: type A occurs with a loss of ridge in an apicocoronal contour (vertical), type B occurs with a loss of ridge contour in a buccolingual dimension (horizontal), and type C is a combination of A and B. In this system the depth of the defect relative to the adjacent ridge is graded as mild (less than 3 mm), moderate (3 to 6 mm), and severe (greater than 6 mm). This depth measurement may be used in either A, B, or C (Allen et al. 1985).

Ridge Expansion—A surgical technique for expanding the maxillary ridge with osteotomes, which allows simultaneous placement of dental implants into the "created" socket. The ridge planned for expansion must have adequate height, because ridge height cannot be achieved with this technique; the labial and lingual plates must not be fused, and they must be separated by an intervening cancellous bone. This last requirement facilitates the placement of the instruments for expansion of the ridge (Sethi and Kaus 2000).

Ridge Preservation—The surgical technique of preventing the collapse of alveolar bone and soft tissue following extraction(s) by placing a variety of osseous regenerative materials into the tooth socket(s) (Christensen 1996). The materials may be autogenous bone grafts, allografts, alloplasts, and/or xenografts with or without barrier membranes (Greenstein et al. 1985; Bahat et al. 1987; Sottosanti 1993; Minsk 2005b). The indications may be to conserve anterior esthetics, facilitate denture/bridge construction, or provide adequate bone height for future implant placement (Christensen 1996).

Rifflizing—The end product of root curettage (planing) of the cementum near the cementoenamel junction (CEJ), as advocated by A.B. Riffle in the 1950s. During root planing near the CEJ, the area of importance to Riffle, all the cementum and part of the enamel/dentin were often removed, leaving the tooth in the shape of an hourglass. This technique became known as rifflizing the root. Riffle stated that the root near the CEJ should have a hard, glassy surface and be velvety to the touch (Riffle 1952, 1953, 1956). This technique and philosophy of root debridement is archaic and is no longer practiced or believed important (Halik 1969). See also radical subgingival curettage.

Riggs' Disease—John Mankey Riggs, an American dentist, was the first practitioner, supposedly, who depended mainly on subgingival curettage for the successful treatment of periodontitis (Riggs 1876). Because his views and ideas on periodontal therapy were so widely accepted, he became recognized as the leading authority in the field, and the disease (periodontitis) became known as Riggs' disease (Adair 1904; Carranza and Shklar 2003). As a pioneer in periodontology John M. Riggs is recognized by his portrait and a reproduction of the March 1876 cover of the *Pennsylvania Journal of Dental Science*, which contains his article, on a plaque awarded by the William J. Gies Foundation. This award is given each year to an individual who has made unusual contributions in the field of periodontology (AAP 1965).

Risk Determinant—This term designates those risk factors that cannot be easily changed or modified by the patient. Some examples are age, race, gender, socioeconomic status, and genetics (AAP 1996a; Newman 1997).

Risk Factor—An environmental, behavioral, or biological factor confirmed by temporal sequence (on the basis of epidemiologic evidence) and known to be associated with disease-related conditions. If absent or removed, the probability of contracting that disease is reduced. Examples of risk factors for periodontal disease are specific microbiota, use of tobacco, defects in neutrophils, HIV infection, and various systemic diseases such as diabetes (AAP 1996a, 1999b; Genco 1996; Page and Beck 1997; Rees 2003; Ronderos and Ryder 2004). See also prognostic factor, periodontal risk calculator (PRC), risk determinant, risk indicator.

Risk Indicator—A probable or putative risk factor, often detected in cross-sectional studies, that has not yet been confirmed by longitudinal studies. Some examples of risk indicators are stress, distress, or coping factors (general adaptation syndrome, or GAS), osteopenia (osteoporosis), frequency of dental visits, HIV, and presence of periodontal pockets (AAP 1996a; Grossi et al. 1994, 1995; Page and Beck 1997; Rees 2003). See also risk factor.

Risk Predictor—Factors that have the ability to predict those individuals who are at high risk for disease but are not part of the causal chain. Examples of risk indicators are elevated levels of prostaglandin E2 in the gingival crevicular fluid and a history of clinical attachment loss (i.e., periodontitis). Individuals with a risk predictor are at higher risk for a disease (Page and Beck 1997). See also risk factor.

Roll Toothbrushing Technique—In this technique of toothbrushing, the bristles are placed parallel to and against the attached gingiva, with the toothbrush head level with the occlusal plane. The wrist is then turned to flex the bristles first against the gingiva and then the facial surface. An arcuate sweeping motion is continued

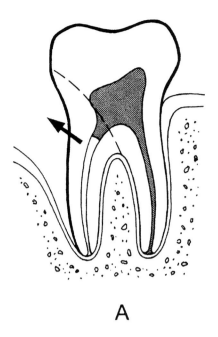
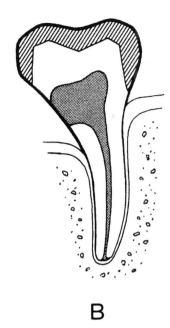

A

B

Fig. R-3

until the occlusal or incisal surface is reached. This press-roll action is repeated at least five times before proceeding to the next site. If performed incorrectly, the patient may miss the gingival third of the tooth and traumatize the alveolar mucosa. This technique is preparational for the modified Stillman, modified Charters, and modified Bass techniques of toothbrushing (Hine 1956; Curtis et al. 1957; Kimmelman 1964; Yankell and Saxer 1999; Ray 2005). See also toothbrushing technique.

Root Amputation—The surgical procedure of removing a root of a multirooted tooth apical to the furcation without removal of the crown portion of the tooth (See Fig. R-3) (Basaraba 1969). The first recorded account of root amputation in the dental literature was made in 1884 by J.N. Farrar of New York City, who had been using this technique nine years prior to reporting his findings (Farrar 1884). Although no mention was made by Farrar about endodontic therapy prior to amputation, William J.

Younger of San Francisco advocated performing root canal therapy prior to root amputation (Younger 1884). G.V. Black, two years later, stated that "a number of cases occur in which a valuable tooth can be saved by the amputations and removal of one of its roots" (Black 1886). See also radectomy, radisectomy, root resection, tooth resection.

Root Biomodification—This term refers to the application of various chemicals such as citric acid, fibronectin, EDTA, or tetracycline to diseased root surfaces for the purpose of (1) removing the smear layer, (2) root demineralization, (3) removal of endotoxins, (4) exposure of collagen fibrils, and (5) preventing the downgrowth of the junctional epithelium in an attempt to enhance new attachment to a pathologically exposed root surface (See Fig. R-4) (Ririe et al. 1980; Polson and Proye 1982; Morris 1980; Miller 1982, 1983, 1985b; Kassab and Cohen 2003). See also citric acid, fibronectin, root demineralization, smear layer.

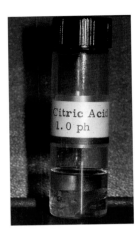

Fig. R-4

Root Curettage—The term *curettage*, as used for instrumentation of soft tissue, has also been referred to as the instrumentation of altered cementum by many authors, thus giving us the term *root curettage*, a procedure used in treating the cemental wall of the pocket as the first step in subgingival curettage (Thebaud 1951; AAP 2001a). See also apoxesis, root planing.

Root Demineralization—Also known as root biomodification. It is postulated that the use of acids on root surfaces induces a process whereby the exposed protein matrix of dentin or cementum can induce formation of cementoblasts and osteoblasts in the periodontal environment, leading to new attachment (Baiorunos and Robbins 1980). See also root biomodification.

Root Planing—A periodontal procedure employed for the removal of contaminated surface cementum or dentin and for making the exposed tooth surface smooth and hard. The objectives of root planing may include the following: (1) securing a biologically acceptable root surface, (2) resolving inflammation, (3) reducing pocket depths, (4) facilitating oral hygiene procedures, (5) improving or maintaining attachment levels, and (6) preparing tissues for surgical procedures. (Ramfjord and

Ash 1979a). Historically, root planing has been broken down into *prophylactic root planing* as performed in routine maintenance or as a preventive measure and *therapeutic root planing* as performed during a treatment procedure (Orban and Manella 1956). See also apoxesis, root curettage, scaling.

Root Resection—This term refers to root amputation or hemisection collectively without reference to the portion of the tooth removed (See Fig. R-5a,b,c,d,e). The following are indications: (1) severe vertical bone loss on multirooted teeth (See Fig. H-1b), (2) furca invasion, (3) unfavorable root proximity, (4) root caries or maintenance problems, (5) hopeless prognosis on bridge abutments, (6) root fractures, (7) root dehiscence, and (8) inadequate endodontic therapy (Basaraba 1969; Langer et al. 1981; Langer 1996). See also radectomy, root amputation, tooth resection.

Root Roof—Also known as *furcation dome*. It consists of that portion of the furcation which is the base of the root trunk and contains the bifurcational ridges (Saadoun 1985). See also bifurcational ridges, furcation dome, root trunk.

Root Separation—This is a synonym for the surgical technique of bisectioning. It is the procedure of splitting a mandibular molar with the retention of both fragments (Saadoun 1985). See also bicuspidization, bisectioning.

Root Trunk—This term refers to the distance from the cementoenamel junction of a multi-rooted tooth to the root's division point or furcation. They have been classified into three categories: (1) short, 3 mm in maxilla and 2 mm in mandible; (2) average, 4 mm in maxilla and 3 mm in mandible; and (3) long, 5 mm in maxilla and 4 mm in mandible (Ochsenbein 1986). They have also been classified according to the ratio of root trunk height to root length, type A being root trunks involving the cervical third of root length, type B being root trunks involving the cervical half of root length, and type C being root

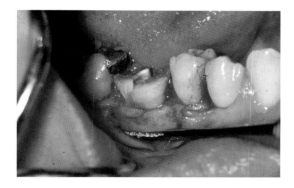

Fig. R-5a: Molar resected

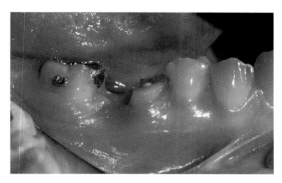

Fig. R-5d: Healing

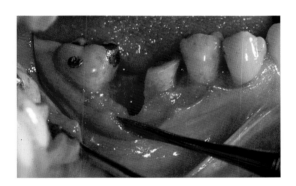

Fig. R-5b: Molar section (distal) removed

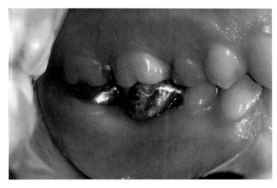

Fig. R-5e: Crown placed on molar (mesial)

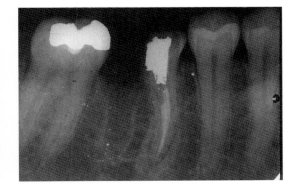

Fig. R-5c: Radiographic image

trunks involving the cervical two-thirds of the root length (Hou and Tsai 1997). See also blowout, root roof.

Rotational Flap—This periodontal flap is useful during periodontal reconstruction or periodontal plastic surgery procedures. It is a flap that moves around a pivot point, where the radius of the arc of rotation is the line of greatest tension (Bahat and Handelsman 1991). See also advanced flap.

"Runner"—The periodontal phenomenon that occurs when a tooth has been orthodontically moved through the alveolar bone and off the "basal bone" (See Fig. R-6). The result is an iatrogenic alveolar dehiscence with accompanying soft tissue

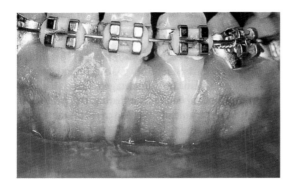

Fig. R-6: (With permission from Blackwell Publishing)

recession. This was referenced in an article of C.L. Nabers, G.R. Spear, and L.E. Beckham and credited to C.T. Rowland, an orthodontist in San Antonio, Texas (Nabers et al. 1960).

Scaling—The removal of all accretions (bacterial plaque, calculus, and stain) from the tooth surface, both supra- and subgingivally (Ramfjord and Kiester 1954; Ramfjord and Ash 1979a; AAP 2001a). See also apoxesis, root planing.

Scalloped Architecture—The contour of the gingiva and bone as it closely follows the cementoenamel junction of the teeth. The difference between marginal and interdental tissue (both gingiva and bone) levels will be greater for the incisors and least for the molars. It is synonymous with the terms *positive architecture* and *physiologic architecture* (Mills and McDonald 1998; AAP 2001a). See also physiologic architecture, positive architecture, reverse architecture.

Schei Ruler—This special ruler, made of plastic, was originally designed to evaluate the effect of oral hygiene on the resorption of alveolar bone. It exhibits 10 radii emanating from a point source, having equal distance between the ten lines. All measurements are taken 1 mm beneath the CEJ from an accurately taken dental radiograph. The ruler is placed over the film and the percentage of bone loss read with the last radius covering the root apex (Schei et al. 1959).

Schmutz Pyorrhea—This is an archaic expression, coined by Bernhard Gottleib, for moderate to severe periodontitis, with the origin of this "filth" pyorrhea being the gums. It was characterized by calculus, in-

Secondary Occlusal Trauma

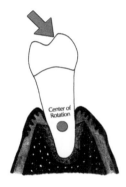

Center of Rotation

Fig. S-1: (With permission from Blackwell Publishing)

fection, pockets, suppuration, and alveolar atrophy (See Fig. N-1) (Gottleib 1925; Held 1989; AAP 2001a; Carranza and Shklar 2003).

Secondary Cuticle—The secondary cuticle is formed by the reduced enamel epithelium (epithelial attachment) as it contacts the cementum. It is Gottleib's "cuticle dentis" and is also known as cuticle B. It is 2 to 10 µ thick (Zander 1953; Werthheimer and Fullmer 1962). See also primary cuticle.

Secondary Occlusal Trauma—The normal occlusal forces that may cause trauma to the attachment apparatus of a tooth or teeth with inadequate support (See Fig. S-1). Otherwise, teeth that have lost so much support that they cannot withstand even the normal occlusal forces are said to be under secondary occlusal trauma (AAP 1989, 2001a). See also primary occlusal trauma.

Secondary Root Coverage—This term, as used during the postsurgical healing of gingival augmentation procedures, is synonymous with *creeping attachment* (Miller 1985b). See also coronal migration, creeping attachment, physiologic regeneration.

Semilunar Coronally Repositioned Flap— This is a surgical procedure to cover a denuded root by coronally positioning the facial tissue which has been relieved through a semilunar incision made parallel to the free gingival margin. A split-thickness flap is employed and positioned in place via finger pressure; no suture material is needed (Tarnow 1986, 1994). The procedure was first reported in 1912; however, a full-thickness flap was employed and sutures were utilized (Rosenthal 1912). See also coronally repositioned flap, incisal repositioning flap.

Sharp Dissection—The procedure of elevating a partial or split-thickness periodontal flap. In this dissection, the gingiva (both attached and unattached) is removed; however, the underlying connective tissue is intentionally left covering the tooth and bone. It is performed with a sharp scalpel or scissors (Staffileno 1960, 1969a; Staffileno et al. 1962, 1966). See also blunt dissection, partial-thickness flap, split-thickness flap.

Sharpey's Fibers—These fibers are the embedded ends of the collagenous connective tissue fibers of the periodontal ligament within the alveolar bone and cementum (See Fig. I-10b) (Orban 1957). They were named after the English anatomist and physiologist William Sharpey, who described them as "connective tissue fiber bundles which penetrated the circumferential lamellae on the surface of bone" (Sharpey 1856). Rudolph Albert Kolliker was the first to use the term *Sharpey's fibers* (Kolliker 1867), while G.V.

Black described them as being an essential part of the suspensory apparatus (Black 1887).

Shick-Ash Plaque Index—This system for measuring and recording plaque is a modification of Ramfjord's periodontal disease index (PDI) (Ramfjord 1959). The Shick-Ash system scores small changes in the amount of plaque present on the gingival halves of the coronal surfaces of the teeth. Following use of a disclosing solution, plaque is scored on both facial and lingual surfaces. Scoring is as follows: 0 = absence of dental plaque on the gingival half of the tooth; 1 = dental plaque covering less than one-third of the gingival half of the tooth; 2 = dental plaque covering one-third or less than two-thirds of the gingival half; and 3 = dental plaque covering two-thirds or more of the tooth surface. Thus, each tooth can receive a facial and a lingual plaque score (Shick and Ash 1961). See also periodontal disease index (PDI).

Silver Point, Calibrated—This device combines the advantages of the millimeter probe and gutta percha point in the diagnosis and prognosis of periodontal disease (See Fig. S-2a,b,c,d). The silver points are soft silver half-round wires, from 4 to 12 mm in length, with ridges every 2 mm. The tip is tapered to enable the point to easily reach the bottom of the pocket, with the first ridge omitted. The silver point is readily visible in the dental radiograph; it has ridges at 4, 6, 8, and 10 mm. The pocket depths can easily be measured on a dental film (Hirschfeld 1953). According to Nathan Friedman, the silver point can be used to indicate the level of the gingiva in the dental film, reveal which portion of the pocket is in soft tissue and which in bone, and show the relationship of the base of the pocket to the alveolar crest (Friedman 1955).

Sinus Lift Graft—This grafting technique was introduced by Hilt Tatum to satisfactorily increase maxillary bone height by placing graft material into the maxillary

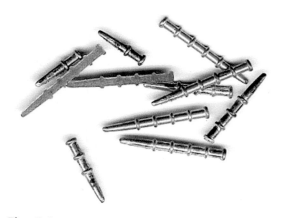

Fig. S-2a: Assorted silver points

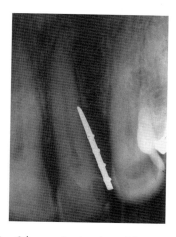

Fig. S-2c: Silver point in place 10-mm pocket

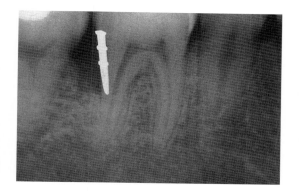

Fig. S-2b: Silver point in place, 7-mm pocket

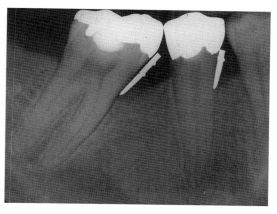

Fig. S-2d: Silver point, 6-mm pocket (molar); silver point, 4-mm pocket (bicuspid)

sinus and under the Schneiderian membrane in preparation for placement of root-form dental implants (Tatum 1986; Minsk 2004). This technique of sinus augmentation has been widely used and reported by many clinicians (Boyne and James 1980; Smiler 1997; Valentini and Abensur 1997). In 1998, a consensus conference report concluded that "the sinus graft should now be considered a highly predictable and effective therapeutic modality" (Shulman and Jensen 1998).

Sliding Flap—This surgery is a mucogingival procedure of transposing a flap of healthy tissue from an adjacent (donor)

site to cover the defective (recipient) site. It is commonly used to cover an isolated root exposure from gingival recession, with a healthy amount of keratinized gingiva (See Fig. L-1a,b,c) (Grupe and Warren 1956). The periodontal literature has been inundated with variations of the original Grupe and Warren procedure, often confusing the reader with redundant terminology. A "letter to the editor" illustrates this confusion (Grupe 1966b). See also contiguous pedicle graft, horizontal gingival pedicle graft, horizontal sliding flap,

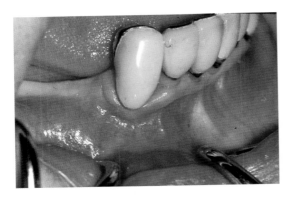

Fig. S-3a: Before autograft

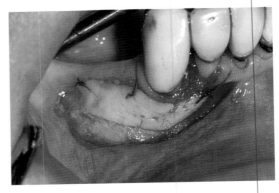

Fig. S-3c: Graft sutured in place

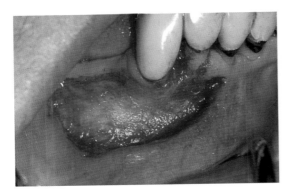

Fig. S-3b: Graft site prepared

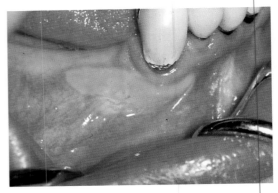

Fig. S-3d: Ten months postoperatively

lateral repositioned flap, lateral sliding flap, modified sliding flap, pedicle flap, pedicle graft.

Sling Suture—This suturing technique permits precise positioning of a flap around individual teeth when different teeth require the flap to be at different levels, especially in the case of apically positioned flaps and in repositioned flaps (Morris 1965a; Dahlberg 1969). See also continuous sling suture, suture.

Smear Layer—This term refers to an amorphous, irregular surface resulting after root planing and found to interfere with connective tissue attachment (Polson et al. 1984). The advocates of root biomodification state that the smear layer is often re-

moved by this method of root conditioning, leaving the pluropotential cells of the periodontal ligament undamaged for improved periodontal healing (Blomlof et al. 1996). See also root biomodification.

Soft Tissue Autograft—Dr. D. Walter Cohen has presented a case for separating soft tissue autografts into contiguous soft tissue autografts and free soft tissue autografts (See Fig. S-3a,b,c,d). Under the former he includes the laterally repositioned flap, double papillae repositioned flap, oblique rotated flap and the apically positioned flap, all being physically connected to a blood supply. On the other hand, once a soft tissue autograft is severed from its blood supply, it becomes a free soft tissue autograft (Cohen 1969). See also apically positioned flap, double-papillae repositioned flap, free soft tissue autograft, lateral repositioned flap, oblique rotated flap.

Soft Tissue Management (STM)—This phase of periodontal treatment addresses the gingival inflammatory component of periodontal disease but has a limited effect on the underlying bone pathology. It is also called *initial therapy*, where soft tissue debridement for inflammatory control is achieved through scaling and root planing. STM is not considered to be an appropriate endpoint therapy for patients with chronic periodontitis (Shapoff 2004). The objective of soft tissue management (STM) is shrinkage of soft tissue, but limited reduction of pocket depth should be expected.

Sonic Instrumentation—This refers to air-turbine units that operate at low frequencies ranging between 3,000 and 8,000 cycles per second (CPS), with a vibratory tip movement that is primarily linear or elliptical in direction (AAP 2000c). See also ultrasonics.

Specific Plaque Hypothesis—This hypothesis states that periodontal disease activity is related to specifically known bacterial species and their products, thus identification and eradication of certain "periodontopathogens" should be the goal in treatment. Examples of these opportunistic periodontal pathogens are *Actinobacillus actinomycetecomitans* (AA), *Bacteroides gingivalis* (BG), *Bacteroides intermedius* (BI), *Eikenella corrodens* (EC), *Fusobacterium nucleatum* (FN), and *Wolinella recta* (WR). The monitoring and control of specific plaque bacteria is based on this hypothesis (Genco et al. 1988). See also nonspecific plaque hypothesis.

Split-Thickness Flap—Half of this periodontal flap consists of the papillary gingiva and also of marginal, attached, and unattached vestibular gingiva dissected from but not stripped from the tooth and bone. This is a procedure designed to "split" the fibrous connective tissue attachment from the tooth without exposing the root. The incision is continued to the unattached gingiva without exposing the vestibular plate of bone. It is achieved by what is referred to as *sharp dissection* (Staffileno 1960, 1969a; Staffileno et al. 1962, 1966). See also blunt dissection, gingival mucosal flap, mucosal flap, partial-thickness flap, sharp dissection.

Stillman's Clefts—These gingival defects have been defined as "small apostrophe-shaped fissures extending apically from the gingival margin to a depth of 5 to 6 mm, usually on the vestibular surface of teeth" (Jablonski 1992). They were originally considered to be due to a regional circulatory disturbance within the gingiva initiated by traumatic occlusion (Stillman 1921; Stillman and McCall 1937). However, research has shown that there is no evidence that such defects are brought about by occlusal disharmonies (Posselt 1959). They may be considered as epithelial downgrowths leading to a splitting of the gingiva (AAP 2001a). See also gingival cleft.

Stillman's Toothbrushing Technique—This technique was originally developed to provide gingival stimulation. The bristles of the brush are placed partly on the gingiva and partly on the cervical portion of the tooth, with the bristles inclined at a 45-degree angle directed apically. Slight pressure is applied to the gingiva-tooth junction with a slight vibratory motion to produce a blanching of the gingiva. The bristles are lifted and replaced in the same area, repeating the pressure-vibratory motion. There is no friction placed upon the gingiva-tooth area, merely pressure to effect a blanching. It is a difficult procedure to perform but was popularized in the eastern United States, with Paul R. Stillman being from New York City (Stillman 1928, 1932; Yankell and Saxer 1999; Ray 2005). See also modified Stillman's toothbrushing technique, toothbrushing technique.

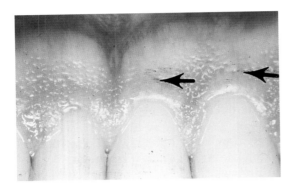

Fig. S-4: Arrows, stippled attached gingiva

Stippling—Balint Orban refers to King's description of normal gingiva as being "matted" in texture, just distant from the dental margin, being associated with the presence of numerous regularly distributed small depressions and giving the tissue an appearance somewhat resembling the peel of an orange (See Fig. S-4). This orange peel appearance is generally called "stippling" (King 1945; Orban 1948a; Greene 1962; AAP 2001a). King referred to it as "surface pitting." The attached gingiva is characterized by high connective tissue ridges elevating the epithelium, the surface of which appears stippled. Between the elevations there are small depressions that correspond to the center of heavier epithelial ridges and show signs of degeneration and hornification in their depth. The degree of stippling varies in different individuals; it had been thought to be an expression of functional adaptation to mechanical impacts (Goldman 1949). See also attached gingival.

Subcrestal Incision—This surgical incision as employed in periodontal flap procedures refers to placement of the scalpel 1 to 2 mm away from the gingival margin and angled toward the crest of bone (Litch et al. 1984). It is believed necessary in order to completely remove the diseased crevicular epithelium during flap preparation (Ramfjord and Nissle 1974). See also extrasulcular incision, submarginal incision, subsulcular incision.

Subepithelial Connective Tissue Graft (SCTG)—The SCTG is surgically transplanted palatal connective tissue (donor) to another area of the mouth (recipient) for the purpose of epithelial keratinization to improve esthetics and/or correct deficiencies of edentulous ridges (See Fig. S-5a,b,c,d). It has been utilized to increase the width of keratinized gingiva (i.e., a free soft tissue graft) (Edel 1974, 1975) and to correct ridge deformities (Langer and Calagna 1980). A benchmark article describing the technique in detail has been published, showing the SCTG in creating root coverage on recession sites where inadequate amounts of lateral attached gingiva precluded the use of a lateral sliding graft (flap) (Langer and Langer 1985).

Subgingival Calculus—Dental calculus that forms apical to the gingival margin, often brown or black, and is very hard and tenacious (See Fig. S-6) (AAP 2001a). Also known as submarginal calculus, its morphology may be crusty, spiny, nodular, ledge, or ring-like, being either finger- or fern-like in formation. It may be deposited in islands or spots and it is even possible for supragingival calculus to form on subgingival deposits when gingival recession occurs (Everett and Potter 1959). Synonyms for subgingival calculus are serumnal, haemotogenic, and or sanguinary calculus (Alexander 1969). See also calculus (dental).

Subgingival Curettage—This procedure is designed to remove calculus deposits, bacterial plaque, materia alba, ulcerated epithelial lining, granulomatous tissue, and occasionally the junctional epithelium (See Fig. S-7a,b). Other benefits of this procedure are to reduce congestion/edema, production of hemorrhage, and institute drainage where periodontal pockets may have closed (i.e., in the event of abscess) (Hirschfeld 1962). See also closed crevicular curettage, closed curettage, curettage, gingival curettage.

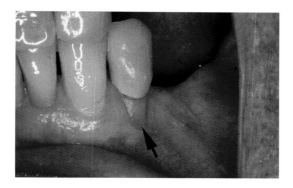

Fig. S-5a: Arrow, note gingival recession

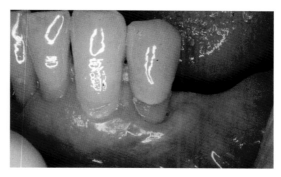

Fig. S-5d: Healing after 4 weeks

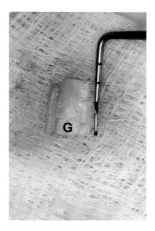

Fig. S-5b: G, SCTG from palate

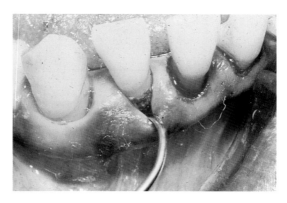

Fig. S-6: (With permission from Elsevier Publishing)

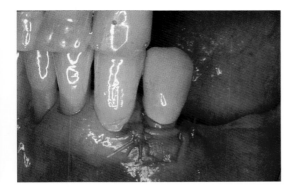

Fig. S-5c: SCTG adapted with gut suture

Submarginal Incision—An inverse bevel incision placed 1 to 2 mm away from the gingival margin and angled toward the bony crest (Litch et al. 1984). See also subcrestal incision.

Subpedicle Connective Tissue Graft—A periodontal plastic procedure for covering root cementum (gingival recession) during periodontal esthetic procedures. It consists of a bilaminar graft composed of a subepithelial connective tissue graft with overlying full-thickness double-pedicle grafts from adjacent papillae (i.e.,

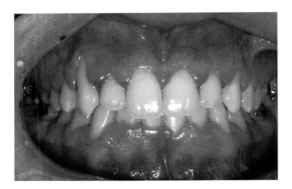

Fig. S-7a: Before treatment, curettage

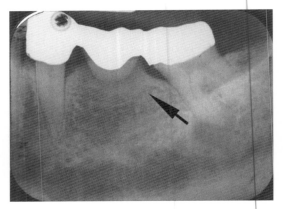

Fig. S-8: Arrow, subpontic osseous hyperplasia (Courtesy of Dr. S. Jin Kim)

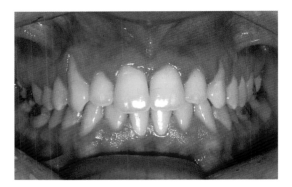

Fig. S-7b: After treatment, curettage

pedicles). It is indicated when a single surgical procedure is desired that will predictably cover denuded root surfaces. It is also appropriate where there is inadequate keratinized gingiva for a pedicle graft and where the prognosis is poor for root coverage with a free soft tissue autograft (Nelson 1987). A similar procedure using partial-thickness double-pedicle grafts to cover the subepithelial connective tissue is also possible (Harris 1992). See also bilaminar graft.

Subpontic Osseous Hyperplasia—This is an ectopic growth of bone occurring on the edentulous ridge beneath the bridge pontic of a fixed partial denture (See Fig. S-8) (Lorenzana and Hallmon 2000). This has

also been referred to as a subpontic osseous proliferation. Both of these terms are a variant of *reactive subpontine exostosis* (Neville et al. 2002). See also exostosis.

Substantivity—The property of a substance (i.e., pharmacologic agent) of binding to the soft and/or hard tissue walls of a periodontal pocket, thereby establishing a drug reservoir. Equilibrium is established between the bound and free drug in the pocket, with eventual dilution in concentration by the flow of the gingival fluid (AAP 2000e, 2001a).

Subsulcular Incision—This incision requires that the surgical scalpel be placed away from the sulcus and aimed at ending near the crest of the alveolar bone. When the amount of attached gingiva is quite narrow on either the labial or facial aspects of the tooth, care must be taken to preserve as much of the keratinized gingiva as possible (Dello Russo 1998). See also extrasulcular incision.

Subtraction Radiography (Digital)—A computerized radiographic enhancement technique that facilitates the detection of osseous changes that are too small to be seen by the naked eye. When two standardized radiographs taken at separate times are aligned, all structures that have not changed are cancelled. This process leaves the area of change readily visible against a neutral gray background. Software can then detect the area of bone loss or gain, color it in shades of red or green, respectively, and superimpose the area on the original radiograph (Jeffcoat 1994). Subtraction radiography is 92 percent sensitive and 97 percent specific in detecting small osseous changes (Jeffcoat et al. 1992) and is able to detect and measure as little as 1 mg of bone-mass change or a change in bone height of 0.1 mm (Jeffcoat 1992).

Sulcular Epithelium—The portion of the gingival epithelium that lines the soft tissue wall of the gingival sulcus (See Fig. J-1). It is nonkeratinized squamous epithelium and extends from the junctional epithelium to the crest of the gingival margin (Innes 1973). See also crevicular epithelium, gingival epithelium.

Sulcular Incision—This surgical incision denotes the placement of the scalpel blade into the gingival sulcus and severing both the epithelial and connective tissue attachment from the tooth (Dello Russo 1998). It is usually followed by the elevation of a full-thickness mucoperiosteal flap (Luebke and Ingle 1964). It is also known as the intracrevicular or intrasulcular incision. As early as 1931, it was described as "placing the blade directly into the sulcus and following the contours of the teeth in the process of flap surgery" (Kirkland 1931). See also crestal incision, crevicular incision.

Sulcus Bleeding Index (SBI)—This index measures bleeding from four gingival units (labial and lingual marginal units and the mesial and distal papillary units) around eight anterior teeth (four maxillary and four mandibular anteriors) using a blunt periodontal probe with a 0.5 mm diameter tip. These units are scored from 0 (healthy appearance of papillary and marginal tissue) to 5 (spontaneous bleeding upon probing with a change in color, marked swelling with or without ulceration). A 30-second period is allowed from probing for the eliciting of bleeding (Muh-lemann and Son 1971). The papillary-marginal index (PM) of Muhlemann and Mazor was renamed the sulcus bleeding index (SBI) so as not to confuse the PM with the papillary marginal attached index (PMA) of Massler and Schour. See also papillary marginal index (PM).

Sulcus Depth—The sulcus depth has been described within the parameters of either a clinical or histological evaluation. The "clinical" sulcus depth does not appear to be limited by the epithelial attachment (i.e., junctional epithelium) and may approach the connective tissue attachment. On the other hand, the "histological" sulcus depth is limited by the coronal border of the junctional epithelium (DeWaal et al. 1986). See also gingival pocket, periodontal pocket.

Supporting Alveolar Bone—That portion of the alveolar process consisting of buccal and lingual cortical plates (compact bone), the intervening cancellous bone (spongy bone) between these plates, and the alveolar bone proper (See Fig. A-4) (Orban 1957). See also alveolar process.

Supportive Periodontal Therapy (SPT)—The American Academy of Periodontology in 1989 preferred this term for periodontal maintenance or periodontal recall (AAP 1989). It consists of the following procedures: (1) updating of medical and dental histories, (2) extra- and intraoral soft tissue examination, (3) dental examination, (4) periodontal evaluation, (5) radiographic review, (6) removal of bacterial plaque and calculus from supra- and subgingival regions, (7) selected root planing if needed, (8) polishing of teeth, and (9) a review of the patient's plaque removal efficiency (AAP 1995). Position papers on supportive periodontal therapy (SPT) have been published (AAP 1998a, 1998c). See also periodontal maintenance (PM), periodontal maintenance therapy (PMT), periodontal recall.

Suprabony Pocket—The suprabony pocket is a pathologic sulcus where the base of the pocket is coronal or occlusal to the alveolar crest. It may further be divided into a gingival or pseudopocket and a periodontal pocket (Carranza and Glickman 1957; Goldman and Cohen 1958). The suprabony pocket may also be referred to as a supra-alveolar or supracrestal pocket. See also gingival pocket, periodontal pocket.

Supracrestal Fiberotomy—A surgical technique for reducing rotational relapse of orthodontically aligned teeth. It is believed that only the free gingival and circumferential transseptal fibers need to be severed to accomplish this. This procedure was described and illustrated by Ross G. Kaplan (Kaplan 1976, 1977). See also circumferential supracrestal fiberotomy (CSF), fiberotomy.

Supragingival Calculus—The calculus covering the coronal surface of the tooth to the crest of the gingival margin (See Fig. S-9). It is usually white or white-yellow and can easily be detached from the tooth surface (Alexander 1969; Jablonski 1992). See also calculus (dental), subgingival calculus, tartar, tooth accumulated material (TAM).

Supraperiosteal Envelope—A surgical procedure for managing areas of gingival recession with deficient amount of keratinized gingiva. The utilization of subepithelial connective tissue grafts (SCTGs) placed into a prepared "envelope" at the recipient site has been shown to correct these mucogingival defects (Allen 1994). This surgical technique is the same as the Raetzke's pouch procedure. See also envelope technique, Raetzke's pouch, subepithelial connective tissue graft (SCTG).

Surgical Curettage—A surgical procedure of elevating a full-thickness mucoperiosteal flap, both buccal and lingual, for the purpose of root planing, removal of all remnants of sulcular epithelium, epithelial attachment (junctional epithelium), and marginal tissue so as to allow healing of connective tissue to tooth and alveolar bone. Following removal of all granulomatous tissue, the flaps are tightly

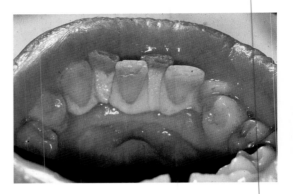

Fig. S-9

adapted. This surgical approach was introduced many years ago and is frequently described by other names (Ingle 1952). See also modified Widman flap (MWF), open-flap curettage.

Suture—A suture is a material used in closing a surgical wound with stitches. Most commonly used materials include silk, catgut, collagen, cotton, synthetic material and polyglycolic acid. This term also refers to the act of uniting or closing wounds (i.e., the application of such materials) (Jablonski 1992; AAP 2001a). The closure of periodontal surgical wounds, using a variety of suture types, utilizes a variety of techniques or approaches as dictated by the surgical objective (Morris 1965a; Levin 1980; Silverstein and Kurtzman 2005). See also anchor suture, circumferential suture, continuous sling periosteal suture, continuous sling suture, continuous suture, cyanoacrylates, horizontal continuous suture, horizontal internal mattress suture, interdental suture, internal mattress suture, interrupted periosteal suture, interrupted suture, mattress suture, periosteal suture, presuturing, sling suture, vertical internal mattress suture, vertical mattress suture, wicking.

Synchronous Burst Hypothesis—The breakdown of periodontal tissues (loss of attachment), which may occur at specific times (e.g., during puberty). It was proposed that the asynchronous multiple burst models be called synchronous burst hypothesis (Zimmerman 1986).

Systemic Periodontitis—This term was coined in 2002 to represent the threat that periodontitis poses to systemic health (Beck and Offenbacher 2002). It was concluded that periodontal disease must be thought of as a disease process that can lead to a systemic disease or condition (outcome) rather than the outcome itself. See also periodontal medicine.

T

"Take"—The "attachment" of a soft tissue autograft over an avascular bed (recipient site). It may be either epithelial in origin (long junctional epithelium) or originate from connective tissue (new attachment) (Pennel et al. 1969). Unfortunately it is often an unpredictable phenomenon. See also bridging, long junctional epithelium, new attachment.

Tartar—This term, a synonym for *calculus*, was introduced to general medicine by Phillipus Aureolus von Hohenheim (Paracelsus), a Renaissance alchemist and chemist, when he likened these stony accretions to the accumulation of minerals seen in wine casks (See Figs. S-6 and S-9) (Wynbrandt 1998). It is said that Paracelsus recognized the extensive formation of tartar on teeth and related this to toothaches (Carranza and Shklar 2003). See also calculus (dental), tooth accumulated material (TAM).

Temporomandibular Disorders (TMD)—This is an all-inclusive term referring to a heterogenous group of psychophysiologic disorders involving the temporomandibular joint (TMJ), all of which cause orofacial pain, masticatory dysfunction, or both (Phillips et al. 2001). Another source states that TMD is a collection of medical/dental conditions affecting the TMJ and/or muscles of mastication and other contiguous tissue components. It includes myofascial pain dysfunction syndrome (MPD), meniscal displacement with or without reduction (internal derangement), degenerative joint disease (osteoarthritis), rheumatoid arthritis and other disorders of systemic origin, facial growth disharmonies, traumatic injuries, and neoplasms (AAP 2001a). Three primary symptoms of TMD are (1) preauricular pain, (2) limited mandibular functioning, and (3) joint sounds, such as clicking, popping, or grinding (Okeson 1997). One of the most common types of temporomandibular disorders (TMD) is myofascial face pain (MFP) (Raphael et al. 2000; Raphael and Marbach 2001). This disorder of the TMJ was adopted by the American Dental Association in 1982, replacing the older, more simplistic concept of TMJ syndrome (Griffiths 1983). See also Costen syndrome, myofascial face pain (MFP), myofascial pain dysfunction syndrome (MPD).

Tension Test—A simple clinical determination of the quantity of attached gingiva surrounding a tooth. When the lips and cheeks are retracted laterally, the attached gingiva is said to be "inadequate" if it pulls away from the tooth. There must be blanching and movement of the marginal gingiva on lip/cheek "tension" (Kopczyk and Saxe 1974; Vincent et al. 1976). See also pull syndrome.

Terminal Hinge Axis—The center of rotation of the condylar heads during the rearmost rotatory opening and closing movements of the mandible (Posselt 1968). See also retruded contact (RC).

Tissue Engineering—This is based on using a combination of growth factors and modulators, scaffolds or matrices, and cells to regenerate lost tissues and organs (Camelo et al. 2003). This approach to bioengineering may be used to promote periodontal (Pini Prato et al. 2000) and peri-implant bone regeneration in a way not previously considered possible (Giannobile 2002). It is very likely that in the near future the major indication for periodontal flap surgery will not be one of debridement or bone removal but of regeneration and repair through tissue engineering (Williams 2003; Williams et al. 2005). An in-depth treatise on the role of bio- or tissue engineering in maxillofacial and periodontal surgery is available (Lynch et al. 1999). See also amelogenins, enamel matrix proteins, growth and differentiation factors, platelet-rich plasma (PRP).

Tooth Accumulated Material (TAM)—The accumulation of different types of accretions on the surfaces of teeth, which may be related to different aspects of periodontal disease. Such accretions may include the acquired salivary pellicle, microbial plaque, dental calculus, food debris (Dawes et al. 1963), and material alba (bacterial and epithelial cells) (WHO 1961). A detailed review and classification of these TAMs has been published (Schwartz and Massler 1969; Schwartz et al. 1971). See also acquired cuticle, calculus (dental), material alba, tartar.

Toothbrushing—According to Maynard K. Hine, the function of the toothbrush is to remove food debris, accumulated microorganisms, and recently deposited calculus from the teeth and to massage the gingival tissues so as to promote a good blood supply and adequate keratinization of the epithelium. Toothbrushing should not irritate or lacerate the gingiva or wear away the tooth substance (Hine 1956). Various methods of toothbrushing have been introduced over the years. See the following toothbrushing techniques for their approach to achieving the above-mentioned goals: Bass, Bell, Charters, circular, Fones, horizontal, Leonard, modified Bass, modified Stillman's, physiologic, roll, Stillman's, vertical, vibratory.

Tooth Lengthening—A surgical procedure to increase the clinical crown of a tooth that has been mutilated by either pathologic or physiologic processes. Pathologic processes may include tooth fracture, dental decay, retrograde or excessive tooth wear or root perforations from endodontic treatment, and restorative posts or pins. Physiologic processes that are benefited by tooth lengthening are altered or delayed passive eruption or overeruption (Rosenberg et al. 1980). See also crown lengthening.

Tooth Mobility—Any degree of perceptible movement of a tooth buccolingually, mesiodistally, or axially when a force is applied to it and the tooth returns to its original position once the pressure is removed (Perlitsh 1980). The horizontal movement of a tooth has been classified by Samuel Charles Miller as being 1, 2, or 3. A movement of 1 is assigned by the first distinguishable sign of movement greater than normal. A degree of 2 is given when movement of the tooth allows the crown to deviate within 1 mm of its normal position in either direction. A mobility of 3 is assigned when movement of a tooth occurs more than 1 mm in any direction or can be rotated or depressed in its socket. He further states that each tooth should be tested by holding it between two rigid instruments; only then can one obtain its true mobility (See Fig. T-1) (Miller 1938). Tooth mobility in a vertical direction (as it depresses in its socket) has been studied (Parfitt 1960; Picton 1963).

Tooth Resection—The removal of furcation from multirooted teeth. Three approaches to tooth resection are (1) root amputation (See Fig. R-3), (2) hemisection (See Fig. H-1), and (3) trisection (Lemmerman 1975).

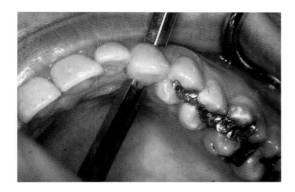

Fig. T-1

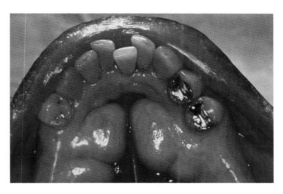

Fig. T-2a

See also radectomy, root amputation, root resection.

Tooth Wear Index (TWI)—This index is designed for use in research and epidemiology for investigating the etiology, prevention, and management of tooth wear problems by monitoring long-time tooth-wear patterns in individual patients. The degree of damage to teeth caused by erosion, attrition, abrasion, and combinations of these conditions. This index is applicable whether or not the cause can be determined. Scoring of all teeth is performed while all tooth surfaces (buccal or labial, lingual or palatal, occlusal, incisal, and cervical) are examined and scored. The criterion for tooth wear (loss) is found in the reference (Smith and Knight 1984).

Torus—An elevation, swelling, or bulging of hard bone either along the midline suture of the hard palate (torus palatinus) or on the lingual aspect of the mandible above the myohyoid line in the region of the premolars (torus mandibularis) (See Figs. T-2a,b and T-3a,b,c) (AAP 2001a; Neville et al. 2002). See also exostosis.

Transgingival Probing—The process of "walking" the periodontal probe along the tissue-tooth interface so as to examine, feel, and predict the underlying osseous topography (See Fig. T-4). This "sounding" process, under local anesthesia, helps the operator to determine flap design and

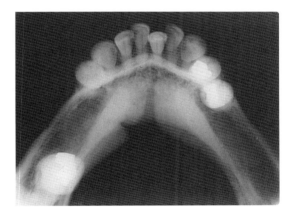

Fig. T-2b: Radiographic image of T-2a

methods of managing bony deformities, be they intrabony defects, craters, dehiscences, and/or fenestrations (See Figs. B-5 and P-7b) (Tibbetts 1969; Greenberg 1976). See also bone sounding.

Transpositional Flap—This periodontal flap is a modification of the laterally positioned papillary flap or oblique rotated flap (Pennel et al. 1965). The modification is produced by extending the incisions of the flap more apically so as to place the turning pivot point of the flap more apically. This produces a greater stretching effect of the flap, which gives it more lateral and incisal movement to cover the de-

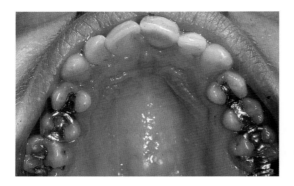

Fig. T-3a

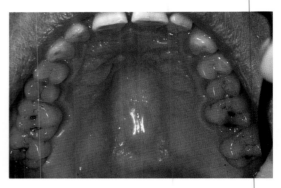

Fig. T-3c

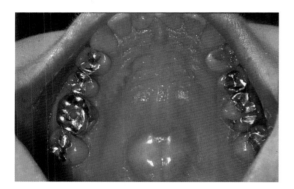

Fig. T-3b

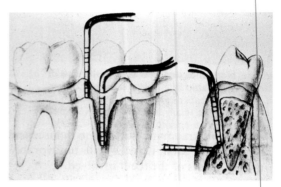

Fig. T-4: (With permission from the American Dental Association)

fect (Bahat et al. 1990). See also oblique rotated flap.

Transseptal Fiber Group—This group of principal fibers of the periodontal ligament extends from the cementum of one tooth over the alveolar crest to insert into the cementum of the adjacent tooth (See Fig. T-5a,b). Their function is to help keep the teeth in alignment, protect the interproximal bone from inflammatory infiltrate, and support the interproximal gingiva. This group is often included in the gingival fiber group (Orban 1957; AAP 2001a). See also gingival fiber group, periodontal ligament.

Trauma from Occlusion—The periodontal tissue injury (i.e., lesion) elicited by traumatic occlusion (i.e., force). Such excessive occlusal forces produce injury confined to the alveolar bone, periodontal ligament, and cementum (Glickman and Smulow 1967). The injuries may consist of thrombosis and/or hyalinization or necrosis of the periodontal ligament with resorption of the alveolar bone and cementum (Muhlemann et al. 1956). See also occlusal trauma.

Trauma from Occlusion Index (TOI)—This index measures trauma from occlusion comprising apparent functional mobility and a radiographically widened periodontal ligament space. TOI-positive teeth have more severe destruction and inflammation of the periodontal tissues while TOI-negative teeth have less (Jin and Cao 1992).

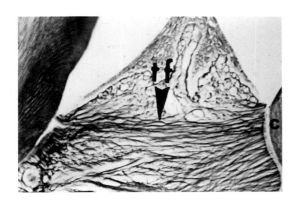

Fig. T-5a: TF, transseptal fibers (molar; C, cementum

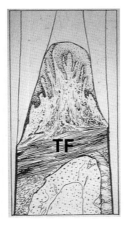

Fig. T-5b: TF, transseptal fibers (bicuspid)

Traumatogenic Occlusion—This term, suggested by Harold Keith Box, refers to the existing intra and extra-occlusal arch tooth relationships. It alludes to the static tooth positions and not to the forces of traumatic occulusion. It was listed as one of the causative factors in the progression of periodontal disease (Box 1930, 1935). See also occlusal trauma, traumatic occlusion.

Traumatic Occlusion—This term refers to the *forces* of occlusion (excessive occlusal forces) that produce the lesion (trauma from occlusion) (Jin and Cao 1992;

Hallmon and Harrel 2004). P.R. Stillman has described it as an abnormal occlusal stress that is capable of producing or has produced an "injury to the periodontium" (Stillman 1921; Stillman and McCall 1922). See also occlusal trauma, trauma from occlusion.

Trench Mouth—The necrotizing ulcerative gingivitis that was found prevalent in mouths of soldiers who lived and worked in garrison and field life in proximity and intimacy during World War II (Schluger 1949b). It is now classified under necrotizing periodontal diseases as necrotizing ulcerative gingivitis (NUG) (Armitage 1999). See also acute necrotizing ulcerative gingivitis, acute ulcerative gingivitis, necrotizing periodontal diseases, necrotizing ulcerative gingivitis (NUG), ulceromembranous gingivitis, Vincent's angina infection.

Trifurcation—This refers to the normal anatomic division of the roots of a tooth, such as a maxillary first molar, into three parts (ADA 1950; AAP 2001a).

Trifurcation Involvement—The extension of a marginal periodontitis with pocket formation into the interradicular area, with concomitant bone loss, in a tooth with three roots (See Fig. H-5, large arrow) (Goldman and Cohen 1968; Ross and Thompson 1978). See also furcation invasion, furcation involvement.

Trisection—The surgical manipulation (sectioning and/or removal) of the roots of a three-rooted tooth, usually a maxillary first molar. It has been explained as a splitting of a maxillary molar into three separate components with removal of one or two of its roots (Greenstein et al. 1984). It has also been described as a splitting of the tooth with or without removal of the root with its accompanying crown portion for a maxillary molar (Saadoun 1985) It has also been mentioned as a splitting of a maxillary molar into three separate roots and their associated crown portion, keeping all three portions of the tooth in situ (Malone and Koth 1989).

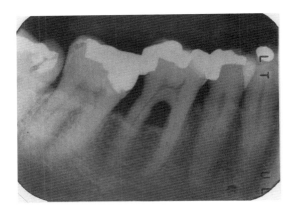

Fig. T-6a: Radiograph of tunneling

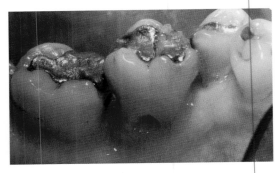

Fig. T-6c: Lingual view

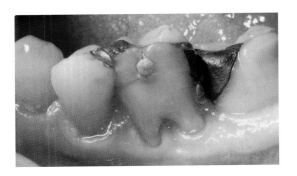

Fig. T-6b: Buccal view

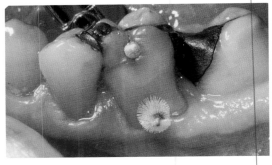

Fig. T-6d: Proximal cleaner through furcation (With permission from the American Dental Association)

Tunneling—A surgical procedure to create a tunnel (through-and-through opening) within a furcated tooth, preparing the furcation by completely opening it to enable postsurgical cleaning (See Fig. T-6a,b,c,d) (Hamp et al. 1975). It is achieved by root resection in maxillary molars and/or either odontoplasty, osteoplasty, ostectomy, and associated soft tissue surgery, as in the mandibular molars, to permit postsurgical access for mechanical plaque removal. This procedure is most applicable to mandibular molars (Highfield 1978; Vandersall and Detamore 2002).

Turesky-Gilmore-Glickman Index—A modified plaque index that reveals and records microbial plaque following the system devised by Gertrude Quigley and John Hein in 1962. The modification consists in the method of recording/reporting plaque severity. A score of 0 is given for each surface scored as low (0 or 1) and a score of 1 for each surface scored as high (2 or more) (Turesky et al. 1970). See also Quigley-Hein plaque index.

U

Ulceromembranous Gingivitis—This is an archaic synonym for necrotizing ulcerative gingivitis (Armitage 1999). It is clinically characterized by necrosis and ulceration of the interdental papilla with possible necrosis of the attached gingiva up to the mucogingival junction (MacPhee and Beagrie 1962) See also acute necrotizing ulcerative gingivitis (ANUG), acute ulcerative gingivitis, necrotizing periodontal diseases, necrotizing ulcerative gingivitis (NUG), trench mouth, Vincent's angina infection.

Ultrasonics, Rotary—Rotary ultrasonics, also known as Rotosonics, is achieved through using a revolving/vibratory bur with an up-and-down motion for the purpose of debriding calculus from a tooth. The bur consists of six sides with six obtuse corners and, while producing 20,000 cycles per second, it is applied circumferentially around the curvature of the tooth (Ellman 1962, 1964).

Ultrasonics, Vibratory—Vibratory ultrasonics are produced by an instrument tip attached to a transducer through which high-frequency current causes vibrations, approximately 25,000 to 30,000 cycles per second. These vibrations, accompanied by a water stream, produce a turbulence that, in turn, removes adherent deposits from the tooth. The working tip of the instrument moves in a reciprocating distance of 0.0015 cm or 1/1000 in. Doran D. Zinner first reported the application of ultrasonics to periodontics for the purpose of calculus removal in the presence of water (Zinner 1955a, 1955b). See recent position paper on sonic and ultrasonic scaling in periodontics (AAP 2000c). See also magnetostrictive, piezoelectric, sonic instrumentation.

Undermining Resorption—When excessive pressure produces a necrosis of the periodontal ligament, the necrotic mass is slowly eliminated by resorption of the bone adjacent to the area of pressure necrosis. This type of bone resorption is known as undermining resorption because the necrotic area is resorbed from the rear, where the tissue is vital (Grant et al. 1988). See also frontal resorption, rear resorption.

Unembellished Gingivectomy—The surgical removal of excess gingival tissue with a 45-degree bevel using a Kirkland gingivectomy knife. It is performed without the factitious addition or embellishment of (1) preliminary scaling; (2) drugs such as silver nitrate, zinc chloride, or trichloracetic acid; or (3) plastic procedures (i.e., gingivoplasty) (Kirkland 1942; Goldman 1950; Glickman 1956).

University of Mississippi Oral Hygiene Index (UM-OHI)—This index is a simple method for recording the presence of plaque. It utilizes a combination of the Patient Hygiene Performance Index

(PHP-I) for its tooth demarcations and the periodontal screening and recording (PSR) with its recording instrument. Twelve sections (six buccal and six lingual sextants) are examined (similar to the PSR) and the tooth surfaces are divided into five sections according to the PHP-I. A score of 0 is given for the absence and a score of 1 is given for the presence of plaque. The highest score for each sextant is recorded and then the examiner moves to the next sextant, as in the PSR. The letters P (proximal) and G (gingival) are added to the sextant score to show sur-faces involved (Silberman et al. 1998). See also Patient Hygiene Performances Index (PHP-I), periodontal screening and recording (PSR).

Unrepositioned Mucoperiosteal Flap—This is a mucoperiosteal flap with inverted beveled incisions followed by osseous resection. It is then returned (i.e., unrepositioned) to its original position for the preservation of attached gingiva, maintenance of vestibular depth, and coverage of bone. It is based on the original operation of Leonard Widman (Widman 1917; Morris 1965b). See also replaced flap.

V

Vertical Bone Loss—In the classification of periodontal pockets, vertical bone loss refers to the loss of interdental bone at an acute angle to the root surface, often called angular bone loss (See Fig. V-1a,b) (Fedi et al. 2000). According to Adolph Berger, the first person to classify and describe vertical bone loss was Oskar Weski in 1921. He described it as "pocket formation occurring parallel to the long axis of the tooth," and Weski is said also to have called it "vertical pyorrhea" (Berger 1927). See also horizontal bone loss.

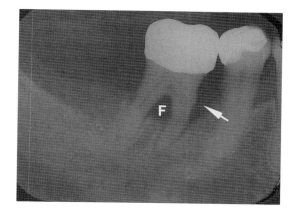

Fig. V-1a: Arrow, vertical bone loss; F, furcation invasion

Vertical Defect Dimension (VDD)—In the placement of immediate dental implants, this term refers to the vertical distance (i.e., dimension) as measured in millimeters from the coronal level of the implant surface to the apex of the bony defect (i.e., socket) (Wilson et al. 1998). See also horizontal defect dimension (HDD); implant, immediate.

Vertical Extrusion—This is a technique of orthodontic movement of erupting teeth in a vertical direction by well-controlled moderate forces. Several benefits can be derived from this procedure. First, teeth that were classified as nonrestorable due to trauma, extensive decay, or periodontal problems can be satisfactorily restored through the coronal movement of the osseous housing and associated attachment apparatus (Ingber 1974; Biggerstaff et al. 1986; Levine 1988). It is a multidiscipli-

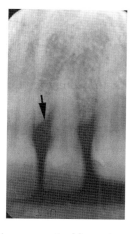

Fig. V-1b: Arrow, vertical bone loss

nary approach to increasing the length or amount of clinical crown with the assistance of orthodontic movement (Ries et al. 1988). Second, orthodontic extrusion (vertical extrusion) has been shown to increase the osseous housing of periodontally hopeless teeth for future placement of dental implants (Salama and Salama 1993; Minsk 2000). See also forced eruption.

Vertical Gingival Pedicle Graft—Also known as the apically repositioned flap described by Nathan Friedman in 1962 (Ratcliff 1966). See also apically repositioned flap.

Vertical Grooving—An osteoplastic procedure to vertically contour the interdental septum so as to blend together the papillae and adjacent areas for deflecting food during mastication (See Fig. R-1) (Ochsenbein 1958; Selipsky 1976). See also festooning, osteoplasty, radicular blending.

Vertical Incision—Vertical incisions are made during periodontal flap surgery for relaxation of the flap in order to gain access to underlying structures. They are placed at the line angles of the teeth and extend through the mucogingival junction to provide maximum mobility of the flap (Johnson, RH 1976). This term is synonymous with *releasing incision* (AAP 2001a).

Vertical Internal Mattress Suture—This suturing technique is applicable in the preservation of esthetics in the "curtain technique" (Frisch et al. 1967). It allows the palatal flap to adapt tightly to the underlying bone while retaining the facial papilla in its original position. Long, thin papillae are best treated with the vertical internal mattress suture, while short, wide papillae are best managed with the horizontal internal mattress suture (Newell and Brunsvold 1985). See also horizontal internal mattress suture, suture.

Vertical Mattress Suture—In this suturing technique, the suture material is kept from under the flap margin and can be used to advantage when the wick effect of the suture would be undesirable. An example of its use would be closing a flap margin over implantation of osseous grafts. Care must be exercised to grasp the attached gingiva with the needle and not the mucosa (Dahlberg 1969; Levin 1980). See also suture, wicking.

Vertical Toothbrushing Technique—With this technique of toothbrushing, the anterior teeth are positioned end-to-end with the bristles of the toothbrush placed at right angles to the facial surfaces of the teeth. The bristles are moved up and down, brushing both maxillary and mandibular teeth with the bristle ends while the gums are massaged with the sides of the bristles. For the lingual surface, the same motion is used with the teeth apart, with the sides of the bristles used to massage the gums (Shick and Ash 1961; Ray 2005). This toothbrushing technique is very similar to the Leonard toothbrushing technique. See also Leonard toothbrushing technique.

Vestibuloplasty—This is an archaic term referring to numerous procedures to deepen the vestibular trough, reposition or increasing the zone of attached gingival, or a combination involving both the alveolar mucosa and the gingival mucosa (Beckham et al. 1962; AAP 2001a). It has been used to refer to the frenectomy, deepening the vestibule, and/or broadening the attached gingiva or gingival repositioning (Glickman 1953). Other names for this procedure are *vestibular deepening* (Friedman 1957), *vestibular trough extension* (Robinson 1957), and *vestibular sulcus extension* (Bergenholtz and Hugoson 1967).

Vibratory Toothbrushing Technique—This involves the placement of the toothbrush horizontal to the long axis of the tooth and with the bristle ends resting on the tooth surfaces. A very short mesiodistal stroke is executed, with pressure applied as the bristle ends enter the embrasures between the teeth covered by the brush. The stroke is short so that it does not carry the bristles beyond the teeth upon which they rested before the stroke was begun

(Sarrazin 1920; Ray 2005). Examples of the vibratory technique used during toothbrushing would be the Bass, Charters, modified Bass, and Stillman techniques of toothbrushing.

Vincent's Angina Infection—This is a discarded term for necrotizing ulcerative gingivitis, which is now classified as one of two necrotizing periodontal diseases (Armitage 1999). It is named after Jean Henri Vincent, a French physician and bacteriologist who stated that the causative organisms for this mouth malady were fusiform and spirochete bacteria (Vincent 1896). See also acute necrotizing ulcerative gingivitis (ANUG), acute ulcerative gingivitis, necrotizing periodontal disease, necrotizing ulcerative gingivitis (NUG), trench mouth, ulceromembranous gingivitis.

Volpe-Manhold Calculus Index (V-M)—This method of measuring calculus formation is limited to the lingual surface of the six mandibular incisors. A periodontal probe, graduated in millimeters, is taped at the 1 and 3 mm markings with colored tape to facilitate the ease of reading. The probe is inserted to the most inferior border of visible calculus in such a manner as to bisect the lingual surface of the lower "incisors" or to reach diagonally through the greatest height of calculus formation. The V-M index is the summation of the millimeter readings of the height of calculus on the lingual surfaces of these six teeth (Volpe and Manhold 1962; Volpe et al. 1965).

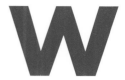

Ward's Wonderpak—The first zinc-oxide eugenol periodontal dressing utilized for wound protection. In addition to zinc-oxide eugenol, it consisted of finely ground crystals of copper sulfate, alcohol, pine oil, and asbestos fibers. According to Ward, the spelling for this periodontal dressing is "Wondrpak" (Ward 1929). See also periodontal dressing.

Wicking—The tracking of bacteria and oral fluids along the suture strands into the wound. It has been shown that less bacterial wicking occurs in a monofilament suture than in a multifilament suture (Lilly 1968; Lilly et al. 1968, 1969, 1972). Although wicking is not a true iatrogenic action, the deleterious side effects of retained multifilament silk suture material are reversible once the affecting agent (i.e., suture) is removed (Manor and Kaffe 1982). See also iatrogenic, suture.

Widman Flap—The Widman flap was originally designed by Leonard Widman for pocket elimination and not for reattachment (i.e., new attachment). There was high flap reflection for root debridement, but the flaps did not cover interproximal bone and it remained exposed postsurgically (Widman 1917, 1918). There is a description of the Widman flap in the current literature (Caffesse 1980; Everett et al. 1971).

Widow's Peak—This term refers to the buccal and/or lingual alveolar bone that remains on the line angles of teeth following traditional ramping of a shallow interproximal crater (See Fig. W-1a,b,c,d,e,f,g) (Schluger 1949a). These line-angled peaks

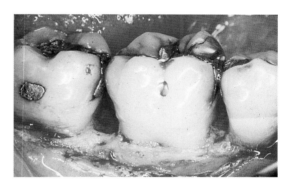

Fig. W-1a: Osseous crater between molars (With permission from the American Dental Association)

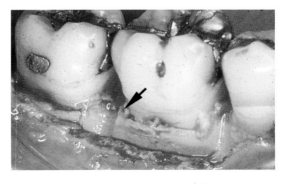

Fig. W-1b: Arrow, widow's peak following grooving of bone

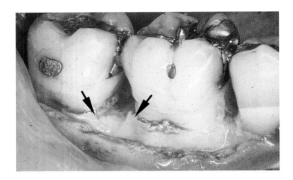

Fig. W-1c: Arrows, widow's peaks prior to osteoplasty

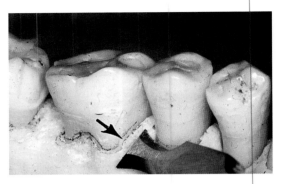

Fig. W-1f: Bone chisel used to remove widow's peaks

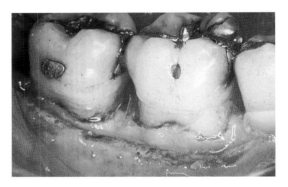

Fig. W-1d: Widow's peak removed with ostectomy (With permission from the Indiana Dental Association)

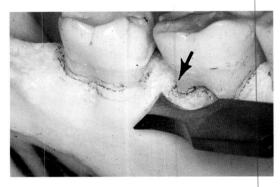

Fig. W-1g: Bone chisel used to remove widow's peaks)

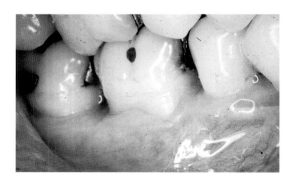

Fig. W-1e: Complete tissue healing following osteoplasty and ostectomy of widow's peaks

of bone are corrected by either buccal or lingual ostectomy to achieve positive architecture and thus to prevent the return of soft tissue pocketing (Selipsky 1976).

Working Side—In the study of occlusion, this term refers to the maxillomandibular occlusion on the chewing or bolus side. It is the opposite of the balancing or nonworking side (Posselt 1968; AAP 2001a). See also balancing side, nonworking side.

Woven Bone—This type of bone is characterized by high cellularity, loosely arranged bundles of collagen fibers, and mineralization, which is highly variable. It is a highly labile type of bone that is easily formed and resorbed. It is observed most frequently during embryogenesis and bone healing in adults. There is no oriented arrangement of collagen fibers characteristic of lamellated bone (Grant et al. 1988). This type of bone is insufficient to accept load-bearing forces of dental implants (Misch 1988). See also bundle bone, lamellar bone.

Xenograft—A tissue graft between members of different species (Mellonig 1992, 1998; AAP 2001a). A classic example of a xenograft used in rebuilding lost alveolar bone is a processed bovine bone called Boplant (Arrocha et al. 1968). Also known as a xenogenic or xenogeneic graft (Wirthlin 1987). See also heterograft.

Z

Zinc Oxide Eugenol Dressing—A periodontal dressing containing 40 to 50 percent free eugenol. Although this periodontal pack caused tissue necrosis and delayed healing, it was popular owing to its obtundent effect on sensitive dentin and connective tissue (Glickman 1960). See also periodontal dressing.

Zinc Oxide Noneugenol Dressing—This periodontal dressing, containing no eugenol, consisted of zinc oxide, various oils and fats, rosin, and a bacteriostatic or fungicidal agent (Baer et al. 1960).

Zooglea—According to Sumter Arnim (Arnim 1964), G.V. Black defined zooglea as mucous membrane secretions that form a slimy gel coating that lines the oral cavity, covering the teeth as well as the mucosa (Black 1911). It forms a nutrient and an environmental media for the development of billions of microbes. Because of the nature of this gel, the adherent masses cannot be effectively removed by water or by antiseptic mouthwashes. The gel also protects the bacterial colonies from the possible neutralizing effects of saliva (Masters 1969). Sumter Arnim refers to zooglea in several of his publications (Arnim and Sandell 1960; Arnim 1966).

Appendix

A

Aas, E
   See gingival hyperplasia – grade

Abbott, BH
   See gindex index

Abdallah, E
   See laminin

Abrams, H
   See iatrogenic

Abrams, L
   See deepithelized connective tissue pedicle graft

Adair, RB
   See Riggs' disease

Adams, DF
   See osseous graft

Ahuja, V
   See Papillon-LeFevre syndrome

Ainamo, A
   See mucogingival junctions

Ainamo, J
   See community periodontal index of treatment needs (CPITN)

Aisenberg, MS
   See acellular cementum; cellular cementum

Albander, JM
   See early onset periodontitis

Alexander, AG
   See subgingival calculus; supragingival calculus

Allen, AL
   See free soft tissue autograft; Raetzke's pouch; supraperiosteal envelope

Allen, EP
   See cosmetic periodontal surgery; crown lengthening; modified Stillman's toothbrushing technique; ridge defects (classification)

Ammons, WF
   See blunt dissection

Angelopoulos, AP
   See gingival hyperplasia – grade

Angle, EH
   See Angle classification of malocclusion

Antczak-Bouckoms, A
   See meta-analysis

Ariaudo, AA
   See periodontoplasty

Armitage, GC
   See aggressive periodontitis; generalized juvenile periodontitis (GJP); gingival crevicular fluid (GCF); hereditary gingival fibromatosis; HIV associated gingivitis (HIV-G); HIV associated periodontitis (HIV-P); juvenile periodontitis; localized juvenile periodontitis (LJP); necrotizing periodontal diseases; Papillon-LeFevre syndrome; periodontal diseases; periodontitis; periodontosis; precocious periodontitis; pregnancy gingivitis; prepubertal periodontitis; prognostic factor; rapidly progressive periodontitis (RPP); refractory periodontitis; trench mouth; ulceromembranous gingivitis; Vincent's angina infection

Arnim, SS
    See circular fiber group; disclosing agent; ligamentum circulare dentis; microcosm; POH; zooglea
Arrocha, R
    See xenograft
Ash, MM
    See periodontal disease index (PDI)
Assaf, ME
    See cinguloradicular groove
Augsburger, RA
    See bicuspidization; hemisection
August, DS
    See radicular lingual groove
Azzi, R
    See electrocoagulation; electrodesiccation; electrofulguration; electrosection; electrosurgery

B

Bacic, M
    See palatal groove
Baer, PN
    See Baer-Sumner fat pack; juvenile periodontitis; periodontosis; zinc oxide noneugenol dressing
Bahat, O
    See advanced flap; periodontal flap; ridge preservation; rotational flap; transpositional flap
Baiorunos, JR
    See root demineralization
Barnes, GP
    See gingival indices; index (pl. indices); irreversible index; periodontal index (pl. indices); reversible index
Barnes, JE
    See new attachment
Barrington, EP
    See envelope flap; full-thickness flap; long junctional epithelium; partial-thickness flap
Basaraba, N
    See hemisection; root amputation; root resection
Bass, CC
    See Bass toothbrushing technique; Modified Bass toothbrushing technique; POH

Baum, BJ
    See fibronectin
Beaumont, RH
    See long junctional epithelium
Beck, JD
    See systemic periodontitis
Becker, NG
    See presuturing
Becker, W
    See biologic width; crown lengthening; gingival morphotype; open probing clinical attachment; open probing new attachment
Beckham, LC
    See gingivectomy; mucoalveolar gingival surgery; vestibuloplasty
Belcher, JM
    See periodontal microsurgery
Bell, DG
    See Bell toothbrushing technique; physiologic toothbrushing technique
Ben-Bassat, Y
    See labiogingival notch
Benjamin, SD
    See periodontosis
Bennet, NG
    See Bennett movement
Bergenholtz, A
    See Edlan-Mejchar technique; radectomy; vestibuloplasty
Berger, A
    See horizontal bone loss; vertical bone loss
Berliner, A
    See Berliner epithelial scalpel
Berman, CL
    See peri-implantitis
Bernimoulin, JP
    See coronally repositioned flap
Beube, FE
    See bone powder; heterogenous bone; interdental resection; interproximal denudation
Bhaskar, SN
    See alveolar process; cyanoacrylates
Bierly, JA
    See osseous filtration
Biggerstaff, RH
    See vertical extrusion
Bjorby, A
    See retention index (RI)

Bjorn, H
See free soft tissue autograft
Bjorndahl, O
See BULL rule; MUDL rule
Black, AD
See epidemiology; epithelial cuff
Black, GV
See calculus (dental); radectomy; root amputation; Sharpey's fibers; zooglea
Block, MS
See onplant
Blomlof, J
See smear layer
Bodecker, CF
See corrosion; gingival crevicular fluid
Bohannon, HM
See fixed long labial mucosal flap; periosteal retention
Bohenkamp, DM
See hemisection
Bosshardt, DD
See cementum
Bowers, GM
See coronectomy; periodontal probe
Box, HK
See periodontium; traumatogenic occlusion
Boyne, PJ
See implant, subperiosteal; sinus lift graft
Brady, JM
See plaque-free zone
Bral, MM
See crevicular epithelium
Branemark, PI
See osseointegration
Brooks, SJ
See amelogenins
Brown, FH
See magnetostrictive; piezoelectric
Brown, IS
See molar uprighting
Brunsvold, MA
See allograft; autogenous bone graft
Bulyhuis, HM
See periodontal probe
Burch, JG
See molar uprighting

Buser, D
See guided bone regeneration (GBR); ridge augmentation
Butler, BL
See plaque assessment scoring system (PASS)
Butler, JH
See juvenile periodontitis; myofascial pain dysfunction syndrome (MPD)

C

Caffesse, RG
See coronally repositioned flap; incisal repositioning flap; modified Widman flap (MWF); periodontal probe; Widman flap
Camelo, M
See tissue engineering
Cameron, CE
See cracked-tooth syndrome
Campbell, PM
See circumferential supracrestal fiberotomy (CSF)
Cantor, MT
See interdental col
Card, SJ
See new attachment
Carlos, JP
See extent and severity index (ESI)
Carlson, NE
See platelet-rich plasma (PRP)
Carnevale, G
See osseous resection
Carranza, FA Jr.
See gomphosis; Karolyi effect; ligamentum circulare dentis; nonspecific plaque hypothesis; osseous resection; osteoplasty; periodontal-endodontic lesion; periodontal probe; periodontosis; primary occlusal trauma; prognosis; pyorrhea alveolaris; radicular blending; Riggs' disease; Schmutz pyorrhea; suprabony pocket; tartar
Carranza, FA Sr.
See osseous resection
Carter, HG
See gingival bleeding index (GBI)

Frisch, J
See curtain technique; horizontal internal mattress suture; vertical internal mattress suture

Frohman, BS
See bruxism; bruxomania

Fullmer, HM
See oxytalan fiber

G

Gage, AA
See cryosurgery

Gantes, BG
See coronally displaced flap

Gara, GG
See osseous graft

Garber, DA
See deepithelized connective tissue pedicle graft

Gargiulo, AW
See biologic width; dentogingival junction; displaced flap; passive eruption

Garnick, J
See rest position

Garrett, S
See coronally positioned flap; periodontal regeneration

Genco, RJ
See risk factor; specific plaque hypothesis

Giannobile, WV
See tissue engineering

Giansanti, JS
See Papillon–Le Fevre syndrome

Gillan, DG
See iontophoresis

Gillette, WB
See flossing clefts; iatrogenic

Glick, M
See HIV-associated gingivitis (HIV-G); necrotizing ulcerative periodontitis (NUP); periodontal medicine

Glickman, I
See bifurcation involvement; bone factor; buttressing bone; calciphylaxis; chronic desquamative gingivitis (CDG); codestructive factor; furcation classification (Glickman); gingival enlargement; peri-

odontal ligament; periodontoclasia; preventive occlusal adjustment; trauma from occlusion; unembellished gingivectomy; vestibuloplasty; zinc oxide eugenol dressing

Goldman, HM
See acellular cementum; cellular cementum; circumferential defect; codestructive factor; complete denudation; crater defect; creeping attachment; frenectomy; furcation classification (Goldman and Cohen); furcation involvement; gingival extension; gingivoplasty; hemiseptum (pl. hemisepta); infrabony defect; interdental grooves; interdental papilla; interproximal crater; local extension of the vestibular trough; mucogingival defect; mucogingival line; mucogingival surgery; odontoplasty; physiologic regeneration; pushback procedure; stippling; suprabony pocket; trifurcation involvement; unembellished gingivectomy

Goodson, JM
See random burst hypothesis

Gorlin, RJ
See hereditary gingival fibromatosis; Papillon–Le Fevre syndrome

Gottlieb, B
See active eruption; cementopathia; diffuse alveolar atrophy; epithel ansatz; epithelial attachment; frontal resorption; periodontosis; rear resorption; Schmutz pyorrhea

Gottsegan, R
See frenectomy; frenum

Grant, DA
See undermining resorption; woven bone

Greenberg, J
See transgingival probing

Greene, AH
See stippling

Greene, JC
See oral hygiene index (OHI); oral hygiene index simplified (OHI-S)

Greenstein, G
See periodontal probe; interdental crest; ridge preservation; trisection

Greenwell, H
See geriatric periodontics; Keyes technique

Luebke, RG
  See mucoperiosteal flap; sulcular incision
Lynch, SE
  See tissue engineering
Lyons, H
  See periodontium

M

Machtei, EE
  See established periodontitis
MacLeod, KM
  See index of gingival architecture form
MacPhee, IT
  See ulceromembranous gingivitis
Magnusson, I
  See long junctional epithelium
Malassez, LC
  See epithelial rests of Malassez
Malone, WFP
  See trisection
Mann, AW
  See long centric
Manor, A
  See iatrogenic; wicking
Manson, JD
  See interdental crater; interproximal crater; lamina dura
Marie, MM
  See bruxomania
Mariotti, A
  See gingivitis
Marks, RG
  See index (pl. indices); papilla bleeding index (PBI); papillary bleeding score (PBS); periodontal index (pl. indices)
Marx, RE
  See platelet-rich plasma (PRP)
Massler, M
  See papillary marginal attached index (PMA); papillary marginal gingivitis index (PMGI)
Masters, DH
  See cervical enamel projection (CEP); zooglea
Matia, JI
  See furcation dome

Matter, J
  See creeping attachment
Mayfield, LJA
  See implant, delayed; implant, late
Maynard, JG
  See gingival augmentation; intracrevicular; mucogingival defect; mucogingival problem
McAllister, BS
  See distraction osteogenesis
McCall, JO
  See pericementum
McFall, WT
  See lateral repositioned flap
McGraw, VA
  See cyanoacrylates
McGuire, MK
  See evidence-based periodontal treatment; prognosis
Meffert, RW
  See biointegration; implant, ailing; implant, failed; implant, failing; implant, vitreous carbon; peri-implantitis
Melcher, AH
  See alveolar bone proper; guided tissue regeneration (GTR); interpapillary fiber group
Mellonig, JT
  See allograft; attachment apparatus; decalcified freeze-dried bone allograft (DFDBA); demineralized freeze-dried bone allograft (DFDBA); freeze-dried bone allograft (FDBA); guided bone regeneration (GBR); heterograft; new attachment; osteoinduction; reattachment; repair; xenograft
Melsen, B
  See orthodontic intrusion
Mercuri, LG
  See myofascial pain dysfunction syndrome (MPD)
Merritt, AH
  See pyorrhea alveolaris
Miller, PD
  See gingival recession; mucogingival surgery; oral plastic surgery; periodontal plastic surgery; periosteal separation; root biomodification; secondary root coverage

gingival rebound; osteoplasty; palatal approach; positive architecture; reverse architecture; root trunk; vertical grooving

O'Connor, TW
See osseous defect

Odrich, RB
See cryosurgery

Ogilvie, AL
See periodontal maintenance (PM); periodontal recall

Okeson, JP
See temporomandibular disorders (TMD)

Older, LB
See heterogenous bone

O'Leary, TJ
See community periodontal index of treatment needs (CPITN); gingival-periodontal index (GPI); Hawthorne effect; microperiodontometer; plaque control record

Olsson, M
See periodontal biotype

Orban, BJ
See alveolar bone proper; alveolar crest fiber group; alveolar mucosa; alveolar process; alveolodental ligament; alveologingival fiber group; apical fiber group; attached epithelial cuff; attached gingiva; cribriform plate; dentogingival fiber group; dentoperiosteal fiber group; epithelial rests of Malassez; free gingiva; free gingival groove; gingiva; gingival epithelium; gingival fiber group; gingival hypertrophy; gingival pocket; gingival sulcus; Hertwig epithelial root sheath; horizontal fiber group; interdental grooves; interdental papilla; interradicular fiber group; localized juvenile periodontitis (LJP); margin of the gingiva; marginal gingiva; mucogingival junction; mucogingival line; oblique fiber group; oral epithelium; oral mucosa; periodontal ligament; periodontal pocket; periodontosis; prosthetic gingival veneer; root planing; Sharpey's fibers; stippling; supporting alveolar bone; transseptal fiber group

Owings, JR
See gingivostomatitis

P

Page, RC
See cementopathia; growth and differentiation factors; periodontal risk calculator (PRC); prepubertal periodontitis; rapidly progressive periodontitis (RPP); risk factor; risk indicator; risk predictor

Papillon, MM
See Papillon-LeFevre syndrome

Paquette, DW
See periodontal medicine

Parfitt, GJ
See tooth mobility

Patur, B
See pedicle flap

Pennel, BM
See free masticatory mucosa graft; oblique rotated flap; transpositional flap

Perlitsh, MJ
See critical mass of alveolar bone support; tooth mobility

Perry, DA
See modified Bass toothbrushing technique

Perry, HO
See gingivostomatitis

Persson, GR
See periodontal risk calculator (PRC)

Pfeifer, J
See lateral repositioned flap

Phillips, JM
See temporomandibular disorders (TMD)

Pick, RM
See laser

Picton, DCA
See tooth mobility

Pihlstrom, PL
See inflammatory index (II)

Pini Prato, GP
See tissue engineering

Podshadley, AG
See patient hygiene performance index (PHP-I)

Pollack, RP
See closed crevicular curettage; curettage; geriatric periodontics; modified distal wedge

Polson, AM
See root biomodification; smear layer

Robinson, PG
   See linear gingival erythema (LGE)
Robinson, RE
   See bone blending; denudation; distal wedge; free mucosal graft; frenulumectomy; lateral repositioned flap; oblique rotated flap; osseous coagulum; periosteal fenestration; vestibuloplasty
Rockoff, SC
   See histologic reattachment
Ronderos, M
   See risk factor
Rosen, PS
   See osseous graft
Rosenberg, ES
   See tooth lengthening
Rosenberg, MM
   See lateral repositioned flap
Rosenberg, RM
   See inflammatory index (II)
Rosenthal, P
   See semilunar coronally repositioned flap
Rosner, D
   See continuous suture
Ross, IF
   See trifurcation involvement
Ross, SE
   See contiguous autogenous transplant; double papillae repositioned flap
Rotstein, I
   See periodontal-endodontic lesion
Rowland, RW
   See necrotizing ulcerative gingivitis (NUG)
Rubach, WC
   See periodontal-endodontic lesion
Rubleman, PA
   See interdental papillae graft; oblique rotated flap
Russell, AL
   See full mouth indices; occlusion feature index (OFI); periodontal index (PI)
Ryan, ME
   See host modulatory therapy (HMT)

S

Saadoun, AP
   See esthetic zone; flute; furcation; interradicular; root roof; root separation; trisection

Saari, JT
   See bony defect; crater defect; inconsistent bony margin; interdental crater; interproximal crater; osseous defect
Saglie, R
   See plaque-free zone
Saklad, M
   See ASA classification
Salama, H
   See vertical extrusion
Salkin, LM
   See periodontal screening and recording (PSR)
Sandler, HC
   See periodontal disease rate (PDR)
Sarrazin, JJ
   See vibratory toothbrushing technique
Saxer, UP
   See papilla bleeding index (PBI); Stillman's toothbrushing technique
Scannapieco, FA
   See periodontal medicine
Schallhorn, RG
   See guided tissue regeneration (GTR); iliac crest autograft; periodontal maintenance (PM); periodontal maintenance therapy (PMT)
Schei, O
   See Schei ruler
Schluger, S
   See hemiseptum (pl. hemisepta); inconsistent bony margin; interproximal crater; osseous resection; positive architecture; trench mouth; widow's peak
Schmid, MO
   See cervical plaque index (CPI)
Schour, I
   See gingivosis; papillary marginal attached index (PMA)
Schroeder, A
   See functional ankylosis
Schroeder, HE
   See junctional epithelium
Schuyler, CH
   See BULL rule; freedom in centric
Schwartz, RS
   See tooth accumulated material (TAM)
Scully, C
   See cyclic neutropenia

Stein, G
    See bundle bone
Stern, IB
    See gingivectomy; junctional epithelium
Stewart, DJ
    See factitial gingival traumatism
Stillman, PR
    See gingival festoons; McCall's festoons; Stillman's clefts; Stillman's toothbrushing technique; traumatic occlusion
Stones, HH
    See new attachment
Sugarman, E
    See pedicle flap
Sugarman, M
    See precocious periodontitis
Sullivan, HC
    See bridging; free soft tissue autograft; gingival recession
Sumner, CF
    See incisal repositioning flap
Suomi, JD
    See dental health center (DHC) index
Swan, RH
    See cervical enamel projection (CEP)
Swenson, HM
    See gingival prosthesis

T

Tagger, M
    See radisectomy
Takei, HH
    See internal bevel incision; mattress suture; papilla preservation technique
Tan, AES
    See disclosing agent
Tandy, RB
    See gingival curettage
Tarnow, DP
    See furcation classification (Tarnow and Fletcher); interdental papilla; interproximal papilla; semilunar coronally repositioned flap
Tatum, H
    See sinus lift graft
Ten Cate, AR
    See cementum; intermediate cementum

Terranova, VP
    See laminin
Thebaud, J
    See root curettage
Theilade, E
    See nonspecific plaque hypothesis
Thoma, KH
    See paradontosis
Tibbetts, LS Jr
    See lingual approach; periodontal microsurgery; periodontal probe; transgingival probing
Tinti, C
    See coronally positioned palatal sliding flap
Turesky, S
    See Quigley-Hein plaque index; Turesky-Gilmore-Glickman index

U

Uitto, V-J
    See gingival crevicular fluid (GCF)
Urist, MR
    See bone morphogenetic protein (BMP); demineralized freeze-dried bone allograft (DFDBA); osteoinduction

V

Valentini, P
    See composite graft; sinus lift graft
Vandersall, DC
    See iatrogenic; tunneling
van der Velden, U
    See periodontal pocket bleeding index (PPBI)
Van Dyke, TE
    See cytokines
Van Kirk, LE
    See malalignment index
Vincent, HJ
    See Vincent's angina infection
Vincent, JW
    See tension test
Volchansky, A
    See delayed passive eruption

Volpe, AR
    See Volpe-Manhold calculus index (V-M)

W

Waerhaug, J
    See attached epithelial cuff; epithelial cuff; plaque-free zone
Wagenberg, BD
    See crown lengthening; preventive treatment visit (PTV)
Walton, RE
    See iontophoresis
Waltzer, RE
    See coronal migration
Wang, H-L
    See periodontal regeneration
Wannenmacher, E
    See periodontosis
Ward, AW
    See Ward's Wonderpak
Watts, TLP
    See confirm bleeding day index
Waugh, ILM
    See periodontal ligament
Weinberg, MA
    See delayed passive eruption; intrabony defect
Weinmann, JP
    See bundle bone; lamellar bone
Weinstein, E
    See gingival crevicular fluid (GCF)
Weiss, CM
    See fibroosseous integration
Wentz, FM
    See occlusal trauma
Wertheimer, FW
    See acquired cuticle; Berliner epithelial scalpel; Nasmyth's membrane; primary cuticle; secondary cuticle
Weski, O
    See horizontal bone loss; paradentium; pyorrhea alveolaris; vertical bone loss
Whinston, GJ
    See mucobuccal fold resection
Whitman, DH
    See platelet-rich plasma (PRP)

Widman, L
    See modified Widman flap; reverse bevel incision; unrepositioned mucoperiosteal flap; Widman flap
Wilderman, MN
    See pedicle flap; pedicle graft; periosteal retention
Williams, RC
    See periodontal diseases; periodontal medicine; tissue engineering
Wilson, RD
    See intracrevicular
Wilson, TG Jr.
    See horizontal defect dimension (HDD); implant, immediate; vertical defect dimension (VDD)
Winkler, JR
    See linear gingival erythema (LGE)
Wirthlin, MR
    See allogenic; osseous surgery; osteoconduction; xenograft
Wise, RJ
    See Clark's rule
Wynbrandt, J
    See tartar

Y

Yankell, SL
    See horizontal toothbrushing technique; roll toothbrushing technique; physiologic toothbrushing technique; Stillman's toothbrushing technique
Younger, WJ
    See root amputation
Yukna, RA
    See alloplast; excisional new attachment procedure (ENAP); long junctional epithelium; repair
Yuodelis, RA
    See external bevel gingivectomy; internal bevel gingivectomy; non-working-side interference

Z

Zamet, JS
    See apically displaced split flap; inverse bevel incision

References

Abbreviation Key

AAID: American Academy of Implant Dentistry
AAO: American Association of Orthodontists
AAP: American Academy of Periodontology
ADA: American Dental Association
ADA/AAP: American Dental Association/ American Academy of Periodontology
AP: Academy of Prosthodontics
WHO: World Health Organization

AAID. Glossary of implant terms. J Oral Implant 1986;12(2):284

AAO. Orthodontic Glossary: Glossary of dentofacial orthopedic terms. St. Louis: American Association of Orthodontists, 1993

AAP. Report of the Committee on Nomenclature of the American Academy of Periodontology. J Periodontol 1937;8:88

AAP. Report of the Committee on Nomenclature of the American Academy of Periodontology. J Periodontol 1947;18:174

AAP. Announcements. J Periodontol 1965;36:86,431

AAP. World Workshop in Periodontics, Ann Arbor, Michigan, June 6-9, 1966

AAP. Report of the Special Committee on the NIH-NIDR study on Periodontal Therapy. Chicago: American Academy of Periodontology, Sept 21, 1984

AAP. Guidelines for Periodontal Therapy. Chicago: American Academy of Periodontology, Oct 1988

AAP. Proceedings of the World Workshop in Clinical Periodontics. Nevins, M, Becker, W, Kornman, K, eds. Chicago: American Academy of Periodontology, July 23-27, 1989

AAP. Position Paper: Periodontal care of the older patient: An informational report. Chicago: American Academy of Periodontology, April 1994

AAP. Current Terminology for Periodontics and Insurance Reporting Manual, 7th ed. Chicago: American Academy of Periodontology, 1995

AAP. Position Paper: epidemiology of periodontal diseases. J Periodontol 1996a;67:935

AAP. Periodontal literature reviews: A summary of current knowledge. Chicago: American Academy of Periodontology, 1996b:39

AAP. Parameters of Care. Chicago: American Academy of Periodontology, 1996c

AAP. Position paper: Lasers in periodontics. J Periodontol 1996d;67:826

AAP. Position paper: The potential role of growth and differentiation factors in periodontal regeneration. J Periodontol 1996e;67:545

AAP. Position paper: Supportive periodontal therapy (SPT). J Periodontol 1998a;69:502

AAP. Position paper: Periodontal Disease as a potential risk factor for systemic diseases. J Periodontol 1998b;69:841

AAP. Position paper: Guidelines for periodontal therapy. J Periodontol 1998c;69:405

AAP. Position paper: Current understanding of the role of microscopic monitoring, baking soda and hydrogen peroxide in the treatment of periodontal disease. J Periodontol 1998d; 69:951

AAP. Consensus report: Necrotizing periodontal diseases. Ann Periodontol 1999a;4(1):78

AAP. Position paper: Tobacco use and the periodontal patient. J Periodontol 1999b;70:1419

AAP. Parameters on placement and management of the dental implant: Supplement on parameters of care. J Periodontol 2000a;71:870

AAP. Position paper: Dental implants in periodontal therapy. J Periodontol 2000b;71:1934

AAP. Position paper: Sonic and ultrasonic scalers in periodontics. J Periodontol 2000c;71:1792

AAP. Parameter on mucogingival conditions: Supplement on parameters of care. J Periodontol 2000d;71:861

AAP. Position paper: The role of controlled drug delivery for periodontitis. J Periodontol 2000e; 71:125

AAP. Position paper: Supplement on parameters of care. J Periodontol 2000f;71:847

AAP. Glossary of Periodontal Terms, 4th ed. Chicago: American Academy of Periodontology, 2001a

AAP. Position paper: Tissue banking of bone allografts used in periodontal regeneration. J Periodontol 2001b;72:834

AAP. The American Academy of Periodontology statement regarding gingival curettage. J Periodontol 2002a;73:1229

AAP. Lasers in periodontics. J Periodontol 2002b; 73:1231

AAP. Position paper: Periodontal maintenance. J Periodontol 2003a;74:1395

AAP. Workshop on contemporary science in clinical periodontics. Ann Periodontol 2003b;8(1): 12–70

AAP. Informational paper: Drug-associated gingival enlargement. J Periodontol 2004;75:1424

AAP. Position paper: Epidemiology of periodontal diseases. J Periodontol 2005a;76:1406

AAP. Position paper: Periodontal regeneration. J Periodontol 2005b;76:1601

Aas, E. Hyperplasia gingivae diphenylhydantoinea. Acta Odont Scand Suppl 1963;21:1

Abbott, BH, Caffesse, RG. The reliability of a colorimetric test in determining gingival inflammation. J Periodontol 1978;49:564

Abdallah, E, Kon, S, Ruben, MP. Biochemical approach to periodontal regeneration: A Review of the literature. J West Soc Periodontol/ Periodontal Abstr 1988;36(2):53

Abrams, H, Barkmeier, WW, Murrin, JR. Gingival sequelae from a retained piece of rubber dam. Report of a case. J Ky Dent Assoc 1978; 30(4):21

Abrams, L. Augmentation of the deformed residual edentulous ridge for fixed prosthesis. Compend Contin Educ Dent 1980;1:205

ADA. Report of the Nomenclature Committee. J Am Dent Assoc 1943;30:1112

ADA. Reports of Councils "A study of Terms: The concept of bifurcation." J Am Dent Assoc 1950;41:250

ADA/AAP. Periodontal screening and recording training program kit. Chicago: American Dental Association, 1992

Adair, RB. Riggs' disease, from the standpoint of a specialist. Dent Cosmos 1904;46:370

Adams, DF. Implant therapy of infrabony pockets. Periodont Abstr 1966;14(2):63

Ahuja, V, Shin, RH, Mudgil, A, Nanda, V, Schoor, R. Papillon-LeFevre syndrome: A successful outcome. J Periodontol 2005;76:1996

Ainamo, A. Influence of age on the location of the maxillary mucogingival junction. J Periodont Res 1978;13:189

Ainamo, J, Ainamo, A. Development of oral health during dental studies in India and Finland. Int Dent J 1978;28:427

Ainamo, J, Barmes, D, Beagrie, G, Cutress, T, Martin, J, Sardo-Infirri, J. Development of the World Health Organization (WHO) Community Periodontal Index of Treatment Needs (CPITN). Int Dent J 1982;32:281

Aisenberg, MS. Histology and physiology of the supporting structures. J Am Dent Assoc 1952;44:628

Albander, JM, Brown, LJ, Loe, H. Clinical features of early-onset periodontitis. J Am Dent Assoc 1997;128:1393

Alexander, AG. Crevicular fluid as a source of the constituents of subgingival calculus. Dent Health 1969;8:1

Allen, AL. Use of the supraperiosteal envelope in soft tissue grafting for root coverage II: Clinical results. Int J Periodont Rest Dent 1994;14(4): 302

Allen, AL, Cohen, DW. King and Pennel's free graft series: A defining moment revisited. Compend Contin Educ Dent 2003;24(9):698

Allen, EP, Gainza, CS, Farthing, GG, Newbold, DA. Improved technique for localized ridge augmentation. A report of 21 cases. J Periodontol 1985;56:195

Allen, EP. Use of mucogingival surgical procedures to enhance esthetics. Dent Clin North Am 1988;32(2):307

Allen, EP. Surgical crown lengthening for function and esthetics. Dent Clin North Am 1993a;37(2):163

Allen, EP. Pedicle flaps, gingival grafts and connective tissue grafts in aesthetic treatment of gingival recession. Pract Periodont Aesthet Dent 1993b;(5):29

Ammons, WF Jr, Smith DH. Flap curettage: Rationale, technique and expectations. Dent Clin North Am 1976;20(1):215

Angelopoulos, AP, Goez, PW. Incidence of diphenylhydantoin gingival hyperplasia. Oral Surg Oral Med Oral Pathol 1972;34:898

Angle, EH. Treatment of Malocclusion of the Teeth. Angles System, 7th ed. Philadelphia: SS White Dental Manufacturing, 1907

Antezak-Bonckoms, A. Meta-analysis of clinical trials in periodontal research. Periodontol 2000, 1993;2:140

AP. Glossary of prosthodontic terms. J Prosthet Dent 1994;71:50

Ariaudo, AA, Tyrrell, HA. Elimination of pockets extending to or beyond the mucogingival junction. Dent Clin North Am 1960;67

Armitage, GC. Periodontal diseases: Diagnosis. Ann Periodontol 1996;1(1):37

Armitage, GC. Development of a classification system for periodontal diseases and conditions. Ann Periodontol 1999;4(1):1

Armitage, GC. Classifying periodontal diseases: A longstanding dilemma. Periodontol 2000, 2002;30:9

Armitage, GC. Periodontal diagnosis and classification of periodontal diseases. Periodontol 2000, 2004a;34:9

Armitage, GC. Analysis of gingival crevice fluid and risk of progression of periodontitis. Periodontol 2000, 2004b;34:109

Arnim, SS, Hagerman, DA. The connective tissue fibers of the marginal gingiva. J Am Dent Assoc 1953;47:271

Arnim, SS. Microcosms of the human mouth. J Tenn Dent Assoc 1959;39:3

Arnim, SS, Sandell, PJ. How to educate high school students in oral hygiene. J Health Phys Edu Rec 1960;31:33

Arnim, SS. The use of disclosing agents for measuring tooth cleanliness. J Periodontol 1963;34:227

Arnim, SS. Microcosms of the mouth Role in periodontal disease. Texas Dent J 1964;82:4

Arnim, SS. How the dentist can help people learn to prevent and control dental disease. North-West Dent 1966;45:3

Arrocha, R, Wittmer, JW, Gargiulo, AW. Tissue response to heterogenous bone implantation in dogs. J Periodontol 1968;39:162

Ash, MM, Gitlin, BN, Smith, WA. Correlation between plaque and gingivitis. J Periodontol 1964;35:424

Assaf, ME, Roller, N. The cingulo-radicular groove: Its significance and management: Two case reports. Compend Contin Educ Dent 1992;13(2):94

Augsburger, RA. Root amputations and hemisections. Gen Dent 1976;24(3):35

August, DS. The radicular lingual groove: An overlooked differential diagnosis. J Am Dent Assoc 1978;96:1037

Azzi, R. Electrosurgery in Periodontics: A literature review. J West Soc Periodontol/Periodontal Abstr 1981;29(1):4

Bacic, M, Karakas, Z, Kaic, Z, Sutalo, J. The association between palatal grooves in upper incisors and periodontal complications. J Periodontol 1990;61:197

Baer, PN, Sumner, CF, Scigliano, J. Studies on a hydrogenated fat zinc bacitracin periodontal dressing. Oral Surg Oral Med Oral Pathol 1960;13:494

Baer, PN. The case for periodontosis as a clinical entity. J Periodontol 1971;42:516

Bahat, O, Deeb, C, Golden, T, Komarnyckyi, O. Preservation of ridges utilizing hydroxyapatite. Int J Periodont Rest Dent 1987;7(6):35

Bahat, O, Handelsman, M, Gordon, J. The transpositional flap in periodontal surgery. Int J Periodont Rest Dent 1990;10(6):473

Bahat, O, Handelsman, M. Periodontal reconstructive flaps: Classification and surgical considerations. Int J Periodont Rest Dent 1991;11(6):481

Baiorunos, JR, Robbins, FE. Root demineralization as a new-attachment procedure. A review of the literature. Int J Periodont Rest Dent 1980;28:84

Barnes, GP, Parks, WA, Lyon, TC, Fultz, RP. Indices used to evaluate signs, symptoms, and etiologic factors associated with diseases of the periodontium. J Periodontol 1986;57:643

Barnes, JE, Schaffer, EM. Subgingival root planing: A comparison using files, hoes and curettes. J Periodontol 1960;31:300

Barrington, EP. The current status of mucogingival surgery. Alpha Omegan 1973;66:17

Barrington, EP. An overview of periodontal surgical procedures. J Periodontol 1981;52:518

Basaraba, N. Root amputation and tooth resection. Dent Clin North Am 1969;13(1):121

Bass, CC. The necessary personal oral hygiene for prevention of caries and periodontoclasia. New Orleans Med Surg 1948;101:52

Bass, CC. An effective method of personal oral hygiene. Louisiana State Med Soc 1954;106:100

Baum, BJ, Wright, WE. Demonstration of fibronectin as a major extracellular protein of human gingival fibroblasts. J Dent Res 1980; 59:631

Beaumont, RH, O'Leary, TJ, Kafrawy, AH. Relative resistance of long junctional adhesions and connective tissue attachments to plaque-induced inflammation. J Periodontol 1984;55:213

Beck, JD, Offenbacher, S. Relationships among clinical measures of periodontal disease and their associations with systemic markers. Ann Periodontol 2002;7:79

Becker, NG. A free gingival graft utilizing a presuturing technique. Periodontics 1967;5:195

Becker, W, Becker, BE, Prichard, JF, Caffesse, R, Rosenberg, E, Gian Grasso, J. Root isolation for new attachment procedures: A surgical and suturing method: Three case reports. J Periodontol 1987;58:819

Becker, W, Becker, BE, Berg, L, Prichard, JF, Caffesse, R, Rosenberg, E. New attachment after treatment with root isolation procedures: Report for treated class III and class II furcations and vertical osseous defects. Int J Periodont Rest Dent 1988;8(3):9

Becker, W, Becker, BE. Keys for successful implant esthetics. Contemp Esthet Rest Pract 1998;2:14

Becker, W, Ochsenbein, C, Becker, BE. Crown lengthening: The periodontal-restorative connection. Compend Contin Educ Dent 1998;19:239

Beckham, LC, Cederbaum, AD, Levy, L, O'Connell, R, Salkind, A. A history of periodontal surgery and suggested changes in terminology and nomenclature. J Periodontol 1962;33:101

Belcher, JM. A perspective on periodontal microsurgery. Int J Periodont Rest Dent 2001;21(2):191

Bell, DG. Home care of the mouth. III Teaching home care to the patient. J Periodontol 1948;19:140

Ben-Bassat, Y, Brin, I. The labiogingival notch. An anatomical variation of clinical importance. J Am Dent Assoc 2001;132:919

Benjamin, SD, Baer, PN. Familial patterns of advanced alveolar bone loss in adolescence (periodontosis). Periodontics 1967;5:82

Bennett, NG. A contribution to the study of the movements of the mandible. Proc R Soc Med (Odontol) 1908;1:79

Bergenholtz, A, Hugoson, A. Vestibular sulcus extension surgery in cases with periodontal disease. J Periodontal Res 1967;2:221

Bergenholtz, A. Radectomy of multirooted teeth. J Am Dent Assoc 1972;85:870

Bergenholtz, A, Hugoson, A. Vestibular sulcus extension surgery in the mandibular front region: The Edlan-Mejchar Method. A five-year follow-up study. J Periodontol 1973;44:309

Berger, A. The surgical treatment of periodontoclasia. J Am Dent Assoc 1927;14:1013

Berliner, A. Elimination of periodontal pockets. Dent Digest 1950;56:397

Berman, CL. Complications: Prevention, recognition, treatment. Dent Clin North Am 1989; 33:635

Bernimoulin, JP, Luscher, R, Muhlemann, HR. Coronally repositioned periodontal flap. Clinical evaluation after one year. J Clin Periodontol 1975;2:1

Beube, FE, Silvers, HF. Influence of devitalized heterogenous bone powder on regeneration of alveolar and maxillary bone in dogs. J Dent Res 1934;14:15

Beube, FE. Interdental tissue resection: An experimental study of a surgical technique which aids in repair of the periodontal tissues to their original contour and function. Am J Orthod Oral Surg 1947;33:497

Bhaskar, SN, Frisch, J, Margetis, PM, Leonard, F. Application of a new chemical adhesive in periodontics and oral surgery. Oral Surg Oral Med Oral Pathol 1966;22:526

Bhaskar, SN, ed. Orbans Oral Histology and Embryology. Maxilla and Mandible (Alveolar Process), 8th ed. St. Louis: Mosby, 1976

Bierly, JA, Sottosanti, JS. Osseous filtration: An improved technique for bone implantation. J Periodontol 1974;45:414

Biggerstaff, RH, Sinks, JH, Carazola, JL. Orthodontic extrusion and biologic width realignment produces methods for reclaiming nonrestorable teeth. J Am Dent Assoc 1986; 112:345

Bjorby, A, Loe, H. The relative significance of different local factors in the initiation and development of periodontal inflammation. Scandinavian Symposium on Periodontology, 1966; abstr 20. J Periodont Res 1967;2:76

Bjorn, H. Free transplantation of gingiva propria. Svensk Tandlak Tidsk 1963a;22:684

Bjorn, H. Free transplantation of gingiva propria. Odontol Rev 1963b;14:323

Bjorndahl, O. Periodontal traumatism. J Periodontol 1958;29:223

Black, A.D. Roentgenographic studies of tissues involved in chronic mouth infections. Dental Summ 1918;38:924

Black, A.D. The pathology and treatment of diseases of the peridental membrane. Dent Cosmos 1920;62:820

Black, G.V. Abrasion and erosion of teeth in The American system of dentistry. Litch, W, ed. Philadelphia: Lea Brothers, 1886:990-992

Black, G.V. A study of histological characteristics of the periosteum and peridental membrane: Dental review (1886-1887). Chicago: Keener, 1887

Black, G.V. Beginnings of pyorrhea alveolaris: Treatment for prevention. Items of Interest 1911;33:420

Block, MS, Hoffman, DR. A new device for absolute anchorage for orthodontics. Am J Orthod Dentofac Orthop 1995;107(3):251

Blomlof, J, Jansson, L, Blomlof, L, Lindskog, S. Root surface etching at neutral pH promotes periodontal healing. J Clin Periodontol 1996; 23:50

Bodecker, CF. Dental erosion: Its possible causes and treatment. Dent Cosmos 1933;75:1056

Bodecker, CF. Local acidity: A cause of dental erosion-abrasion. Ann Dent 1945;4:50

Bohannon, HM. Studies in the alteration of vestibular depth I: Complete denudation. J Periodontol 1962a;33:120

Bohannon, HM. Studies in the alteration of vestibular depth II: Periosteal retention. J Periodontol 1962b;33:354

Bohannon, HM. The fixed long labial mucosal flap in vestibular alteration. Periodontics 1963a;1:13

Bohannon, HM. Studies in the alteration of vestibular depth III: Vestibular incision. J Periodontol 1963b;34:209

Bohnenkamp, DM, Garcia, LT. Fixed restoration of sectional mandibular molar teeth. Compend Contin Educ Dent 2004;25(11):920

Bosshardt, DD, Selvig KA. Dental cementum: The dynamic tissue covering the root. Periodontol 2000, 1997;13:41

Bowers, GM. A study of the width of attached gingiva. J Periodontol 1963;34:201

Bowers, GM, Chadroff, B, Carnevale, R, Mellonig, J, Corio, R, Emerson, J, Stevens, M, Romberg, E. Histologic evaluation of new attachment apparatus formation in humans Part I. J Periodontol 1989;60:664

Box, HK. Traumatic occlusion and traumatogenic occlusion. Oral Health 1930;20:642

Box, HK. Experimental traumatogenic occlusion in sheep. Oral Health 1935;25:9

Box, HK. Twelve Periodontal Studies. Toronto, Canada: University of Toronto Press, 1940

Boyne, PJ, James, RA. Grafting of the maxillary sinus floor with autogenous marrow and bone. J Oral Surg 1980;38:613

Boyne, PJ, James, RA. Advances in subperiosteal implant reconstruction. Dent Clin North Am 1986;30(2):259

Brady, JM. A plaque-free zone on human teeth: scanning and transmission electron microscopy. J Periodontol 1973;44:416

Bral, MM, Stahl, SS. Keratinizing potential of human crevicular epithelium. J Periodontol 1977;48:381

Branemark, PI. Introduction to osseointegration. In Branemark, PI, Zarb, G, Albrektsson, T. eds. Tissue Integrated Prosthesis: Osseointegration in Clinical Dentistry. Chicago: Quintessence, 1995:11

Brooks, SJ, Robinson, C, Kirkham, J, Bonass, WA. Biochemistry and molecular biology of amelogenin proteins of developing dental enamel. Arch Oral Biol 1995;40:1

Brown, FH, Lubow, RM, Cooley, RL. A review of applied ultrasonics in periodontal therapy. J West Soc Periodontol/Periodontal Abstr 1987;35(2):53

Brown, IS. The effect of orthodontic therapy on certain types of periodontal defects: I. Clinical findings. J Periodontol 1973;44:742

Brunsvold, MA, Mellonig, JT. Bone grafts and periodontal regeneration. Periodontol 2000, 1993;1:80

Bulyhuis, HM, Barendregt, DS, Timmeran, MF, Loos, BG, vander Velden, U. Probe penetration in relation to the connective tissue attachment: Influence of the tine shape and probing force. J Clin Periodontol 1998;25:417

Burch, JG, Bagci, B, Sabulski, D, Landrum, C. Periodontal changes in furcations resulting from orthodontic uprighting of mandibular molars. Quintessence Int., 1992;23:509

Buser, D, Dula, K, Belser, U, Hert, H-P, Berthold, H. Localized ridge augmentation using guided bone regeneration: I. Surgical procedure in the maxilla. Int J Periodont Rest Dent 1993;13(1):29

Butler, BL, Morejon, O, Low, SR. An accurate time-efficient method to assess plaque accumulation. J Am Dent Assoc 1996;127:1763

Butler, JH. A familial pattern of juvenile periodontitis. J Periodontol 1969;40:115

Butler, JH, Folke, LEA, Bandt, CL. A descriptive survey of signs and symptoms associated with myofascial pain-dysfunction syndrome. J Am Dent Assoc 1975;90:635

Caffesse, RG, Guinard, EA. Treatment of localized gingival recessions: Part II: coronally repositioned flap with a gingival graft. J Periodontol 1978;49:357

Caffesse, RG. Longitudinal evaluation of periodontal surgery. Dent Clin North Am 1980; 24:751

Camelo, M, Nevins, ML, Schenk, RK, Lynch, SE, Nevins, M. Periodontal regeneration in human class II furcations using purified recombinant human platelet-derived growth factor-BB (rh PDGF-BB) with bone allograft. Int J Periodont Rest Dent 2003;23(3):213

Cameron, CE. The cracked tooth syndrome: Additional findings. J Am Dent Assoc 1976;93:971

Campbell, PM, Moore JW, Matthews, JL. Orthodontically corrected midline diastemas. A histological study and surgical procedure. Am J Orthod 1975;67:139

Cantor, MT, Stahl, SS. The effects of various interdental stimulators upon the keratinization of the interdental col. Periodontics 1965;3:243

Card, SJ, Caffesse, RG, Smith, BA. A historical perspective of current new attachment procedures. J West Soc Periodontol/Periodontal Abstr 1987;35(3):93

Carlos, JP, Wolfe, MD, Kingman, A. The extent and severity index: A simple method for use in epidemiologic studies of periodontal disease. J Clin Periodontol 1986;13:500

Carlson, NE, Roach, RB Jr. Platelet-rich plasma. Clinical applications in dentistry. J Am Dent Assoc 2002;133:1383

Carnevale, G, Kaldahl, WB. Osseous resective surgery. Periodontol 2000, 2000;22:59

Carranza, FA Jr. Letter to the editor. J Periodontol 1956;27:65

Carranza, FA Jr, Glickman, I. Some observations on the microscopic features of infrabony pockets. J Periodontol 1957;28:33

Carranza, FA Jr. Glickman's Clinical Periodontology, 7th ed. Philadelphia: Saunders, 1990

Carranza, FA Jr, Newman, MG. Clinical Periodontology, 8th ed. Philadelphia: Saunders, 1996

Carranza, FA Jr, Shklar, G. History of Periodontology. Chicago: Quintessence, 2003.

Carter, HG, Barnes, GP. The gingival bleeding Index. J Periodontol 1974;45:801

Caton, JG, Polson, AM. The interdental bleeding index: A simplified procedure for monitoring gingival health. Compend Contin Educ Dent 1985;6:88

Caton, J. Periodontal diagnosis and diagnostic aids. In Proceedings of the World Workshop in Clinical Periodontics, Nevins, M, Becker, W, Kornman, K, eds. Chicago: AAP, 1989:I-1,I-32

Caton, J, Bouwsman, O, Polson, A, Espeland, M. Effects of personal oral hygiene and subgingival scaling on bleeding interdental gingiva. J Periodontol 1989;60:84

Chace, R. The maintenance phase of periodontal therapy. J Periodontol 1951;22:234

Chace, R. Gingivectomy and inter-dental resection. J Periodontol 1954;25:246

Chace, R Jr, Keyes, PH. Salt, soda and hydrogen peroxide: Is it enough? Florida Dent J 1981;52(2):13

Charters, WJ. Immunizing both hard and soft mouth tissue to infection by correct stimulation with the toothbrush. J Am Dent Assoc 1928;15:87

Charters, WJ. Eliminating mouth infections with the toothbrush and other stimulating instruments. Dent Digest 1932;38:130

Chavrier, C. The elastic system fibers in healthy human gingiva. Arch Oral Biol 1990;35(Suppl): 223

Cho, MI, Lin, WL, Genco, RJ. Platelet derived growth factor modulated guided tissue regenerative therapy. J Periodontol 1995;66:522

Cho, MI, Garant, PR. Development and general structure of the periodontium. Periodontol 2000, 2000;24:9

Christensen, GJ. Ridge preservation: Why not? Am Dent Assoc 1996;127:669

Ciancio, SG, Cunat, JJ, Mather, ML, Harvey, DH. A comparison of plaque accumulation in bonded vs. banded teeth. J Dent Res 1985;64: 359 (abstr 1664)

Ciancio, SG. Medications' impact on oral health. J Am Dent Assoc 2004;135:1440

Cieszynski, A. Bemerkungen zur radical chirurgischeen Behandlung der sogennanten Pyorrhea Alveolaris. Dtsch Monattschr Zahnheilk 1914;32:575

Clark, CF. A method of ascertaining the relative position of unerupted teeth by means of film radiographs. Proc R Soc Med (Odontol) 1910;3:87

Cohen, B. Morphological factors in the pathogenesis of periodontal disease. Br Dent J 1959;107:31

Cohen, DW, Morris, AL. Periodontal manifestations in cyclic neutropenia. J Periodontol 1961;32:159

Cohen, DW, Chacker, FM. Criteria for selection of one treatment plan over another. Dent Clin North Am 1964; March:3

Cohen, DW, Ross, SE. The double papillae repositioned flap in periodontal therapy. J Periodontol 1968;39:65

Cohen, DW. Periodontics: Reflections and projections. Alpha Omegan 1969;62(3):173

Cohen, DW, Freedman, L, Shapiro, JA. A longitudinal investigation of the periodontal changes during pregnancy. J Periodontol 1969;40:563

Cohen, DW, Slavkin, HC. Periodontal diseases and systemic disease. In: Periodontal Medicine. Rose, LF, Genco, RJ, Cohen, DW, Mealey, BL, eds. Hamilton, Ont., Canada: B.C. Decker, 2000: chap 1

Cohen, DW. Guest editorial: Periodontal Medicine in the next millennium. Int J Periodont Rest Dent 2000;20(1):6

Cohen, ES. Atlas of Cosmetic and Reconstructive Surgery, 2nd ed. Philadelphia: Lea & Febiger, 1989

Coolidge, ED. The thickness of the human periodontal membrane. J Am Dent Assoc 1937; 24:1260

Cordero, FF. Vocabulary in Periodontology: Part I. The concept of "paradentium." Periodontics 1966;4:137

Corn, H. Periosteal separation: Its clinical significance. J Periodontol 1962;33:140

Corn, H. Edentulous area pedicle grafts in mucogingival surgery. Periodontics 1964;2:229

Corn, H. Mucogingival surgery and associated problems. In: Periodontal Therapy, 4th ed. Goldman, HM, Cohen, DW, eds. St. Louis: Mosby, 1968:692

Corn, H. Reconstructive mucogingival surgery. In: Periodontal Therapy, 6th ed. Goldman, HM, Cohen, DW, eds. St. Louis, Mosby, 1980:848

Cortellini, P, Prato, GP, Tonetti, MS. The modified papilla preservation technique. A new surgical approach for interproximal regeneration procedures. J Periodontol 1995;66:261

Cortellini, P. The simplified papilla preservation flap. A novel surgical approach for the management of the soft tissues in regenerative procedures. Int J Periodont Rest Dent 1999; 19:589

Cortellini, P, Tonetti, MS. Focus on intrabony defects: Guided tissue regeneration. Periodontol 2000, 2000;22:104

Coslet, JG, Vanarsdall, R, Weisgold, A. Diagnosis and classification of delayed passive eruption of the dentogingival junction in the adult. Alpha Omegan 1977;70:24

Costen, JB. A Syndrome of ear and sinus symptoms dependent upon disturbed function of the temporomandibular joint. Ann Otol Rhin and Laryng 1934;43:1

Crane, AB, Kaplan, H. The Crane-Kaplan operation for the prompt elimination of pyorrhea alveolaris. Dent Cosmos 1931;73:643

Cupit, GW. A Consideration of the "periodontium" or the membrane which holds a tooth in its socket. Am Dent J 1904;3:619

Curtis, GH, McCall, CM, Overaa, HI. Clinical study of the effectiveness of the roll and Charters' methods of brushing teeth. J Periodontol 1957;28:277

Dabelsteen, I. The use of Balneotherapy in removing dental plaques and cleansing periodontal pockets. Tandlaegebladet 1964;68:107 [abstr of article in Periodont Abstr 1965;13(3):141]

Dahlberg, WH. Incision and suturing: Some basic considerations about each in periodontal flap surgery. Dent Clin North Am 1969;13(1):149

Daly, LE, Bourke, GJ. Interpretation and uses of Medical Statistics. 5th ed. Edinburgh, Scotland: Blackwell Science, 2000

D'Amico, A. The canine teeth: Normal functional relation of the natural teeth of man. J South Calif State Dent J 1958;26:6,49,127, 175,194,239

D'Amico, A. Application of the concept of the functional relation of the canine teeth. J South Calif State Dent J 1959;27:39

Darle, C. Guest Editorial- Honoring a Pioneer. Int J Periodont Rest Dent 2003;23(4):311

Daskalogiannakis, J. Glossary of Orthodontic Terms. Chicago: Quintessence, 2000

Davies, DM, Picton, DCA, Alexander, AG. An objective method of assessing the periodontal condition in human skulls. J Periodont Res 1969;4:74

Davies, GN. Dental conditions among the Polynesians of Pukapuka (Danger Island). J Dent Res 1956;35:734

Davis, RK, Baer, PN, Palmer, JH. A preliminary report on a new therapy for dilantin gingival hyperplasia. J Periodontol 1963;34:17

Dawes, C, Jenkins, GN, Tonge, CH. The nomenclature of the integuments of the enamel of teeth. Br Dent J 1963;15:65

De La Rosa, RM, Sturzenberger, OP. Clinical reduction of gingivitis through the use of a mouthwash containing two quaternary ammonium compounds. J Periodontol 1976;47:535

Dello Russo, NM. Spotlight on excellence: Interview with R. Earl Robinson. Periodontal Insights 1995;2(2):11

Dello Russo, NM. Flap design and suturing in periodontal surgery. In: Periodontal Therapy—Clinical Approaches and Evidence of Success. Nevins, M, Mellonig, JT, eds. Chicago: Quintessence, 1998;1:187

DeWaal, H, Kon, S, Ruben, MP. Periodontal Probing. J West Soc Periodontol Periodont Abstr 1986;34(1):5

Diem, CR, Bowers, GM, Moffett, WC. Bone blending: A technique for osseous implants. J Periodontol 1972;43:295

Dobell, C. Anton van Leeuwenhoek and his "little animals." New York: Harcourt, 1932. New York: Dover, 1960.

Douglas, GL. Mucogingival repairs in periodontal surgery. Dent Clin North Am 1976;20(1):107

Drum, W. Uber Parafunktionen insbesondere uber die ubewusste (Karolyi) Parafunction des Gebisses. Zahnarztl Rdsch 1950;59:257,287

Dunkin, RT. Microbial index as a method of measuring effectiveness of mechanical toothbrush. J Periodontol 1966;37:391

Dunning, JM, Leach, LB. Gingival-bone count: A method for epidemiological study of periodontal disease. J Dent Res 1960;39:506

Easley, JR. Methods of determining alveolar osseous form. J Periodontol 1967;38:112

Easley, JR, Drennan, GA. Morphological classification of the furca. J Can Dent Assoc 1969;35:104

Edel, A. Clinical evaluation of free connective tissue grafts used to increase the width of keratinized gingiva. J Clin Periodontol 1974;1:185

Edel, A. The use of a free connective tissue graft to increase the width of attached gingiva. Oral Surg Oral Med Oral Pathol 1975;39:341

Edlan, A, Mejchar, B. Plastic surgery of the vestibulum in periodontal therapy. Int Dent J 1963;13:593

Edmunds, RS, Simmons TA, Cox, CF, Avery, JK. Light and ultrastructural relationship between oxytalan fibers in the periodontal ligament of the guinea pig. J Oral Pathol 1979;8:109

Edwards, JG. A surgical procedure to eliminate rotational relapse. Am J Orthod 1970;57:35

Elfenbaum, A. Alveolar lamina dura: Radiographic interpretation. Dent Radiogr Photogr 1958;31(2):21

Elliott, JR, Bowers, GM. Alveolar dehiscence and fenestration. Periodontics 1963;1:245

Ellman, IA. Rotary ultrasonics for preventive periodontics. NY State Dent J 1962;28:404

Ellman, IA. Comparative safety of the rotosonic scaler and the curet. J Periodontol 1964;34:410

El Mostehy, MR, Stallard, RE. Intermediate cementum. J Periodont Res 1968;3:24

Emmings, FG, Koepf, SW, Gage, AA. Cryotherapy for benign lesions of the oral cavity. J Oral Surg 1967;25:320

Emslie, RD. The #621 periodontal probe. Int Dent J 1980;30:287

Ennever, J, Sturzenberger, OP, Radike, AW. The calculus surface index method for scoring clinical calculus studies. J Periodontol 1961;32:54

Eskow, RN, Kapin, SH. Furcation invasions: Correlating a classification system with therapeutic considerations: Part I. Examination, diagnosis and classification. Compend Contin Educ Dent 1984a;5(6):479

Eskow, RN, Kapin, SH. Furcation invasions: Correlating a classification system with therapeutic considerations: Part II. Periodontal and restorative considerations in furcation management. Compend Contin Educ Dent 1984b;5(7):527

Everett, FG, Kunkel, PW. Abrasion through the use of dental floss. J Periodontol 1953;24:186

Everett, FG, Jump, EB, Holder, TD, Williams, GC. The intermediate bifurcation ridge: A study of the morphology of the bifurcation of the lower first molar. J Dent Res 1958;37:162

Everett, FG, Potter, GR. Morphology of submarginal calculus. J Periodontol 1959;30:29

Everett, FG, Fixott, HC. Use of an incorporated grid in the diagnosis of oral roentgenograms. Oral Surg Oral Med Oral Pathol 1963;16:1061

Everett, FG, Hall WB, Bennett, JS. Retrocuspid papillae. Periodontics 1965;3:81

Everett, FG. The case of the disappearing clefts. J Periodontol 1968;39:296

Everett, FG, Waerhaug, J, Widman, A. Leonard Widman—Surgical treatment of pyorrhea alveolaris. J Periodontol 1971;42:571

Everett, FG, Kramer, GM. The disto-lingual groove in the maxillary lateral incisor: A periodontal hazard. J Periodontol 1972;43:352

Evian, CI, Cutler, SA, Rosenberg, ES, Shah, RK. Altered passive eruption: The undiagnosed entity. J Am Dent Assoc 1993;12:107

Ewen, SJ, Sorrin, S. Ultrasonics and periodontal therapy. Dent Clin North Am 1964; March:145

Ewen, SJ. Bone swaging. J Periodontol 1965;36:57

Farrar, JN. Radical and heroic treatment of alveolar abscess by amputation of roots of teeth. Dent Cosmos 1884;26:79

Farshchian, F, Kaiser, DA. Restoration of the split molar: Bicuspidization. Am J Dent 1988;1(1):21

Fedi, PF, Vernino, AR, Gray, JL. The Periodontic Syllabus, 4th ed. Philadelphia: Lippincott Williams & Wilkins, 2000

Fialkoff, B, Fry, HR. Acid demineralization in periodontal therapy. J West Soc Periodontol/ Periodontal Abstr 1982;30(2):52

Firkin, BG, Whiteworth, JA. Dictionary of Medical Eponyms, 2nd ed. New York: Parthenon, 1996

Fischman, SL. Current status of indices for plaque. J Clin Periodontol 1986;13:371

Fish, EW. Etiology and prevention of periodontal breakdown. Dent Progr 1961;1:234

Flocken, JE. Electrosurgical management of soft tissues and restorative dentistry. Dent Clin North Am 1980;24(2):247

Fones, AC. Instructions for the home care of the mouth. Dent Items Int 1915;37:356

Foss, CL, Grupe, HE, Orban, B. Gingivosis. J Periodontol 1953;24:207

Francetti, L, del Fabbro, M, Testori, T, Weinstein, RL. Chlorhexidine spray versus chlorhexidine mouthwash in the control of dental plaque after periodontal surgery. J Clin Periodontol 2000;27:425

Friedman, N. Periodontal osseous surgery: Osteoplasty and osteoectomy. J Periodontol 1955;26:257

Friedman, N. Mucogingival surgery. Texas Dent J 1957;75:358

Friedman, N. Mucogingival surgery: The apically repositioned flap. J Periodontol 1962a;33:328

Friedman, N. Etiology of marginal gingivitis and periodontitis. Alpha Omegan 1962b;55:107

Friedman, N, Levine, HL. Mucogingival surgery: Current status. J Periodontol 1964;35:5

Frisch, J, Jones, RA, Bhaskar, SN. Conservation of maxillary anterior esthetics: A modified surgical approach. J Periodontol 1967;38:11

Frohman, BS. The application of psychotherapy to dental problems. Dent Cosmos 1931;73:1117

Fullmer, HM, Lillie, RD. The oxytalan fiber: A previously undescribed connective tissue fiber. J Histochem Cytochem 1958;6:425

Fullmer, HM. A histochemical study of periodontal disease in the maxillary alveolar process of 135 autopsies. J Periodontol 1961;32:206

Gage, AA, Koepf, SW, Wehrle, D, Emmings, FG. Cryotherapy for cancer of the lip and oral cavity. Cancer 1965;8:1646

Gantes, BG, Garrett, S. Coronally displaced flaps in reconstructive periodontal therapy. Dent Clin North Am 1991;35:495

Gara, GG, Adams, DF. Implant therapy in human intrabony pockets: A review of the literature. J West Soc Periodontol/Periodontal Abstr 1981;29(2):32

Garber, DA, Rosenberg, ES. The edentulous ridge in fixed prosthodontics. Compend Contin Educ Dent 1981;(4):212

Gargiulo, AW, Wentz, FM, Orban, B. Dimensions and relations of the dentogingival junction in humans. J Periodontol 1961;32:261

Gargiulo, AW. Research in periodontal therapy. Dent Clin North Am 1969;13:203

Garnick, J, Ramfjord, SP. Rest position: An electromyographic and clinical investigation. J Prosthet Dent 1962;12:895

Garrett, S, Gantes, B, Zimmerman, G, Egelberg, J. Treatment of mandibular class III periodontal furcation defects. Coronally positioned flaps with and without expanded polytetrafluorethylene membranes. J Periodontol 1994;65:592

Garrett, S, Bogle, G. Periodontal regenerations: Review of flap management. Periodontol 2000, 1993;1:100

Genco, RJ, Zambon, JJ, Christersson, LA. The role of specific bacteria in periodontal infections. Adv Dent Res 1988;2:245

Genco, RJ. Current view of risk factors for periodontal disease. J Periodontol 1996;67:1041

Giannobile, WV. Guest editorial: What does the future hold for periodontal tissue engineering? Int J Periodont Rest Dent 2002;22(1):7

Giansanti, JS, Hrabak, RP, Waldron, CA. Palmar-plantar hyperkeratosis with concomitant periodontal destruction (Papillon-LeFevre syndrome). Oral Surg Oral Med Oral Pathol 1973;36:40

Gillam, DG, Newman, HN. Iontophoresis in the treatment of cervical dentinal sensitivity: A review. J West Soc Periodontol/Periodontal Abstr 1990;38:129

Gillette, WB, Van House, RL. Ill effects of improper oral hygiene procedures. J Am Dent Assoc 1980;101:476

Glick, M, Muzyka, BC, Lurie, D, Salkin, LM. Oral manifestations associated with HIV-related disease as markers for immune suppression and AIDS. Oral Surg Oral Med Oral Pathol 1994;72:344

Glick, M. View: Exploring our role as health care providers. The oral-medical connection. J Am Dent Assoc 2005;136:716

Glickman, I. The bone factor in periodontoclasia. Bull Mass Dent Soc 1944;20:14

Glickman, I, Morse, A, Robinson, L. The systemic influence upon bone in periodontoclasia. J Am Dent Assoc 1944;31:1435

Glickman, I. The experimental basis for the "bone factor" concept in periodontal disease. J Periodontol 1949;20:7

Glickman, I. Bifurcation involvement in periodontal disease. J Am Dent Assoc 1950a; 40:528

Glickman, I. A basic classification of gingival enlargement. J Periodontol 1950b;21:131

Glickman, I. Clinical Periodontology. Philadelphia: Saunders, 1953:795

Glickman, I. The results obtained with an unembellished gingivectomy technic in a clinical study in humans. J Periodontol 1956;29:247

Glickman, I. The complete-mouth gingivectomy: A hospital procedure. Dent Clin North Am 1960;March:3

Glickman, I. Inflammation and trauma from occlusion, Co-destructive factors in chronic periodontal disease. J Periodontol 1963;34:5

Glickman, I, Smulow, JB. Chronic desquamative gingivitis: Its nature and treatment. J Periodontol 1964;35:397

Glickman, I. Buttressing bone formation in the periodontium. J Periodontol 1965;36:365

Glickman, I, Selye, H, Smulow, J. Reduction by calciphylaxis of the effects of chronic dihydrotachysterol overdose upon the periodontium. J Dent Res 1965;44:734

Glickman, I, Smulow, JB. Further observations on the effects of trauma from occlusion in humans. J Periodontol 1967;38:280

Glickman, I. Role of occlusion in the etiology and treatment of periodontal disease. J Dent Res 1971;50:199

Glickman, I. The periodontal ligament. In: "Clinical Periodontology," 4th ed. Philadelphia: Saunders, 1972:32

Goldman, HM. Abstracts of current periodontal literature. J Periodontol 1949;20:59

Goldman, HM. The development of physiologic gingival contour by gingivoplasty. Oral Surg Oral Med Oral Pathol 1950;3:879

Goldman, HM. Periodontia, 3rd ed. St. Louis: Mosby, 1953:552

Goldman, HM. Gingival vascular supply in induced occlusal traumatism. Oral Surg Oral Med Oral Pathol 1956;9:939

Goldman, HM, Schluger, S, Fox, L. Alterations in the mucobuccal fold. In: Periodontal Therapy, 2nd ed. St. Louis: Mosby, 1956:301

Goldman, HM. Histologic structure of the attachment apparatus. Alpha Omegan 1957;51:102

Goldman, HM. Therapy of the incipient bifurcation involvement. J Periodontol 1958;29:112

Goldman, HM, Cohen, DW. The infrabony pocket: Classification and treatment. J Periodontol 1958;29:272

Goldman, HM, Schluger, S, Fox, L, Cohen, DW. Periodontal Therapy, 2nd ed. St. Louis: Mosby, 1956

Goldman, HM, Schluger, S, Fox, L, Cohen, DW. Periodontal Therapy, 3rd ed. St. Louis: Mosby, 1964

Goldman, HM, Cohen, DW. Periodontal Therapy, 4th ed. St. Louis: Mosby, 1968

Goodson, JM, Tanner, ACR, Haffajee, AD, Sornberger, GC, Socransky, SS. Patterns of progression and regression of advanced destructive periodontal disease. J Clin Periodontol 1982;9:472

Gorlin, RJ, Cohen, MM, Hennekam, RCM. Syndrome of the Head and Neck, 4th ed. New York: Oxford University Press, 2001

Gottleib, B. Zur Aetiologie und Therapie der alveolar Pyorrhea (Etiology and Therapy of Alveolar Pyorrhea). Zeitschr Stomat 1920;18:59

Gottleib, B. Der Epithelansatz am Zahne. Dtsch Monaschr Zahnheilk 1921;39:142

Gottleib, B. Schmutzpyorrhea, parodontal pyorrhea and alveolar atrophy. Berlin and Vienna: Urban and Schwarzenberg, 1925

Gottleib, B. The formation of the pocket: Diffuse atrophy of alveolar bone. J Am Dent Assoc 1928;15:462

Gottleib, B, Orban, B. Active and passive continuous eruption of the teeth (abstr). J Dent Res 1933;13:214

Gottleib, B. Some histologic facts useful in orthodontic practice. J Ortho Oral Surg 1942;28:167

Gottleib, B. The new concept of periodontoclasia. J Periodontol 1946;7:7

Gottsegan, R. Frenum position and vestibular depth in relation to gingival health. Oral Surg Oral Med Oral Pathol 1954;7:1069

Grant DA, Stern, IB, Listgarten, MA. Periodontics, St. Louis: Mosby, 1988

Greenberg, J, Laster, L, Listgarten, MA. Transgingival probing as a potential estimator of alveolar bone level. J Periodontol 1976;47:514

Greene, AH. A study of the characteristics of stippling and its relation to gingival health. J Periodontol 1962;33:176

Greene, JC, Vermilion, JR. The oral hygiene index: A method for classifying oral hygiene status. J Am Dent Assoc 1960;61:172

Greene, JC, Vermilion, JR. The simplified oral hygiene index. J Am Dent Assoc 1964;68:7

Greenstein, G, Polson, A, Iker, H, Meitner, S. Associations between crestal lamina dura and periodontal status. J Periodontol 1981;52:362

Greenstein, G, Caton, J, Polson, A. Trisection of maxillary molars: A clinical technique. Compend Contin Educ Dent 1984;5:624

Greenstein, G, Jaffin, RA, Hilsen, KL, Berman, CL. Repair of anterior deformity with durapatite. J Periodontol 1985;56:200

Greenstein, G. Advances in periodontal disease diagnosis. Int J Periodont Rest Dent 1990;10:351

Greenstein, G. Current interpretations of periodontal probing evaluation: Diagnostic and therapeutic implications. Compend Contin Educ Dent 2005;26(6):381

Greenwell, H, Bissada, NF, Mayberry, JE, De Marco, TJ. Clinical and microbiologic effectiveness of the Keyes' method of oral hygiene on human periodontitis treated with and without surgery. J Am Dent Assoc 1983;106:457

Greenwell, H, Bissada, NF. Factors influencing periodontal therapy for the geriatric patient. Dent Clin North Am 1989;33:91

Griffiths, RH. Report of the Presidents' Conference on the examination, diagnosis, and management of temporomandibular disorders. J Am Dent Assoc 1983;106:75

Grippo, JO. Abfractions: A new classification of hard tissue lesions of teeth. J Esthet Dent 1991; 3(1):14

Grippo, JO, Simring, M, Schreiner, S. Attrition, abrasion, corrosion and abfraction revisited. A new perspective on tooth surface lesions. J Am Dent Assoc 2004;135:1109

Grossi, SG, Zambon, JJ, Ho, AW, Kock, G, Dunford, RG, Machtei, EE, Norderyd, OM, Genco, RJ. Assessment of risk for periodontal disease. I Risk indicators for attachment loss. J Periodontol 1994;65:260

Grossi, SG, Genco, RJ, Machtei, EE, Ho, AW, Koch, G, Dunford, R, Zambon, JJ, Hausmann, E. Assessment of risk for periodontal disease. II Risk indicators for alveolar bone loss. J Periodontol 1995;66:23

Grossman, FD, Fedi, PF Jr. Navy periodontal screening examination. J Am Soc Prev Dent 1974;3:41

Grossman, LI. Root resection. In: Endodontic Practice, 10th ed. Philadelphia: Lea & Febiger, 1981

Grupe, HE, Warren, RF Jr. Repair of gingival defects by a sliding flap operation. J Periodontol 1956;27:92

Grupe, HE. Horizontal sliding flap operation. Dent Clin North Am 1960;March:43

Grupe, HE. Modified technique for the sliding flap operation. J Periodontol 1966a;37:491

Grupe, HE. Letter to the editor. Periodontics 1966b;4:213

Guinard, EA, Caffesse, RG. Treatment of localized gingival recession: Part III. Comparison of results obtained with lateral sliding and coronally repositioned flaps. J Periodontol 1978; 49:457

Halik, FJ. The role of subgingival curettage in periodontal therapy. Dent Clin North Am 1969;13(1):19

Hall, WB. Pure mucogingival problems. Chicago: Quintessence, 1984:97

Hallmon, WW, Waldrop, TC, Houston, GD, Hawkins, BF. Flossing clefts: Clinical and histologic observations. J Periodontol 1986;57:501

Hallmon, WW, Harrel, SK. Occlusal analysis, diagnosis and management in the practice of periodontics. Periodontology 2000, 2004;34:151

Hammarstrom, L. Enamel matrix, cementum development and regeneration. J Clin Periodontol 1997;24:658

Hammarstrom, L, Heijl, K, Gestrelius, S. Periodontal regeneration in a buccal dehiscence model in monkeys after application of enamel matrix proteins. J Clin Periodontol 1997; 24:669

Hammerle, CH, Jung, RE. Bone augmentation by means of barrier membranes. Periodontol 2000, 2003;33:36

Hamp, SE, Nyman, S, Lindle, J. Periodontal treatment of multi-rooted teeth: Results after 5 years. J Clin Periodontol 1975;2:126

Hancock, EB, Wirthlin, MR. An evaluation of the Navy Periodontal Screening Examination. J Periodontol 1977;48:63

Hancock, EB, Mayo, CV, Schwab, RR, Wirthlin, MR. Influence of interdental contacts on periodontal status. J Periodontol 1980;51:445

Hardekoph, JD, Dunlop, RM, Ahl, DR, Pelleu, GP. The "Furcation Arrow." A reliable radiographic image? J Periodontol 1987;58:258

Harris, RJ. The connective tissue and partial thickness double pedicle graft: A predictable method of obtaining root coverage. J Periodontol 1992;63:477

Hase, MP, Reade, PC. The oral leukocyte migration rate index as a method of assessing periodontal disease in an individual. J Periodontal Res 1979;14:153

Haskell, EW, Stanley, HR. Vital root resection on a maxillary first molar. Oral Surg Oral Med Oral Pathol 1972;33:92

Hasler, JF, Schultz, WF. Factitial gingival traumatism: Case report. J Periodontol 1968;39:362

Hassell, TM. Tissues and cells of the periodontium. Periodontol 2000, 1993;3:9

Hattler, AB. Mucogingival surgery: Utilization of interdental gingiva as attached gingiva by surgical displacement. Periodontics 1967;5:126

Hawley, CE, Staffileno, H. Clinical evaluation of free gingival grafts in periodontal surgery. J Periodontol 1970;41:105

Hegedus, Z. The rebuilding of the alveolar process by bone transplantation. Dental Cosmos 1923;65:736

Heins, PJ, Canter, SR. The furca involvement: A classification of bony deformities. Periodontics 1968;6:84

Heins, PJ. Osseous resection: An evaluation after twenty years. Dent Clin North Am 1969;13:75

Held, AJ. Periodontology. From Its Origin up to 1980: A survey. Boston: Birkhauser, 1989.

Hellden, L, Robertson, PB, Rosania, D, Hock, J. Evaluation of a colorimetric essay as a measure of gingival inflammation. J Periodontol 1980; 51:279

Herschfeld, JJ. Varaztad H. Kazanjian, the dentist who became the pioneer in plastic surgery. Bull Hist Dent 1984;32:97

Hiatt, WH. The repositioned alveolar ridge mucosal flap. J Periodontol 1967;5:132

Hiatt, WH. Incomplete crown-root fracture in pulpal-periodontal disease. J Periodontol 1973; 44:369

Highfield, JE. Periodontal treatment of multi-rooted teeth. Aust Dent J 1978;23:91

Hildebrand, CN. Crown lengthening for optimum restorative success. Compend Contin Educ Dent 2003;24(8):620

Hine, MK. The Tooth Brush. Int Dent J 1956;6:15

Hirschfeld, I. Interdental canals. J Am Dent Assoc 1927;14:617

Hirschfeld, I. Food impaction. J Am Dent Assoc 1930;17:1504

Hirschfeld, I. The toothbrush: its use and abuse. Brooklyn, NY: Dental Items of Interest Publishing Company, 1939. [Serially published in Dental Items of Interest, vols 53 (1931) through 60 (1938)]

Hirschfeld, I. The retrocuspid papillae. Am J Orthod Oral Surg 1947;33:447

Hirschfeld, L. A calibrated silver point for periodontal diagnosis and recording. J Periodontol 1953;24:94

Hirschfeld, L. The role of subgingival curettage in periodontal therapy. Alpha Omegan 1962;55: 115

Hoexter, D. Aesthetics and Dentistry: Part 3. A new technique for cosmetic periodontal surgery. Dent Today 1999;18(12):78

Holden, MJ, Smith, BA. Citric acid and fibronectin in periodontal therapy. J West Soc Periodontol/Periodontal Abstr 1983;31(2):45

Holbrook, T, Ochsenbein, C. Complete coverage of the denuded root surface with a one-stage gingival graft. Int J Periodont Rest Dent 1983;3(3):9

Holmstrup, P, Westergaard, J. HIV infections and periodontal diseases. Periodontology 2000, 1998;18:37

Holmstrup, P. Non-plaque-induced gingival lesions. Ann Periodontol 1999;4(1):20

Hou, GL, Tsai, CC. Relationship between palato-radicular grooves and localized periodontitis. J Clin Periodontol 1993;20:678

Hou, GL, Tsai, CC. Types and dimensions of root trunks correlating with diagnosis of molar furcation involvement. J Clin Periodontol 1997; 24:129

Hurt, WC. Freeze-dried bone homografts in periodontal lesions in dogs. J Periodontol 1968; 39:89

Ilizarov, GA. The principles of the Ilizarov method. Bull Hosp Joint Distr Orthop Inst 1988;48:1

Ingber, JS. Forced eruption: Part I. A method of treating one and two wall intrabony defects. Rationale and case report. J Periodontol 1974;45:199

Ingber, JS, Rose, LF, Coslet, JG. The "Biologic width": A concept in periodontics and restorative dentistry. Alpha Omegan 1977;70:62

Ingle, JI. Periodontal curettement in the premaxilla. J Periodontol 1952;23:143

Innes, PB. The ultrastructure of the connective tissue underlying the sulcular epithelium. N Z Dent J 1973;69:185

Ivancie, GP. Experimental and histological investigation of gingival regeneration in vestibular surgery. J Periodontol 1957;28:259

Jablonski, S. Jablonski's Dictionary of Dentistry. Malabar, FL: Krieger, 1992

Jacobs, SG. Radiographic localization of unerupted maxillary anterior teeth using the vertical tube shift technique: The history and application of the method with some case reports. Am J Orthod Dentofacial Orthop 1999; 116(4):415

Jeffcoat, MK. Radiographic methods for the detection of progressive alveolar bone loss. J Periodontol 1992;63:367

Jeffcoat, MK, Reddy, MS, van den Berg, R, Martens, E. Quantitative digital subtraction radiography for the assessment of peri-implant bone changes. Clin Oral Implants Res 1992;3:22

Jeffcoat, MK. Current concepts in periodontal disease testing. J Am Dent Assoc 1994;125:1071

Jeffcoat, MK, McGuire, MK, Newman, MG. Evidence-based periodontal treatment. Highlights from the 1996 World Workshop in Periodontics. J Am Dent Assoc 1997;128:713

Jemt, T. Regeneration of gingival papillae after single-implant treatment. Int J Periodont Rest Dent 1997;17(4):326

Jin, LJ, Cao, CF. Clinical diagnosis of trauma from occlusion and its relation with severity of periodontitis. J Clin Periodontol 1992;19:92

Johansen, JR, Gjermo, P, Bellini, HT. A system to classify the need for periodontal treatment. Acta Odontol Scand 1973;31:297

John, V, Warner, NA, Blanchard, SB. Periodontal-endodontic interdisciplinary treatment: A case report. Compend Contin Educ Dent 2004; 25(8):601

Johnson, BD, Engel, D. Acute necrotizing ulcerative gingivitis: A review of diagnosis, etiology, and treatment. J Periodontol 1986;57:141

Johnson, RH. Basic flap management. Dent Clin North Am 1976;20(1):3

Johnson, RL. Principles in Periodontal osseous resection. Dent Clin North Am 1976;20(1):35

Jovanovic, SA. Diagnosis and treatment of peri-implant disease. In: Clinical Periodontology. Carranza, FA Jr, Newman, MG, eds. Philadelphia: Saunders, 1996

Kapin, SH, Eskow, RN. Furcation invasions: Correlating a classification system with therapeutic considerations: Part III. Sectioning teeth in the treatment of furcation invasions. Compend Contin Educ Dent 1984a;5(8):612

Kapin, SH, Eskow, RN. Furcation invasions: Correlating a classification system with therapeutic considerations: Part IV. Restoration of sectioned teeth. Compend Contin Educ Dent 1984b;5(9):734

Kaplan, H, Milobsky, L. A surgical procedure for periodontal pocket elimination: Revised Crane-Kaplan Technique. Oral Surg Oral Med Oral Pathol 1951;4:546

Kaplan, RG. Clinical experience with circumferential supracrestal fiberotomy. Am J Orthod 1976;70:146

Kaplan, RG. Supracrestal fiberotomy. J Am Dent Assoc 1977;95:1127

Karolyi, M. Beobachtungen uber Pyorrhea alveolaris. Virschr Zahnheilk 1901;17:279

Kassab, M, Cohen, RE. The effect of root modification and biomodification on periodontal therapy. Compend Contin Educ Dent 2003;24(1):31

Kassolis, JD, Rosen PS, Reynolds, MA. Alveolar ridge and sinus augmentation utilizing platelet-rich plasma in combination with freeze-dried bone allograft: Case report. J Periodontol 2000;71:1654

Kazanjian, VH. Surgical operations as related to satisfactory dentures. Dent Cosmos 1924;66:387

Kazanjian, VH. Surgery as an aid to more efficient service with prosthetic dentures. J Am Dent Assoc 1935;22:556

Kennedy, JE, Cohen, DW. Guest editorial: Periodontal medicine in the next millennium. Int J Periodont Rest Dent 2000;20(3):222

Kerr, DA. The cementum: Its role in periodontal health and disease. J Periodontol 1961;32:183

Keyes, PH, Wright, WE, Howard, SA. The use of phase-contrast microscopy and chemotherapy in the diagnosis and treatment of periodontal lesions: An initial report, I. Quintessence Int. 1978a;1:53

Keyes, PH, Wright, WE, Howard, SA. The use of phase contrast microscopy and chemotherapy in the diagnosis and treatment of periodontal lesions: An initial report, II. Quintessence Int. 1978b;2:69

Keyes, PH. Microbiologically modulated periodontal therapeutics: An introduction. Quintessence Int. 1982;13(2):1321

Keyes, PH, Rams, TE. A rationale for the management of periodontal disease: Rapid identification of microbial "therapeutic targets" with phase contrast microscopy. J Am Dent Assoc 1983;106:803

Kimmelman, BB. Teaching toothbrushing techniques: Aids and observations. NY State Dent J 1964;30:237

King, JD. Gingival disease in Dundee. Dent Rec 1945;65:9

King, KO, Pennell, BM. Evaluation of attempts to increase the width of attached gingiva. Paper presented before the Philadelphia Society of Periodontology, April 15, 1964.

Kirkland, O. The suppurative periodontal pus pocket, its treatment by modified flap operation. J Am Dent Assoc 1931;18:1462

Kirkland, O. Gingivectomy as conservative treatment of periodontoclasia. NY State J Dent 1942;12:235

Klavan, B. The replaced flap. J Periodontol 1970;41:406

Klein, H, Palmer, CE, Knutson, JW. Studies on dental caries: Part 1. Dental status and dental needs of elementary school children. Public Health Rep 1938;53:751

Klinge, B, Hultin, M, Berglundh, T. Peri-implantitis. Dent Clin North Am 2005;49(3):661

Klinkhamer, JM. Quantitative evaluation of gingivitis and periodontal disease: I. The orogranulocytic migratory rate. Periodontics 1968a; 6:207

Klinkhamer, JM. Quantitative evaluation of gingivitis and periodontal disease: II. The mobil mucus phase of oral secretions. Periodontics 1968b;6:253

Knocht, A, Zohn, H, Deasy, M, Chang, KM. Assessment of periodontal status with PSR and traditional clinical periodontal examination. J Am Dent Assoc 1995;126:1658

Knocht, A, Zohn, H, Deasy, M, Chang, KM. Screening for periodontal disease: Radiographs vs. PSR. J Am Dent Assoc 1996;127:749

Kobayashi, LY, Ash, MM Jr. A clinical evaluation of an electric toothbrush used by orthodontic patients. Angle Ortho 1964;34:209

Kogon, SL. The prevalence, location and conformation of palato-radicular grooves in maxillary incisors. J Periodontol 1986;57:231

Kohler, CA, Ramfjord, SP. Healing of gingival mucoperiosteal flaps. Oral Surg Oral Med Oral Pathol 1960;13:89

Kois, JC. Altering gingival levels: The restorative connections: Part I. Biologic variables. J Esthet Dent 1994;6(1):3

Kolliker, RA. Handbrich der Gewebelehre des Menschen. Leipzig, Ger.: Wilhelm Engelman, 1867:95

Kon, S, Novaes, AB, Ruben, MP, Goldman, HM. Visualization of the microvascularization of the healing periodontal wound: II. Curettage. J Periodontol 1969;40:96

Kopczyk, RA, Saxe, SR. Clinical signs of gingival inadequacy: The tension test. J Dent Child 1974;41:352

Kowolik, MJ, Nisbet, T. Smoking and acute ulcerative gingivitis: A study of 100 patients. Br Dent J 1983;154:241

Kozlovsky, A, Tal, H, Yechezkiely, N, Mozes, O. Facial radicular groove in a maxillary central incisor, Case report. J Periodontol 1988;59:615

Kramer, GM, Schwarz, MS. A technique to obtain primary intention healing in pocket elimination adjacent to an edentulous area. Periodontics 1964;2:252

Kramer, GM, Kohn, JD. A classification of periodontal surgery: An approach based on tissue coverage. Periodontics 1966;4:80

Kramer, GM, Nevins, M, Kohn, JD. The utilization of periosteal suturing in periodontal surgical procedures. J Periodontol 1970;4:457

Kronfeld, R. Histologic study of the influences of function on the human periodontal membrane. J Am Dent Assoc 1931;18:1242

Lane, JJ. Gingival fenestration. J Periodontol 1977;48:225

Langer, B, Calagna, L. The subepithelial connective tissue graft. J Prosthet Dent 1980;44:363

Langer, B, Stein, SD, Wagenberg, B. An evaluation of root resections. A 10 year study. J Periodontol 1981;52:719

Langer, B, Langer, L. Subepithelial connective tissue graft technique for root coverage. J Periodontol 1985;56:715

Langer, B, Langer, L. The overlapped flap: A surgical modification for implant fixture installation. Int J Periodont Rest Dent 1990;10(3):209

Langer, B. Root Resections revisited: Guest editorial. Int J Periodont Rest Dent 1996;16(3):200

Larato, DC. Periodontal bone defects in the juvenile skull. J Periodontol 1970a;41:473

Larato, DC. Intrabony defects in the dry human skull. J Periodontol 1970b;41:496

Larato, DC. Furcation involvement: Incidence and distribution. J Periodontol 1970c;41:499

Larato, DC. Alveolar plate fenestrations and dehiscences of the human skull. Oral Surg Oral Med Oral Pathol 1970d;29:816

Larato, DC. Simulated natural gingival restorations for teeth with root exposure after periodontal surgery. J Periodontol 1970e;41:21

Larato, DC. Relationship of food impaction to interproximal intrabony lesions. J Periodontol 1971;42:237

Larato, DC. Palatal exostosis of the posterior maxillary alveolar process. J Periodontol 1972; 43:486

Lee, KW, Lee, EC, Poon, KY. Palato-gingival grooves in maxillary incisors: A possible predisposing factor to localized periodontal disease. Br Dent J 1968;124:14

Lekholm, U, Zarb, GA. Patient selection and preparation. In: Tissue-Integrated Prosthesis Osseointegration in Clinical Dentistry. Branemark, PI, Zarb, GA, Albrektsson, T, eds. Chicago: Quintessence, 1985

Lemmerman, K. Tooth resection. Periodont Abstr 1975;23:109

Leonard, HJ. Periodontoclasia. J Am Dent Assoc 1936;23:2032

Leonard, HJ. Conservative treatment of periodontoclasia. J Am Dent Assoc 1939;26:1308

Levin, MP. Periodontal suture materials and surgical dressings. Dent Clin North Am 1980; 24(4):767

Levine, RA. Forced eruption: Part III. Esthetic treatment of non-restorable teeth. Compend Contin Educ Dent 1988;9:136

Lie, T. Periodontal Surgery for the maxillary anterior area. Int J Periodont Rest Dent 1992; 12(1):73

Lilly, GE. Reaction of oral tissues to suture materials. Oral Surg Oral Med Oral Pathol 1968;26:128

Lilly, GE, Armstrong, JH, Salem, JE, Cutcher, JL. Reaction of oral tissues to suture materials, Part II. Oral Surg Oral Med Oral Pathol 1968;26:592

Lilly, GE, Salem, JE, Armstrong, JH, Cutcher, JL. Reaction of oral tissues to suture materials, Part III. Oral Surg Oral Med Oral Pathol 1969;28:432

Lilly, GE, Cutcher, JL, Jones, JC, Armstrong, JH. Reaction of oral tissues to suture materials, Part IV. Oral Surg Oral Med Oral Pathol 1972;33:152

Lindhe, J, Socransky, SS, Nyman, S, Haffajee, A, Westfelt, E. "Critical probing depths" in periodontal therapy. J Clin Periodontol 1982; 9:323

Lindhe, J. Textbook of Clinical Periodontology, 2nd ed. Copenhagen: Munksgaard, 1989

Linkow, LI. Endosseous blade vent implants: A two-year report. J Prosthet Dent 1970;23:441

Listgarten, MA. Changing concepts about the dento-gingival junction. J Can Dent Assoc 1970;36:70

Listgarten, MA. Microorganisms and dental implants. J Periodontol 1999;70:220

Litch, JM, O'Leary, TJ, Kafrawy, AH. Pocket epithelium removal via crestal and subcrestal scalloped internal bevel incisions. J Periodontol 1984;55:142

Litonjua, LA, Bush, PJ, Andreana, S, Tobias, TS, Cohen, RE. Effects of occlusal load on cervical lesions. J Oral Rehabil 2004;31:225

Little, RM. The irregularity index: A quantitative score of mandibular anterior alignment. Am J Orthod 1975;68:554

Liu, W, J-L, Solt, CW. A surgical procedure for the treatment of localized gingival recession in conjunction with root surface citric acid conditioning. J Periodontol 1980;51:505

Loe, H, Silness, J. Periodontal disease in pregnancy: I. Prevalence and severity. Acta Odont Scand 1963;21:532

Loe, H. Periodontal changes in pregnancy. J Periodontol 1965;36:209

Loe, H. The gingival index, the plaque index, and the retention index. J Periodontol 1967;38:610

Loe, H, Brown, LJ. Early onset periodontitis in the United States of America. J Periodontol 1991;62:608

Loesche, WJ. Clinical and microbiological aspects of chemotherapeutic agents used according to the specific plaque hypothesis. J Dent Res 1979;58:2404

LoFrisco, C, Bramson, JB. Periodontal screening and recording: perceptions and effects on practice. J Am Dent Assoc 1993;124:226

Lorenzana, ER, Hallmon, WW. Subpontic osseous hyperplasia: A case report. Quintessence Int., 2000;31:57

Luebke, RG, Ingle, JI. Geometric nomenclature for mucoperiosteal flaps. Periodontics 1964;2:301

Lynch, SE, Genco, RJ, Marx, RE. Tissue Engineering: Applications in Maxillofacial Surgery and Periodontics. Chicago: Quintessence, 1999

Lyons, H, Kerr, DM, Hine, MK. Report from the 1949 Nomenclature Committee of the American Academy of Periodontology. J Periodontol 1950;21:40

Machtei, EE, Christersson, LA, Grossi, SG, Dunford, R, Zambon, JJ, Genco, RJ. Clinical criteria for the definition of "established periodontitis." J Periodontol 1992;63:206

MacLeod, KM, Betz, PK, Ratcliff, PA. An index of gingival architectural form. J Periodontol 1965;36:413

MacPhee, IT, Beagrie, GS. Treatment of ulceromembranous gingivitis. Br Dent J 1962;113:107

Magnusson, I, Runstad, L, Ny, S, Lindhe, J. A long junctional epithelium: a locus minoris resistentiae in plaque infection. J Clin Periodontol 1983;10:333

Malassez, LC. Sur l'existence de debris epitheliaux autour de la racine des dents chez l'homme adulte et a l'etat normal (debris epitheliaux parodentaires). Arch Physiol (Paris) 1885;5:129

Malone, WFP, Koth, DL. Tylman's Theory and Practice of Fixed Prosthodontics, 8th ed. St. Louis: Ishyakee Euro America, 1989

Mann, AW, Pankey, LD. Oral rehabilitation utilizing the Pankey-Mann instrument and a functional bite technique. Dent Clin North Am 1959;March, 215

Manor, A, Kaffe, I. Unusual foreign body reaction to a braided silk suture: A case report. J Periodontol 1982;53:86

Manson, JD. The lamina dura. Oral Surg Oral Med Oral Pathol 1963;16:432

Manson, JD, Nicholson, K. The distribution of bone defects in chronic periodontitis. J Periodontol 1974;45:88

Marie, MM, Pietkiewicz, M. Bruxomania (gritting of the teeth). Dent Cosmos 1907;49:525

Mariotti, A. Dental plaque-induced gingival diseases. Ann Periodontol 1999;4(1):7

Marks, RG, Magnusson, I, Taylor, M, Clouser, B, Maruniak, J, Clark, WB. Evaluation, reliability and reproducibility of dental indices. J Clin Periodontol 1993;20:54

Marx, RE, Carlson, ER, Eichstaedt, RM, Schimmele, SR, Strauss, JE, Georgeff, KR. Platelet-rich plasma: Growth factor enhancement for bone grafts. Oral Surg Oral Med Oral Pathol Oral Radiol Endod 1998;85:638

Massler, M, Schour, I. The P-M-A index of gingivitis. J Dent Res 1949;28:634

Massler, M. The P-M-A Index for the assessment of gingivitis. J Periodontol 1967;38:592

Masters, DH, Hoskins, SW Jr. Projection of cervical enamel into molar furcations. J Periodontol 1964;35:49

Masters, DH. Oral hygiene procedures for the periodontal patient. Dent Clin North Am 1969;13:3

Matia, JI, Bissada, NF, Maybury, JE, Ricchetti, P. Efficiency of scaling of the molar furcation area with and without surgical access. Int J Periodontics Restorative Dent 1986;6(6):25

Matter, J, Cimasoni, G. Creeping attachment after free gingival grafts. J Periodontol 1976;47:574

Mayfield, LJA. Immediate, delayed, and late submerged and transmucosal implants. In: Proceedings of the 3rd European Workshop on Periodontology: Implant Dentistry. Lang, NP, Karring, T, Lindhe, J, eds. Berlin: Quintessence, 1999:520-534

Maynard, JG Jr, Wilson, RD. Physiologic dimension of the periodontium fundamental to successful restorative dentistry. J Periodontol 1979;50:170

Maynard, JG Jr. Mucogingival considerations for the adolescent patient. In: Periodontal Therapy—Clinical Approaches and Evidence of Success. Nevins, M, Mellonig, JT, eds. Chicago: Quintessence, 1998.

McAllister, BS, Gaffaney, TE. Distraction osteogenesis for vertical bone augmentation prior to oral implant reconstruction. Periodontol 2000, 2003;33:54

McCall, JO. Traumatic occlusion. J Am Dent Assoc 1939;26:519

McFall, WT. Laterally repositioned flap-Criteria for success. Periodontics 1967;5:89

McGraw, VA, Caffesse, RG. Cyanoacrylates in periodontics. J West Soc Periodontol/Periodontal Abstr 1978;26:4

McGuire, MK. Prognosis versus actual outcome: A long term survey of 100 treated periodontal patients under maintenance care. J Periodontol 1991;62:51

McGuire, MK, Newman, MG. Evidence-based periodontal treatment: I. A strategy for clinical decisions. Int J Periodont Rest Dent 1995;15(1):71

McGuire, MK. Prognosis vs outcome: Predicting tooth survival. Compend Contin Educ Dent 2000;21(3):217

Meffert, RM. Vitreous carbon: Where are we now? Chicago Dent Soc Rev 1977;30(3):22

Meffert, RM, Block, MS, Kent, JN. What is osseointegration? Int J Periodont Rest Dent 1987;7(4):9

Meffert, RM. How to treat ailing and failing implants. Implant Dent 1992;1:25

Meffert, RM. Periodontitis vs peri-implantitis: The same disease? The same treatment? Crit Rev Oral Biol Med 1996;7:278

Melcher, AH. The interpapillary ligament. Dent Prac Dent Rec 1962;12:461

Melcher, AH. On the repair potential of periodontal tissues. J Periodontol 1976;47:256

Mellonig, JT, Bowers, GM, Bright, RW, Lawrence, JJ. Clinical evaluations of freeze-dried bone allograft in periodontal osseous defects. J Periodontol 1976;47:125

Mellonig, JT. Alveolar bone induction: Autografts and allografts. Dent Clin North Am 1980; 24:719

Mellonig, JT. Histologic evaluation of freeze-dried bone allografts in periodontal osseous defects (abstr 388). J Dent Res 1981;60

Mellonig, JT. Regenerating bone in clinical periodontics. J Am Dent Assoc 1990;121:497

Mellonig, JT. Autogenous and allogenic bone grafts in periodontal therapy. Crit Rev Oral Biol Med 1992;3:333

Mellonig, JT. Bone allografts in periodontal therapy. Clin Orthop 1996;324:116

Mellonig, JT. Periodontal regeneration: Bone Grafts. In: Periodontal Therapy—Clinical Approaches and Evidence of Success. Nevins, M, Mellonig, JT, eds. Chicago: Quintessence, 1998

Mellonig, JT, Nevins, M, Sanchez, R. Evaluation of a bioabsorbable physical barrier for guided bone regeneration: Part I. material alone. Int J Periodont Rest Dent 1998;18(2):129

Mellonig, JT. Enamel matrix derivative for periodontal reconstructive surgery: Technique and clinical and histologic case report. Int J Periodont Rest Dent 1999;19(1):9

Melsen, B, Agerbaek, N, Ericksen, J, Terp, S. New attachment through periodontal treatment and orthodontic intrusion. Am J Orthod Dentofac Orthop 1988;94:104

Mercuri, LG, Olson, RF, Laskin, DM. The Specificity of response to experimental stress in patients with myofascial pain dysfunction syndrome. J Dent Res 1979;58:1866

Merritt, AH. A brief history of periodontology. J Dent Res 1921;3:149

Miller, PD Jr. Root coverage using a free soft tissue autograft following citric acid application: Part I. Technique. Int J Periodont Rest Dent 1982;2(1):65

Miller, PD Jr. Root coverage using the free soft tissue autograft following citric acid application: II. Treatment of the carious root. Int J Periodon Rest Dent 1983;3(5):39

Miller, PD Jr. A classification of marginal tissue recession. Int J Periodont Rest Dent 1985a;5(2):9

Miller, PD Jr. Root coverage using the free soft tissue autograft following citric acid application: III. A successful and predictable procedure in areas of deep-wide recession. Int J Perioodont Rest Dent 1985b;5(2):15

Miller, PD Jr. Regenerative and reconstructive periodontal plastic surgery: Mucogingival surgery. Dent Clin North Am 1988;32:287

Miller, PD Jr. Concept of periodontal plastic surgery. Pract Periodont Aesthet Dent 1993;5:15

Miller, PD Jr, Allen, EP. The development of periodontal plastic surgery. Periodontol 2000, 1996;11:7

Miller, PD Jr. Current Techniques in Periodontal Plastic Surgery, paper presented before the Indiana Society of Periodontists, March 29, 2003

Miller, SC. Textbook of Periodontia. Philadelphia: Blakiston, 1938

Miller, WD. The Microorganisms of the Human Mouth. Philadelphia: SS White, 1890

Miller, WD. Experiments and observations on the wasting of tooth tissue variously designated as erosion, abrasion, chemical abrasion, denudation, etc. Dent Cosmos 1907;49(1):1;49(2): 109;49(3):225

Mills, MP, McDonnell, HT. Osseous surgery: The resection approach in periodontal therapy. In: Periodontal Therapy—Clinical Approaches and Evidence of Success. Nevins, M, Mellonig, JT, eds. Chicago: Quintessence, 1998

Minsk, L. Orthodontic tooth extrusion as an adjunct to periodontal therapy. Compend Contin Educ Dent 2000;21:768

Minsk, L. Maxillary-sinus-elevation procedures for endosseous dental implants. Compend Contin Educ Dent 2004;25:672

Minsk, L. Factors determining the timing of implant placement after tooth extraction. Compend Contin Educ Dent 2005a;26:400

Minsk, L. Extraction-site ridge preservation. Compend Contin Educ Dent 2005b;26(4):272

Mirko, P, Miroslav, S, Lubor, M. Significance of the labial frenum attachment in periodontal disease in man: Part I. Classification and epidemiology of the labial frenum attachment. J Periodontol 1974;45:891

Misch, CE. Bone character: Second vital implant criterion. Dent Today 1988;7(5):39

Misch, CE. Density of bone: Effect on treatment plans, surgical approach, healing and progressive bone loading. Int J Oral Implant 1990;6(2):23

Misch, CE, Dietsh-Misch, F, Hoar, J, Beck, G, Hazen, R, Misch, CM. A bone quality-based implant system: First year of prosthetic loading. J Oral Implant 1999;25(3):185

Misch, CE. Density of bone: Effect on surgical approach and healing. In: Contemporary Implant Dentistry. St Louis: Mosby, 1999:371

Misch, CE. Bone density: A key determinant for clinical success. In: Dental Implant Prosthetics. Philadelphia: Elsevier, 2005:130-141

Mombelli, A, Lang, NP. The diagnosis and treatment of peri-implantitis. Periodontol 2000, 1998;17:63

Morris, ML. Suturing techniques in periodontal surgery. Periodontics 1965a;3:84

Morris, ML. The unrepositioned muco-periodontal flap. Periodontics 1965b;3:147

Morris, ML. The effect of root decalcification on the formation of "functionally" oriented collagen fibers. J Periodontol 1980;51:171

Moskow, BS, Bressman, E. Localized gingival recession. Dent Radiogr Photogr 1965;38(1):3,19

Moskow, BS. Calculus attachment in cemental separations. J Periodontol 1969;40:125

Moskow, BS. Some observations on radicular enamel. J Periodontol 1971;42:92

Moskow, BS, Canut, PM. Studies on root enamel: Enamel pearls. A review of their morphology, localization, nomenclature, occurrence, classification, histogenesis, and incidence. J Clin Periodontol 1990;17:275

Muhlemann, HR. Periodontometry: A method for measuring tooth mobility. Oral Surg Oral Med Oral Pathol 1951;4:120

Muhlemann, HR. Tooth mobility V. Tooth mobility changes through artificial trauma. J Periodontol 1954;25:202

Muhlemann, HR, Hertzog, H, Vogel, A. Occlusal trauma and tooth mobility. Schweiz Monatschr Zahnheilk 1956;66:527

Muhlemann, HR, Mazor, ZS. Gingivitis in Zurich school children. Helv Odont Acta 1958;2(1):3

Muhlemann, HR. Ten years of tooth-mobility measurements. J Periodontol 1960;31:110

Muhlemann, HR, Villa, PR. The marginal line Calculus Index. Helv Odont Acta 1967;11:175

Muhlemann, HR, Son, S. Gingival sulcus bleeding: A leading symptom in initial gingivitis. Helv Odont Acta 1971;15:107

Munch-Hansen, E. Om Balneoteropiens Anuerdelse i den moderne Parodontoterape (about the use of balneotherapy in modern periodontal therapy). Tandlaegebladet 1953;57:22

Murphy, KG. Post operative healing complications associated with Gore-Tex periodontal material: Part I. Incidence and characterization. Int J Periodont Rest Dent 1995a; 15(4):363

Murphy, KG. Postoperative healing complications associated with Gore-Tex periodontal material: Part II: Effect of complications on regeneration. Int J Periodont Rest Dent 1995b;15(6):549

Murray, PA. HIV Disease as a risk factor for periodontal disease. Compend Contin Educ Dent 1994a;15(8):1052

Murray, PA. Periodontal diseases in patients infected by human immunodeficiency virus. Periodontol 2000, 1994b;16:50

Nabers, CL. Repositioning the attached gingiva. J Periodontol 1954;25:38

Nabers, CL, Spear, GR, Beckham, LC. Alveolar Dehiscence. Texas Dent J 1960;78(1):4

Nabers, CL, O'Leary, TJ. Autogenous bone transplants in the treatment of osseous defects. J Periodontol 1965;36:5

Nabers, CL, O'Leary, TJ. Autogenous bone graft: Case report. Periodontics 1967;5:251

Nagao, M. Comparative studies of the curve of Spee in mammals, with a discussion of its relation to the form of the fossa mandibularis. J Dent Res 1919;1:159

Nelson, SW. The subpedicle connective tissue graft: A bilaminar reconstructive procedure for the coverage of denuded root surfaces. J Periodontol 1987;58:95

Nery, EB, Davies, EE. The historical development of mucogingival surgery. J West Soc Periodontol/Periodontal Abstr 1976;24(4):149

Nery, EB, Corn, H, Eisenstein, IL. Palatal exostosis in the molar region. J Periodontol 1977;48:663

Neville, BW, Damm, DD, Allen, CM, Bouquot, JE. Oral and Maxillofacial Pathology, 2nd ed. Philadelphia: Saunders, 2002

Nevins, M, Skurow, HM. The intracrevicular restorative margin, the biologic width, and maintenance of the gingival margin. Int J Periodont Rest Dent 1984;4(3):31

Nevins, M, Cappetta, EG. The biologic width: Preventing postsurgical recession. In: Periodontal Therapy—Clinical Approaches and Evidence of Success. Nevins, M, Mellonig, JT, eds. Chicago: Quintessence, 1998

Nevins, M, Mellonig, JT. The advantages of localized ridge augmentation prior to implant placement: A staged event. Int J Periodont Rest Dent 1994;14(2):97

Newell, DH, Brunsvold, MA. A modification of the "curtain technique" incorporating an internal mattress suture. J Periodontol 1985;56:484

Newell, DH. The role of the prosthodontist in restoring root resected molars: A study of 70 molar root resections. J Prosthet Dent 1991;65:7

Newell, DH. The diagnosis and treatment of molar invasions. Dent Clin North Am 1998; 42:301

Newman, MG. Genetic risk for severe periodontal disease. Compend Contin Educ Dent 1997; 18(9):881

Newman, MG. Editorial. Periodontal medicine and risk assessment: A critical connection for implant therapy in partially edentulous patients. Int J Periodont Rest Dent 1998;13:449

Newman, PS. The effects of the inverse bevel flap procedure on gingival contour and plaque accumulation. J Clin Periodontol 1984;11:361

Noble, HW. The evolution of the periodontium. In: Biology of the Periodontium. Melcher, AH, Bowers, WH, eds. New York: Academic Press, 1969:1

Norberg, O. Ar en uhadning utav vevnadsforbust otankbar vid kuvrgisk behandling alveolar pyorrheoe. Svensk Tandlak Tidsk 1926;19:171

Nordland, PW, Tarnow, DP. A classification system for loss of papillary height. J Periodontol 1998;69:1124

Novak, MJ. Necrotizing ulcerative periodontitis. Ann Periodontol 1999;4(1):74

Noyes, FB, Schour, I, Noyes, HJ. A Textbook of Dental Histology and Embryology, 5th ed. Philadelphia: Lea & Febiger, 1938:113

Noyes, HJ. The anatomy of the frenum labii in newborn infants. Angle Orthop 1935;5:3

Nyman, S, Gottlow, J, Karring, T, Lindhe, J. The regenerative potential of the periodontal ligament. An experiment study in the monkey. J Clin Periodontol 1982a;9:257

Nyman, S, Lindhe, J, Karring, T, Rylander, H. New attachment following surgical treatment of human periodontal disease. J Clin Periodontol 1982b;9:290

Ochsenbein, C. Osseous resection in periodontal surgery. J Periodontol 1958;29:15

Ochsenbein, C. Newer concepts of mucogingival surgery. J Periodontol 1960;31:175

Ochsenbein, C, Bohannon, HM. The palatal approach to osseous surgery: I. Rationale. J Periodontol 1963;34:60

Ochsenbein, C. The double flap procedure. Periodontics 1963;1:17

Ochsenbein, C, Bohannon, HM. The palatal approach to osseous surgery: II. Clinical application. J Periodontol 1964;35:54

Ochsenbein, C, Ross, S. A reevaluation of osseous surgery. Dent Clin North Am 1969;13:87

Ochsenbein, C. A primer for osseous surgery. Int J Periodont Rest Dent 1986;6(1):8

O'Connor, TW, Biggs, NL. Interproximal bony contours. J Periodontol 1964;35:326

Odrich, RB, Kelman, CD. Cryotherapy: A new and experimental approach to the treatment of periodontal disease. Periodontics 1967;5:313

Ogilvie, AL. Recall and maintenance of the periodontal patient. Periodontics 1967;5:198

Okeson, JP. Current terminology and diagnostic classification schemes. Oral Surg Oral Med Oral Pathol Oral Radiol Endod 1997;83:61

Older, LB. The use of heterogenous bovine bone implants in the treatment of periodontal pockets: An experimental study in humans. J Periodontol 1967;38:539

O'Leary, TJ, Gibson, WA, Shannon, IL, Schuessler, CF, Nabers, CL. A screening examination for detection of gingival and periodontal breakdown and local irritants. Periodontics 1963; 1:167

O'Leary, TJ, Rudd, KD. An instrument for measuring horizontal tooth mobility. Periodontics 1963;1:249

O'Leary, TJ. The periodontal screening examination. J Periodontol 1967;38:617

O'Leary, TJ. Oral hygiene agents and procedures. J Periodontol 1970;41:625

O'Leary, TJ, Drake, RB, Naylor, JE. The plaque control record. J Periodontol 1972;43:38

Olsson, M, Lindhe, J. Periodontal characteristics in individuals with varying form of the upper central incisors. J Clin Periodontol 1991;18:78

Orban, B, Weinmann, JP. Diffuse atrophy of the alveolar bone (periodontosis). J Periodontol 1942;13:31

Orban, B. Classification and nomenclature of Periodontal diseases. J Periodontol 1942;13:88

Orban, B. Surgical gingivectomy. J Am Dent Assoc 1945;32:701

Orban, B, Sicher, H. The oral mucosa. J Dent Educ 1946;10:94, 163

Orban, B. Clinical and histologic study of the surface characteristics of the gingiva. Oral Surg Oral Med Oral Pathol 1948a;1:827

Orban, B. Gingivectomy vs conservative treatment of periodontal disease. J South Cal State Dent Assoc 1948b;15(4):15

Orban, B. The epithelial network in the periodontal membrane. J Am Dent Assoc 1952;44:632

Orban, B, Manella, VB. A macroscopic and microscopic study of instruments designed for root planing. J Periodontol 1956;27:120

Orban, BJ, Bhatia, H, Kollar, JA, Wentz, FM. The epithelial attachment (The attached epithelial cuff). J Periodontol 1956;27:167

Orban, BJ. Oral Histology and Embryology, 4th ed. Philadelphia: Mosby, 1957

Owings, JR Jr. An atypical gingivostomatitis: A report of four cases. J Periodontol 1969;40:538

Page, RC, Schroeder, HE. Periodontitis in man and other animals: A comparative review. Basel: Karger, 1982

Page, RC, Altman, LC, Ebersole, JL, Vandesteen, GE, Dahlberg, WH, Williams, BL, Osterberg, SK. Rapidly progressive periodontitis. A distinct clinical condition. J Periodontol 1983a;54:197

Page, RC, Bowen, T, Altman, L, Vandesteen, E, Ochs, H, Mackenzie, P, Osterberg, S, Engel, LD, Williams, BL. Prepubertal periodontitis: I. Definition of a clinical disease entity. J Periodontol 1983b;54:257

Page, RC, Baab, DA. A new look at the etiology and pathogenesis of early-onset periodontitis. Cementopathia revisited. J Periodontol 1985; 56:748

Page, RC. Periodontal therapy: Prospects for the future. J Periodontol 1993;64:744

Page, RC, Beck, JD. Risk assessment for periodontal disease. Int Dent J 1997;47:61

Page, RC, Krall, EA, Martin, J, Mancl, L, Garcia, RI. Validity and accuracy of a risk calculator in predicting periodontal disease. J Am Dent Assoc 2002;133:569

Page, RC, Martin, JA, Loeb, CF. Use of Risk assessment in attaining and maintaining oral health. Compend Contin Educ Dent 2004;25:657

Papillon, MM, LeFevre, P. Deux cas de keratodermie palmaire et plantaire symetrique familiamle. (maladie de Meleda) chez le frere et la soeur. Coexistance dans les deux cas d'alterations dentaires graves. [Two cases of symmetrical familial (Meleda's malady) palmar and plantar keratosis of brother and sister. Coexistence in two cases with serious dental changes.] Bull Soc Fr Dermatol Syph 1924;31:82

Paquette, DW. The periodontal-cardiovascular link. Compend Contin Educ Dent 2004;25:681

Parfitt, GJ. Measurement of the physiological mobility of individual teeth in an axial direction. J Dent Res 1960;39:608

Patur, B, Glickman, I. Gingival pedicle flaps for covering root surfaces denuded by chronic destructive periodontal disease: A clinical experiment. J Periodontol 1958;29:50

Pennel, BM, Higgason, JD, Towner, JD, King, KO, Fritz, BD, Salder, JF. Oblique rotated flap. J Periodontol 1965;36:305

Pennel, BM, Tabor, JC, King, KO, Towner, JD, Fritz, BD, Higgason, JD. Free masticatory mucosa graft. J Periodontol 1969;40:162

Perlitsh, MJ. A systematic approach to the interpretation of tooth mobility and its clinical implications. Dent Clin North Am 1980;24:177

Perry, DA, Beemsterboer, PL. Plaque control for the periodontal patient. In: Periodontology for the Dental Hygienist. Perry, DA, Beemsterboer, PL, Taggert, EJ, eds. Philadelphia: Saunders, 2001

Perry, HO, Deffner, NF, Sheridan, PJ. Atypical gingivostomatitis: Nineteen cases. Arch Dermatol 1973;107:872

Persson, GR, Mancl, LA, Martin, J, Page, RC. Assessing periodontal disease risk. A comparison of clinicians' assessment versus a computerized tool. J Am Dent Assoc 2003;134:575

Pfeifer, J, Heller, R. Histologic evaluation of full and partial thickness lateral repositioned flaps. A pilot study. J Periodontol 1971;42:331

Phillips, JM, Gatchel, RJ, Wesley, AL, Ellis III, E. Clinical implications of sex in acute temporomandibular disorders. J Am Dent Assoc 2001;132:49

Pick, RM, Powell, GL. Lasers in dentistry: Soft tissue procedures. Dent Clin North Am 1993; 37:281

Picton, DCA. Vertical mobility of cheek teeth during biting. Arch Oral Biol 1963;8:109

Pihlstrom, PL, Ramfjord, SP. Periodontal effect of non-function in monkeys. J Periodontol 1971; 42:748

Pini Prato, GP, Rotundo, R, Magnani, C, Soranzo, C. Tissue engineering technology for gingival augmentation procedures: A case report. Int J Periodont Rest Dent 2000;20(6):553

Podshadley, AG, Haley, JV. A method for evaluating oral hygiene performance. Public Health Rep 1968;83:259

Pollack, RP. Modified distal wedge procedure. J Periodontol 1980;51:513

Pollack, RP. Curettage: A new look at an old technique. Int J Periodont Rest Dent 1984;4(5):25

Pollack, RP. An analysis of periodontal therapy for the 65-year-old patient. Gerodontics 1986;2:135

Pollack, RP. Guest editorial: Considerations of the aging population. Int J Periodont Rest Dent 1991;11(4):256

Polson, AM, Proye, MP. Effect of root surface alterations on periodontal healing: II. Citric acid treatment to denuded root. J Clin Periodontol 1982;9:441

Polson, AM, Frederick, GT, Ladenheimer, S, Hanes, PJ. The production of a root smear layer by instrumentation and its removal by citric acid. J Periodontol 1984;55:443

Pontoriero, R, Lindhe, J, Nyman, S, Karring, T, Rosenberg, E, Sanavi, F. Guided tissue regeneration in degree II Furcation-involved mandibular molars. A clinical study. J Clin Periodontol 1988;15:247

Posselt, U. An analyzer for mandibular positions. J Prosthet Dent 1957;7:368

Posselt, U. Occlusal disharmonies and their effect on periodontal disease. Int Dent J 1959;9:367

Posselt, U, Wolff, IB. Treatment of bruxism by bite guards and bite plates. J Can Dent Assoc 1963;29:773

Posselt, U. Physiology of Occlusion and Rehabilitation, 2nd ed. Oxford, England: Blackwell Scientific, 1968

Poulton, DR, Aaronson, SA. The relationship between occlusion and periodontal status. Am J Orthod 1961;47:690

Prichard, JF. Advanced Periodontal Disease/ Surgical Prosthetic Management, 2nd ed. Philadelphia: Saunders, 1972

Prichard, JF. Present state of the interdental denudation procedure. J Periodontol 1977;48:566

Prichard, JF. The diagnosis and management of vertical bony defects. J Periodontol 1983; 54:29

Prinz, H. Chronic diffuse desquamative gingivitis. Dent Cosmos 1932;74:331

Pruzansky, S. Applicability of electromyographic procedures as a clinical aid in the detection of occlusal disharmony. Dent Clin North Am 1960;(March):117

Pugh, CE, Smerke, JW. Rationale for fixed prostheses in the management of advanced periodontal disease. Dent Clin North Am 1969; 13:243

Quigley, GA, Hein, JW. Comparative cleansing efficiency of manual and power brushing. J Am Dent Assoc 1962;65:26

Raetzke, PB. Covering localized areas of root exposure employing the "envelope" technique. J Periodontol 1985;56:397

Ramfjord, SP. Gingivectomy: Its place in periodontal therapy. J Periodontol 1952a;23:30

Ramfjord, SP. Reattachment in periodontal therapy. J Am Dent Assoc 1952b;45:513

Ramfjord, SP, Kiester, G. The gingival sulcus and the periodontal pocket immediately following scaling of the teeth. J Periodontol 1954;25:167

Ramfjord, SP. Indices for prevalence and incidence of periodontal disease. J Periodontol 1959;30:51

Ramfjord, SP. Bruxism: A clinical and electromyographic study. J Am Dent Assoc 1961;62:21

Ramfjord, SP, Ash, MM. Occlusion. Philadelphia: Saunders, 1966

Ramfjord, SP, Costich, ER. Healing after exposure of periosteum on the alveolar process. J Periodontol 1968;39:199

Ramfjord, SP, Nissle, RR. The modified Widman flap. J Periodontol 1974;45:601

Ramfjord, SP. Present status of the modified Widman flap. J Periodontol 1977;48:558

Ramfjord, SP, Ash, MM. Scaling and tooth planing. In: Periodontology and Periodontics. Philadelphia: Saunders, 1979a:362

Ramfjord, SP, Ash, MM. Treatment of Intrabony pockets and furcation involvement—Bone Implants. Periodontology and Periodontics. Philadelphia: Saunders, 1979b:653

Ramfjord, SP, Ash, MM. Examination and Diagnosis in Periodontology and Periodontics. Philadelphia: Saunders, 1979c:297

Ramfjord, SP. Root planing and curettage. Int Dent J 1980;30:93

Rams, TE, Keyes, PH, Wright, WE, Howard, SA. Long-term effects of micro-biologically modulated periodontal therapy on advanced adult periodontitis. J Am Dent Assoc 1985;111:429

Rams, TE, Listgarten, MA, Slots, J. Utility of radiographic crestal lamina dura for predicting periodontitis disease activity. J Clin Periodontol 1994;21:571

Raphael, KG, Marbach, JJ, Klausner, J. Myofascial face pain: Clinical characteristics of those with regional and widespread pain. J Am Dent Assoc 2000;131:161

Raphael, KG, Marbach, JJ. Widespread pain and the effectiveness of oral splints in myofascial face pain. J Am Dent Assoc 2001;132:305

Ratcliff, PA, Raust, GT. Interproximal denudation: A conservative approach to osseous surgery. Dent Clin North Am 1964;March:121

Ratcliff, PA. An analysis of repair systems in periodontal therapy. Periodont Abstr 1966;14(2):57

Ray, TS. Oral Infection Control. In: Troothbrushes and Toothbrushing in Clinical Practice of the Dental Hygienist, 9th ed. Wilkins, EM, ed. Philadelphia: Lippincott, Williams & Wilkins, 2005:402

Raybin, M. Disclosing solutions: Their importance and uses. Dental Outlook 1943;30:159

Raybin, M. Disclosing solutions. Dent Items Int 1945;67:235

Reddie, AH. Biologic principles of bone induction. Orthop Clin North Am 1987;18:207

Rees, TD, Biggs, NL, Collings, CK. Radiographic interpretation of periodontal osseous defects. Oral Surg Oral Med Oral Pathol 1971;32:141

Rees, TD. Periodontal Risk Factors and Indicators. Periodontol 2000, 2003;32:9

Rehwinkle, FH. Pyorrhea alveolaris. Dent Cosmos 1877;19:572

Rethman, M. Periodontal terminology: Letter to the editor. J Periodontol 1993;64:583

Ricchetti, PA. A furcation classification based on pulp chamber-furcation relationship and vertical radiographic bone loss. Int J Periodonts Rest Dent 1982;2(5):51

Ries, BJ, Johnson, GK, Nieberg, LG. Vertical extrusion using a removable orthodontic appliance. J Am Dent Assoc 1988;116:521

Riffle, AB. The cementum during curettage. J Periodontol 1952;23:170

Riffle, AB. The dentin: Its physical characteristics during curettage. J Periodontol 1953;24:232

Riffle, AB. Radical subgingival curettage. J Periodontol 1956;27:102

Riggs, JM. Suppurative inflammation of the gums and absorption of the gums and alveolar process. Penn J Dent Sci 1876;3:99 (reprinted in J Periodontol 1941;12:82)

Ririe, CM, Crigger, M, Selvig, KA. Healing of periodontal connective tissue following surgical wounding and application of citric acid in dogs. J Periodontal Res 1980;15:314

Risch, JR, White, JG, Swenson, HM. The esthetic labial gingival prosthesis. J Ind Dent Assoc 1977;56(3):15

Ritchey, B, Orban, B. The crests of the interdental alveolar septa. J Periodontol 1953a;24:75

Ritchey, B, Orban, B. Cysts of the gingiva. Oral Surg Oral Med Oral Pathol 1953b;6:765

Robinson, PG, Winkler, JR, Palmer, G, Westenhouse, J, Hilton, JF, Greenspan, JS. The diagnosis of periodontal conditions associated with HIV infection. J Periodontol 1994;65:236

Robinson, RE. The use of a stent in a periodontal frenectomy. J Calif State Dent Assoc 1956;26:32

Robinson, RE. Mucogingival junction surgery. J Calif State Dent Assoc 1957;33:379

Robinson, RE. Periodontal fenestration in mucogingival surgery. J West Soc Periodontol/Periodontal Abstr 1961;9:107

Robinson, RE. Utilizing an edentulous area as a donor site in the lateral repositioned flap. Periodontics 1964;2:79

Robinson, RE. The distal wedge operation. Periodontics 1966;4:256

Robinson, RE. The free mucosal graft in the edentulous mouth. J Calif Dent Assoc 1967;43:552

Robinson, RE. Osseous Coagulum for bone induction. J Periodontol 1969;40:503

Rockoff, SC, Rockoff, HS, Sackler, AM. Reattachment: A case in point. J Periodontol 1958;29:261

Ronderos, M, Ryder, MI. Risk assessment in clinical practice. Periodontol 2000, 2004;34:120

Rosen, PS, Reynold, MA, Bowers, GM. The treatment of intrabony defects with bone grafts. Periodontol 2000, 2000;22:88

Rosenberg, ES, Garber, DA, Evian, CI. Tooth lengthening procedures. Compend Contin Educ Dent 1980;1:161

Rosenberg, MM. A laterally repositioned flap involving a non-vital tooth: Case report. Periodontics 1963;1:164

Rosenberg, RM, Ash, MM. The effect of root roughness on plaque accumulation and gingival inflammation. J Periodontol 1974;45:146

Rosenthal, P. Re-covering the exposed necks of teeth by autoplasty. Dent Cosmos 1912;54:377

Rosner, D. Clinical annotation: A continuous simultaneous interdental suture technique. J Periodontol 1977;48:792

Ross, IF, Thompson, RH. A long term study of root retention in the treatment of maxillary molars with furcation involvement. J Periodontol 1978;49:238

Ross, SE, Malamed, EH, Amsterdam, M. The contiguous autogenous transplant: Its rationale, indications and technique. Periodontics 1966;4:246

Ross, SE, Crosetti, HW, Gargiulo, A, Cohen, DW. The double papillae repositioned flap—An alternative: I. Fourteen years in retrospect. Int J Periodont Rest Dent 1986;6(6):47

Rotstein, I, Simon, JHS. Diagnosis, prognosis and decision-making in the treatment of combined periodontal-endodontic lesions. Periodontol 2000, 2004;34:165

Rowland, RW. Necrotizing ulcerative gingivitis. Ann Periodontol 1999;4(1):65

Rubach, WC, Mitchell, DF. Periodontal disease, accessory canals and palpal pathosis. J Periodontol 1965;36:34

Rubelman, PA. Interdental papillae grafts. Alpha Omegan 1977;70:66

Russell, AL. A system of classification and scoring for prevalence surveys of periodontal disease. J Dent Res 1956;35:350

Ryan, ME. Clinical applications for host modulatory therapy. Compend Contin Educ Dent 2002;23(11A):1071

Ryan, ME. Nonsurgical approaches for the treatment of periodontal diseases. Dent Clin North Am 2005;49(3):611

Saadoun, AP. Management of furcation involvement. J West Soc Periodontol/Periodontal Abstr 1985;33(3):91

Saadoun, AP. The key to peri-implant esthetics: hard and soft-tissue management. Dent Impl Update 1997;8:41

Saari, JT, Hurt, WC, Biggs, NL. Periodontal bony defects on the dry skull. J Periodontol 1968;39:278

Saglie, R, Johansen, JR, Rollefsen, T. Plaque-free zones in human teeth in periodontitis. J Clin Periodontol 1975;2:190

Saklad, M. Grading of patients for surgical procedures. Anesthesiology 1941;2:281

Salama, H, Salama, M. The role of orthodontic extrusive remodeling in the enhancement of soft and hard tissue profiles prior to implant placement: A systematic approach to the management of extraction site defects. Int J Periodont Rest Dent 1993;13(4):313

Salkin, LM, Cuder, R, Rush, R. A look at the PSR impact on one dental practice. J Am Dent Assoc 1993;124:230

Sandler, HC, Stahl, SS. Measurement of periodontal disease prevalence. J Am Dent Assoc 1959;58:93

Sarrazin, JJ. The toothbrush and methods of cleaning the teeth. J Am Dent Assoc 1920;7:155

Saxer, UP, Muhlemann, HR. Motivation und Aufklarung. Schweiz Monatschr Zahnheilkd 1975;85:905

Scannapieco, FA. Systemic effects of periodontal diseases. Dent Clin North Am 2005;49(3):533

Schallhorn, RG. The use of autogenous hip marrow biopsy implants for bone crater defects. J Periodontol 1968;39:145

Schallhorn, RG. Postoperative problems associated with iliac transplants. J Periodontol 1972;43:3

Schallhorn, RG, Snider, LE. Periodontal maintenance therapy. J Am Dent Assoc 1981;103:227

Schallhorn, RG, McClain, PK. Combined osseous composite grafting, root conditioning, and guided tissue regeneration. Int J Periodont Rest Dent 1988;8(4):9

Schei, O, Waerhaug, J, Lovdal, A, Arno, A. Alveolar bone loss as related to oral hygiene. J Periodontol 1959;30:7

Schluger, S. Osseous resection: A basic principle in periodontal surgery. Oral Surg Oral Med Oral Pathol 1949a;2:316

Schluger, S. Necrotizing ulcerative gingivitis in the army. Incidence, communicability, and treatment. J Am Dent Assoc 1949b;38:174

Schmid, MO, Balmelli, OP, Saxer, UP. Plaque-removing effect of a toothbrush, dental floss, and a toothpick. J Clin Periodontol 1976;3:157

Schour, I, Massler, M. Gingival disease in Postwar Italy (1945): I. Prevalence of gingivitis in various age groups. J Am Dent Assoc 1947;35:475

Schroeder, A, van der Zypen, E, Stich, H, Sutter, F. The reactions of bone connective tissue, and epithelium to endosteal implants with titanium-sprayed surfaces. J Maxilla Fac Surg 1981;9:15

Schroeder, HE, Listgarten, MA. The fine structure of the developing epithelial attachment of human teeth. In: Monographs in Developmental Biology, vol 2. Basel, Switzerland: Karger, 1971

Schuyler, CH. Fundamental principles in the correction of occlusal disharmony, natural and artificial. J Am Dent Assoc 1935;22:1193

Schuyler, CH. Correction of occlusal disharmony of the natural dentition. NY State Dent J 1947;13:445

Schuyler, CH. Freedom in Centric. Dent Clin North Am 1969;13:681

Schwartz, RS, Massler, M. Tooth accumulated materials: A review and classification. J Periodontol 1969;40:407

Schwartz, RS, Massler, M, LeBeau, LJ. Gingival reactions to different types of tooth accumulated materials. J Periodontol 1971;42:144

Scully, C, MacFadyen, E, Campbell, A. Oral manifestations in cyclic neutropenia. Brit J Oral Surg 1982;20:96

Seibert, JS. Reconstructive periodontal surgery: Case report. J Periodontol 1970;41:113

Seibert, JS. Soft tissue grafts in periodontics. In: Clinical Transplantation in Dental Specialties. Robinson, PJ, Guernsey, LH, eds. St. Louis: Mosby. 1980:107

Seibert, JS. Reconstruction of deformed, partially edentulous ridges, using full thickness onlay grafts: Part I. Technique and wound healing. Compend Contin Educ Dent 1983a;4(5):437

Seibert, JS. Reconstruction of deformed, partially edentulous ridges, using full thickness onlay grafts: Part II. Prosthetic/periodontal interrelationships. Compend Contin Educ Dent 1983b;4(6):549

Seibert, JS. Reconstruction of the partially edentulous ridge: Gateway to improved prosthetics and superior aesthetics. Pract Periodont Aesthet Dent 1993;5(5):47

Seibert, JS, Louis, JV. Soft tissue ridge augmentation utilizing a combination onlay-interpositional graft procedure: A case report. Int J Periodont Rest Dent 1996;16(4):311

Selipsky, H. Osseous surgery: How much need we compromise? Dent Clin North Am 1976;20:79

Selye, H. The general adaptation syndrome and the diseases of adaptation. J Clin Endocrinol 1946;6:117

Selye, H. Report on "Calciphylaxis": Annual meeting of the American Academy of Periodontology. J Periodontol 1964;35:85

Serres, A. Study of the Anatomy and Physiology of the Teeth. Paris: Meguignon, 1817

Sethi, A, Kaus, T. Maxillary ridge expansion with simultaneous implant placement: 5 year results of an ongoing clinical study. Int J Oral Maxillofac Impl 2000;15:491

Seymour, RA, Smith, DG, Turnbull, DN. The effects of phenytoin and sodium valproate on the periodontal health of adult epileptic patients. J Clin Periodontol 1985;12:413

Shanelec, DA, Tibbetts, LS. A perspective on the future of periodontal microsurgery. Periodontol 2000, 1996;11:58

Shapoff, CA. Understanding the limitations of dental radiographs: Implications for soft-tissue management programs. Compend Contin Educ Dent 2004;25(5):338

Sharpey, W. Quains's Elements of Anatomy, 6th ed. New York: Longman's, Green, 1856

Shetty, V, Han, TJ. Alloplastic materials in reconstructive periodontal surgery. Dent Clin North Am 1991;35:521

Shick, RA, Ash, MM Jr. Evaluation of the vertical method of toothbrushing. J Periodontol 1961;32:346

Shick, RA. Maintenance phase of periodontal therapy. J Periodontol 1981;52:576

Shulman, LB, Jensen, OT. Sinus graft consensus conference: Special Supl. Int J Oral Maxfac Impl 1998;13:5

Shuman, IE. Bipolar versus monopolar electrosurgery. Clinical applications. Dent Today 2001;20:74

Sicher, H. Bau und Function des Fixationsapparatus der Meerschweinchenmolaren. Zeitschr Stomat 1923;21:580

Sicher, H. Tooth eruption: The axial movement of continuously growing teeth. J Dent Res 1942;21:201

Sicher, H. Oral Anatomy. St. Louis: Mosby, 1949:185

Sicher, H. The principal fibers of the periodontal membrane. The Bur 1954a;55(3):2

Sicher, H. Position and movement of the mandible. J Am Dent Assoc 1954b;48:620

Sicher, H. Changing concepts of the supporting dental structures. Oral Surg Oral Med Oral Pathol 1959;12:31

Silberman, SL, LeJeune, RC, Serio, FG, Devidos, M, Davidson, L, Vernon, K. A method for determining patient oral care skills: The University of Mississippi Oral Hygiene Index. J Periodontol 1998;69:1176

Silness, J, Loe, H. Periodontal disease in pregnancy: II. Correlation between oral hygiene and periodontal condition. Acta Odont Scand 1964;22:121

Silness, J. Periodontal conditions in patients treated with dental bridges. J Periodontal Res 1970;5:60

Silverstein, LH, Kurtzman, GM. A review of dental suturing for optimal soft-tissue management. Compend Contin Educ Dent 2005;26:163

Silverton, JF, Burgett, FG. Probing of pockets related to the attachment level. J Periodontol 1976;47:281

Simon, JHS, Glick, DH, Frank, AL. The relationship of endodontic-periodontic lesions. J Periodontol 1972;43:202

Simonton, FV. Examination of the mouth with special reference to pyorrhea. J Am Dent Assoc 1925;12:287

Simring, M, Goldberg, M. The pulpal pocket approach: Retrograde periodontitis. J Periodontol 1964;35:22

Singer, SL, Goldblatt, T, Hallam, A, Winters, JC. Hereditary gingival fibromatosis with a recessive mode of inheritance: Case reports. Aust Dent J 1993;38(6):427

Skillen, WG, Mueller, E. Epithelium and the physiologic pocket. J Am Dent Assoc 1927;14:1149

Smiler, DG. The sinus lift graft: Basic technique and variations. Pract Periodont Aesthet Dent 1997;9:885

Smith, BGN, Knight, JK. An index for measuring the wear of teeth. Br Dent J 1984;156:435

Smith, RG. Gingival recession: Reappraisal of an enigmatic condition and a new index for monitoring. J Clin Periodontol 1997;24:201

Smith, TS. Anatomic and physiologic conditions governing the use of the toothbrush. J Am Dent Assoc 1940;27:874

Smukler, H, Tagger, M. Vital root amputation. A Clinical and histologic study. J Periodontol 1976;47:324

Socransky, SS, Haffajee, AD. Dental biofilms: Difficult therapeutic targets. Periodontol 2000, 2002;28:12

Solomon, C, Chaflin, H, Kellert, M, Weseley, P. The endodontic-periodontal lesion: A rationale approach to treatment. J Am Dent Assoc 1995;126:473

Sottosanti, JS. Aesthetic extractions with calcium salfate and the principles of guided tissue regeneration. Pract Periodont Aesthet Dent 1993;5(5):61

Spee, FG. Die Verschiebungsbahn des Unterkiefers am Schadel (Orientation of the mandibular path related to the skull). Arch Anat Physiol 1890.

Sperber, GH, Buckingham, J. Odonto-eponymology: Historical dental names. J Hist Dent 2000; 48(3):127

Staffileno, H. A histologic study of healing of split thickness gingival flap surgery in dogs. Master's thesis. Chicago: Loyola University, 1960

Staffileno, H, Wentz, FM, Orban, B. Histologic study of healing of split thickness flap surgery in dogs. J Periodontol 1962;33:56

Staffileno, H. Management of gingival recession and root exposure problems associated with periodontal disease. Dent Clin North Amer 1964;March:111

Staffileno, H, Levy, S, Gargiulo, A. Histologic study of cellular mobilization and repair following a periosteal retention operation via split thickness mucogingival flap surgery. J Periodontol 1966;37:117

Staffileno, H. Palatal flap surgery: Mucosal flap (split thickness) and its advantages over the mucoperiosteal flap. J Periodontol 1969a; 40:547

Staffileno, HJ. Surgical management of the furca invasion. Dent Clin North Am 1969b;13:103

Stahl, SS, Morris, AL. Oral health conditions among army personnel at the Army Engineer Center. J Periodontol 1955;26:180

Stahl, SS. Morphology and healing pattern of human interdental gingiva. J Am Dent Assoc 1963;67:48

Stahl, SS, Cantor, H, Zwig, E. Fenestrations of the labial alveolar plate in human skulls. Periodontics 1963;1:99

Stallard, RE, Diab, MA, Zander, HA. The attaching substance between enamel and epithelium: A product of the epithelial cells. J Periodontol 1965;36:130

Stambaugh, RV, Dragoo, M, Smith, DM, Carasali, L. The limits of subgingival scaling. Int J Periodont Rest Dent 1981;1(5):31

Stambaugh, RV. A clinician's 3-year experience with perioscopy. Compend Contin Educ Dent 2002;23(11A):1061

Stambaugh, RV, Myers, G, Ebling, W. Endoscope visualization of the subgingival dental sulcus and tooth surfaces. J Periodontol 2002;73:374

Stein, G, Weinmann, JP. Die physiologische Wanderung der Zahne (The physiologic wandering of teeth). Zeitshc Stomatol 1925;8:733

Stern, IB, Everett, FG, Robicsek, K. S. Robicsek—A pioneer in the surgical treatment of periodontal disease. J Periodontol 1965;36:265

Stern, IB. Current concepts of the dento-gingival junction: The epithelial and connective tissue attachments to the teeth. J Periodontol 1981; 52:465

Stewart, DJ, Kernohan, DC. Self-inflicted gingival injuries. Gingivitis artifacta, factitial gingivitis. Dent Pract 1972;22:418

Stillman, PR. Early clinical evidences of disease in the gingiva and pericementum. J Dent Res 1921;3:xxv

Stillman, PR, McCall, JO. A textbook of Clinical Periodontia. New York: Macmillan, 1922

Stillman, PR. Stimulation of the gingiva. J Am Dent Assoc 1928;15:1077

Stillman, PR. A philosophy of the treatment of periodontal disease. Dent Digest 1932;38:315

Stillman, PR, McCall, JO. A Textbook of Clinical Periodontics, 2nd ed. New York: Macmillan, 1937

Stones, HH. The reaction and regeneration of cementum in various pathological conditions. Proc R Soc Med 1934;27:728

Sugarman, E. A clinical and histological study of the attachment of grafted tissue to bone and teeth. J Periodontol 1969;40:381

Sugarman, M. Precocious periodontitis: A clinical entity and a treatment responsibility. J Periodontol 1977;48:397

Sullivan, HC, Atkins, JH. Free autogenous gingival grafts: III. Utilization of grafts in the treatment of gingival recession. Periodontics 1968; 6:152

Sumner, CF. Surgical repair of recession on the maxillary cuspid: Incisally repositioning the gingival tissues. J Periodontol 1969;40:119

Suomi, JD, Greene, JC, Vermillion, JR, Chang, JJ, Leatherwood, EC. The effect of controlled oral hygiene procedures on the progression of periodontal disease in adults: Results after two years. J Periodontol 1969;40:416

Swan, RH, Hurt, WC. Cervical enamel projections as an etiologic factor in furcation involvement. J Am Dent Assoc 1976;93:342

Swenson, HM, Hansen, NM. The periodontist and cosmetic dentistry. J Periodontol 1961; 32:82

Tagger, M, Smukler, H. Microscopic study of the pulps of human teeth following vital root resection. Oral Surg Oral Med Oral Pathol 1977;44:96

Takei, HH, Han, TJ, Carranza, FA Jr, Kenney, EB, Lekovic, V. Flap technique for periodontal bone implants: Papilla preservation technique. J Periodontol 1985;56:204

Takei, HH, Yamada, H, Han, T. Maxillary anterior esthetics: Preservation of the interdental papilla. Dent Clin North Am 1989;33:263

Takei, HH. Surgical techniques for reconstructive periodontics. Dent Clin North Am 1991;35(3): 531

Takei, HH, Carranza, FA Jr. The periodontal flap. In: Clinical Periodontology, 8th ed. Philadelphia: Saunders, 1996:592

Tan, AES. Disclosing agents in plaque control: A review. J West Soc Periodontol/Periodontal Abstr 1981;29(3):81

Tandy, RB. Gingival Curettage. Periodontal Abstracts 1970;18:100

Tarnow, D, Fletcher, P. Classification of the vertical component of furcation involvement. J Periodontol 1984;55:283

Tarnow, DP. Semilunar coronally repositioned flap. J Clin Periodontol 1986;13:182

Tarnow, DP, Wagner, AW, Fletcher, P. The effect of the distances from the contact point to the crest of bone on the presence or absence of the interproximal dental papilla. J Periodontol 1992; 63:995

Tarnow, DP. Solving restorative esthetic dilemmas with the semilunar coronally positioned flap. J Esthet Dent 1994;6(2):61

Tatum, H Jr. Maxillary and sinus implant reconstructions. Dent Clin North Am 1986; 30(2):207

Ten Cate, AR. The development of the periodontium: A largely ectomesenchymally derived unit. Periodontol 2000, 1997;13:9

Terranova, VP, Aumailley, M, Sulton, LH, Martin, GR, Kleinman, HK. Regulation of cell attachment and cell numbers by fibronectin and laminin. J Cell Physiol 1986;127:473

Thebaud, J. Some microscopic aspects of the curetted surface of the cementum after the subgingival curettage. J Can Dent Assoc 1951; 17:127

Theilade, E. The non-specific theory in microbial etiology of inflammatory periodontal diseases. J Clin Periodontol 1986;13:905

Thoma, KH, Goldman, HM. Classification and histopathology of parodontal disease. J Am Dent Assoc 1937;24:1915

Thoma, KH, Goldman, HM. Wandering and elongation of the teeth and pocket formation in parodontosis. J Am Dent Assoc 1940;27:335

Tibbetts, LS Jr. Use of diagnostic probes for detection of periodontal disease. J Am Dent Assoc 1969;78:549

Tibbetts, LS Jr, Ochsenbein, C, Loughlin, DM. Rationale for the lingual approach to mandibular osseous surgery. Dent Clin North Am 1976;20(1):61

Tibbetts, LS Jr, Shanelec, DA. An overview of periodontal microsurgery. Curr Opin Perio 1994;2:187

Tibbetts, LS Jr, Shanelec, D. Periodontal microsurgery. Dent Clin North Am 1998;42(2):339

Tinti, C, Parma-Benfenoti, S. Coronally positioned palatal sliding flap. Int J Periodont Rest Dent 1995;15(3):299

Turesky, S, Gilmore, ND, Glickman, I. Reduced plaque formation by the chloromethyl analogue of vitamin C. J Periodontol 1970; 41:41

Uitto, V-J. Gingival crevicular fluid. Periodontol 2000, 2003;31:9-167

Urist, MR. Bone: Formation by autoinduction. Science 1965;150:893

Urist, MR, Silverman, BF, Buring, K, Dubric, FL, Rosenberg, JM. The bone induction principle. Clin Orthop 1967;53:243

Urist, MR, Strates, BS. Bone morphogenetic protein. J Dent Res 1971;50:1392

Urist, MR, Sisto, K, Brownell, M, Malinin, TI, Lietze, A, Huo, VK, Prolo, DJ, Oklund, S, Finerman, GAM, DeLange, RJ. Human bone morphogenetic protein (hBMP). Proc Soc Exp Biol Med 1983;173:194

Valentini, P, Abensur, D. Maxillary sinus elevation for implant placement with demineralized freeze-dried bone and bovine bone (BioOss): A clinical study of 20 patients. Int J Periodont Rest Dent 1997;17(3):233

Vandersall, DC. Localized periodontitis induced by rubber elastic: Report of a case. J Am Dent Assoc 1971;83:1326

Vandersall, DC. Problems and Dangers in Adult Tooth Movement. In: Adult Tooth Movement in General Dentistry. Schlossberg, A, ed. Philadelphia: Saunders, 1975:195

Vandersall, DC, Slade, DL. The missing orthodontic elastic band: A periodontic-orthodontic dilemma. J Am Dent Assoc 1978;97:661

Vandersall, DC, Detamore, RJ. The mandibular molar class III furcation invasion. A review of treatment options and a case report of tunneling. J Am Dent Assoc 2002;133:55

van der Velden, U, DeVries, JH. Introduction of a new periodontal probe: The pressure probe. J Clin Periodontol 1978;5:188

van der Velden, U. Probing force and the relationship of the probe tip to the periodontal tissues. J Clin Periodontol 1979;6:106

van der Velden, U. The influences of probing force on the reproducibility of the depth measurements. J Clin Periodontol 1980;7:414

Van Dyke, TE, Lester, MA, Shapira, L. The role of the host response in periodontal disease progression: Implications for future treatment strategies. J Periodontol 1993;64:792

Van Kirk, LE, Pennell, EH. Assessment of malocclusion in population groups. Am J Orthod 1959;45:752; Am J Public Health 1959;49:1157

Vincent, HJ. Sur l'etiologic et sur les lesions anatomopathologiques de la pouriture d'hopital. Ann Inst Pasteur 1896;10:488

Vincent, JW, Machen, JB, Levin, MP. Assessment of attached gingiva using the tension test and clinical measurements. J Periodontol 1976; 47:412

Volchansky, A, Cleaton-Jones, P. The position of the gingival margins expressed by clinical crown height in children ages 6-16 years. J Dent 1976;4:116

Volpe, AR, Manhold, JH. A method of evaluation the effectiveness of potential calculus inhibiting agents. NY State Dent J 1962;7:289

Volpe, AR, Manhold, JH, Hazen, SP. In vivo calculus assessment: Part I. A method and its examiner reproducibility. J Periodontol 1965;36:292

Waerhaug, J. The gingival pocket. Odont Tidscrift 1952;60 (Suppl)

Waerhaug, J. The dimension of instruments for removal of subgingival calculus. J Periodontol 1954;25:281

Waerhaug, J. The angular bone defect and its relationship to trauma from occlusion and downgrowth of subgingival plaque. J Clin Periodontol 1979;6:61

Wagenberg, BD, Eskow, RN, Langer, B. Exposing adequate tooth structure for restorative dentistry. Int J Periodont Rest Dent 1989;9:323

Wagenberg, BD. Surgical tooth lengthening: Biologic variables and esthetic concerns. J Esthet Dent 1998;10:30

Wagenberg, BD. Considerations in treatment planning of the periodontal patient. Dent Today 2005;(March):108

Walton, RE, Leonard, LA, Sharawy, M, Gangarosa, LP. Effects on pulp and dentin of iontophoresis of sodium fluoride on exposed roots in dogs. Oral Surg Oral Med Oral Pathol 1979;48:545

Waltzer, RE, Halik, FJ. Repositioning of the frenum in periodontal involvement. J Okla Dent Assoc 1954;43:10

Wang, HL, Cooke, J. Periodontal regeneration techniques for treatment of periodontal diseases. Dent Clin North Am 2005;49(3):637

Wannenmacher, E. Umschau auf dem Gebiet der Paradentose. (Survey of paradentoses). Ztrbl Zahn, Mund Kieferheilk 1936;4:161

Wannenmacher, E. Umschau auf dem Gebiet der paradentose. Ztrbl Zahn Mund Kieferheilk 1938;6:81

Ward, AW. Postoperative care in the surgical treatment of pyorrhea. J Am Dent Assoc 1929; 16:635

Watts, TLP, Lennon, MA, Davies, RM. Gingival bleeding in an experimental clinical trial design. J Clin Periodontol 1979;6:15

Waugh, ILM. The alveolo-dental membrane: Its minute structure from a practical viewpoint. Dent Cosmos 1904;46:744

Weinberg, MA, Eskow, RN. An overview of delayed passive eruption. Compend Contin Educ Dent 2000a;21:511

Weinberg, MA, Eskow, RN. Osseous defects: Proper terminology revisited. J Periodontol 2000b;71:1928

Weinmann, JP, Sicher, H. Bone and Bones: Fundamentals of Bone Biology, 2nd ed. St. Louis: Mosby, 1955

Weinstein, E, Mandel, ID. The fluid of the gingival sulcus. Periodontics 1964;2:147

Weiss, CM. Tissue integration of dental endosseous implants: Description and comparative analysis of the fibro-osseous integration and osseous integration systems. J Oral Impl 1986;12(2):169

Wentz, FM, Jarabek, J, Orban, B. Experimental occlusal trauma imitating cuspal interferences. J Periodontol 1958;29:117

Wertheimer, FW. Effectiveness of "Berliner epithelial scalpel" in removing the epithelial lining of periodontal pockets. J Periodontol 1954;25:264

Wertheimer, FW, Fullmer, HM. Morphologic and histochemical observations on the human dental cuticle. J Periodontol 1962;33:29

Weski, O. Die chronischen marginalen Entzundungen des Alveolarfortsatzes mit besonderer Berucksichtigung der alveolar-Pyorrhoe. Vjschr Zahnheilk 1921;37:1

Weski, O. New denomination of the so-called alveolar pyorrhea. Dent Cosmos 1932;74:200

Whinston, GJ. Frenotomy and mucobuccal fold resection utilized in periodontal therapy. NY State Dent J 1956;22:495

Whitman, DH, Berry, RL, Green, DM. Platelet gel: An autologous alternative to fibrin glue with applications in oral and maxillofacial surgery. J Oral Maxillofac Surg 1997;55:1294

WHO Periodontal Disease: Report of an Expert Committee on dental health. Int Dent J 1961;11:544

WHO Epidemiology, Etiology and Prevention of Periodontal Disease (Tech Rep Ser 621). Geneva: World Health Organization, 1978

Widman, L. The operative treatment of alveolar pyorrhea. Br Dent J 1917;37:105

Widman, L. The operative treatment of pyorrhea alveolaris: A new surgical method. (Revised in Br Dent J 1920;1:293.) Svensk Tandlak Tidsk Suppl 1918;16:3

Wilderman, MN. Repair after a periosteal retention procedure. J Periodontol 1963;34:487

Wilderman, MN, Wentz, FM. Repair of a dentogingival defect with a pedicle flap. J Periodontol 1965;36:218

Wilderman, MN. Periodontal surgery: Mucogingival and osseous. Int Dent J 1967;17:519

Williams, RC. Periodontal disease. New Engl J Med 1990;322:373

Williams, RC, Offenbacher, S. Periodontal medicine. Periodontol 2000, 2000;23:9

Williams, RC. The future of periodontology. In: History of Periodontology. Carranza, FA, Shklar, G, eds. Chicago: Quintessence, 2003

Williams, RC, Cochran, DL, Lynch, SE. Tissue engineering: What does it mean? Why is it important? Compend Contin Educ Dent 2005; 26:54

Wilson, RD, Maynard, JG Jr. Intracrevicular restorative dentistry. Int J Periodont Rest Dent 1981;1(4):35

Wilson, TG Jr, Weber, HP. Classification of and therapy for areas of deficient bony housing prior to dental implant placement. Int J Periodont Rest Dent 1993;13(5):451

Wilson, TG Jr, Schenk, R, Buser, D, Cochran, D. Implants placed in immediate extraction sites: A report of histologic and histometric analysis of human biopsies. Int J Oral Maxillofac Implants 1998;13(3):333

Winkler, JR, Murray, PA, Grossi, M, Hammerla, C. Diagnosis and management of HIV-associated periodontal lesions. J Am Dent Assoc 1989; 119:255

Wirthlin, MR. Resective and Regenerative Osseous surgery. J West Soc Periodontol/ Periodontal Abstr 1987;35(1):5

Wise, RJ. Periodontal diagnosis and management of the impacted maxillary cuspid. Int J Periodont Rest Dent 1981;1(2):57

Wynbrandt, J. The Excruciating History of Dentistry. New York: St Martin's Press, 1998

Yankell, SL, Saxer, UP. Toothbrushing and Toothbrushing Techniques in Primary Preventive

Dentistry, 5th ed. Norwalk, CT: Appleton & Lange, 1999:77

Younger, WJ. Pyorrhea alveolaris. J Am Med Assoc 1884;23:790

Yukna, RA, Bowers, GM, Lawrence, JJ, Fedi, PF. A clinical study of healing in humans following the excisional new attachment procedure. J Periodontol 1976;47:696

Yukna, RA. A clinical and histologic study of healing following the excisional new attachment procedure in rhesus monkeys. J Periodontol 1976;47:701

Yukna, RA, Lawrence, JJ. Gingival surgery for soft tissue new attachment. Dent Clin North Am 1980;24:705

Yukna, RA. Synthetic bone grafts in periodontics. Periodontol 2000, 1993;1:92

Yuodelis, RA, Mann, WV Jr. The prevalence and possibly role of non-working contacts in periodontal disease. Periodontics 1965;3:219

Yuodelis, RA, Smith, DH. Correction of periodontal abnormalities as a preliminary phase in oral rehabilitation. Dent Clin North Am 1976;20:181

Zamet, JS. A comparison of unembellished gingivectomy with the inverse bevel flap procedure incorporating osseous contouring. Dent Pract Dent Rec 1967;17:387

Zamet, JS. A clinical comparison of the apically repositioned flap procedure with the apically displaced split-flap procedure. Dent Pract Dent Rec 1969;20(4):121

Zander, HA. The attachment of calculus to root surfaces. J Periodontol 1953;24:16

Zander, HA. Review of Glickman: "Role of occlusion in the etiology and treatment of periodontal disease." J Dent Res 1971;50:205

Zaner, DJ, Yukna, RA. Particle size of periodontal bone grafting materials. J Periodontol 1984; 55:406

Zemsky, JL. Surgical treatment of periodontal disease with author's open-view operation for advanced cases of dental periclasia. Dent Cosmos 1926;68:465

Zimmerman, SO. Discussion: Attachment level changes in destructive periodontal changes. J Periodontol 1986;13:473

Zingale, JA. Observations on free gingival autografts. J Periodontol 1974;45:748

Zinner, DD. Ultrasonic studies in dentistry: A preliminary report. Proc of Fourth Annual Conference on Ultrasonic Therapy. Library of Congress No. 55:12257. 1955a;(Aug):6

Zinner, DD. Recent ultrasonic studies, including periodontia, without the use of an abrasive (abstr M-37). J Dent Res 1955b;34:748

Zubery, Y, Kozlowsky, A, Tal, H. Histologic assessment of a contiguous autogenous transplant in a human intrabony defect: A case report. J Periodontol 1993;64:66

Zwarych, PD, Quigley, MB. The intermediate plexus of the periodontal ligament: History and further observations. J Dent Res 1965; 44:383